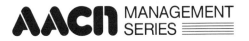

# PERSONNEL MANAGEMENT

IN

# CRITICAL CARE NURSING

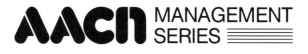

AACn MANAGEMENT SERIES

# PERSONNEL MANAGEMENT
## IN
# CRITICAL CARE NURSING

EDITED BY

## Suzette Cardin, RN, MS, CCRN

*Nurse Manager*
*Coronary Care Unit/Coronary Observation Unit*
*UCLA Medical Center*
*Assistant Clinical Professor*
*UCLA School of Nursing*
*Los Angeles, California*

## Cathy Rodgers Ward, RN, MS, CCRN

*Nurse Manager*
*Cardiothoracic Intensive Care Unit/Intermediate Care Unit*
*UCLA Medical Center*
*Assistant Clinical Professor*
*UCLA School of Nursing*
*Los Angeles, California*

## WILLIAMS & WILKINS
Baltimore • Hong Kong • London • Sydney

*Editor*: Susan M. Glover
*Associate Editor*: Marjorie Kidd Keating
*Copy Editor*: Susan S. Vaupel
*Design*: Norman W. Och
*Illustration Planning*: Wayne Hubbel
*Production*: Raymond E. Reter

Copyright © 1989
Williams & Wilkins
428 Preston Street
Baltimore, Maryland 21202, USA

*Printed in the United States of America*

**Library of Congress Cataloging-in-Publication Data**

Personnel management in critical care nursing / edited by Suzette Cardin [and] Cathy Rodgers Ward.
      p.    cm.—(AACN management series)
    ISBN 0-683-01451-X
     1. Intensive care nursing—Planning. 2. Nursing services—Personnel administration.  I. Cardin, Suzette.  II. Ward, Cathy Rodgers.  III. Series.
RT120.I5P36    1989
362.1′73′068—dc19

89-5273
CIP

89 90 91 92 93
1 2 3 4 5 6 7 8 9 10

*To*
*visionary*
*nurse managers*

*and to*
*our husbands*

*Edward Robert Barden*
*and*
*Robert Tyson Ward*

# Foreword

*Personnel Management in Critical Care Nursing* is AACN's first book in a series of management books for critical care nurses. The idea for this series grew out of the work of AACN's Management Special Interest Group (SIG). They first developed a document on "Role Expectations for the Critical Care Nurse Manager," which described the clinical practice, personnel, and the fiscal and environmental aspects of the nurse manager's role in a critical care unit. The Management SIG delineated the areas of role function specific to management in critical care and recognized that additional resources were needed to support the achievement of these expectations.

*Personnel Management in Critical Care Nursing* was developed as a resource for critical care managers in meeting the responsibilities of personnel management in critical care nursing. This book is a unique contribution to nursing management literature because the authors have provided information specific to critical care. The content addresses decentralization, mentoring, selecting qualified staff, shared governance, and professional development. AACN's Scope of Practice, Position Statements, and Nursing Care Standards are integrated throughout the book creating an excellent reference for application to practice. A talented array of authors, whose positions range from vice president to first-line management, have contributed their knowledge and expertise. The strength of this book lies not only in the emphasis on critical care but also in the opportunities and tools provided to apply the information on management principles and theory.

We have learned over time that a positive practice environment contributes directly to work satisfaction and retention. In this type of environment, there is a high likelihood that professional concepts will be consistently demonstrated in the care of critically ill patients. Leadership and motivation skills, comfort with decentralized decision making, and providing consistent and timely feedback are just a few of the cornerstones for effective personnel management. Clearly, the nurse manager and, specifically, the way the nurse manager's role is implemented are a crucial force in defining the practice environment for those directly providing care to patients.

The most challenging responsibilities of the nurse manager's role involve aspects of personnel management such as motivating, mentoring, and encouraging professional development. These concepts are usually the most difficult to learn. Providing leadership and guidance through effective personnel management contributes to the delivery of quality care to the critically ill patient and at the same time contributes to a satisfactory professional experience for both the nurse manager and the critical care nurse. *Personnel Management in Critical Care Nursing* is an outstanding resource for critical care managers and nurses, as they work together to make the key difference in critical care nursing.

Linda D. Searle, RN, MN, CNA
President, AACN
Director of Nursing
Santa Monica Hospital
Medical Center
Santa Monica, California

# Preface

Recognizing the tendency for many critical care nurses to leap from the clinically excellent to the managerially inept, this text is designed to provide first-line managers with strategies for success as managers of critical care nursing personnel. Personnel management is viewed as an interactive, dynamic, and open process between the critical care nurse manager and the staff of the critical care setting.

Effective personnel management occurs through an integration of the nursing process with the management process, utilizing applicable management theory and professional standards to formulate a critical care nursing management model. In this book the critical care nurse manager is guided through this framework in a logical progression; the chapters have been organized according to this nursing management process. The steps of this process as well as the chapter titles are stated in verbs to indicate the action orientation of the text.

## Integrative Model for Critical Care Personnel Management

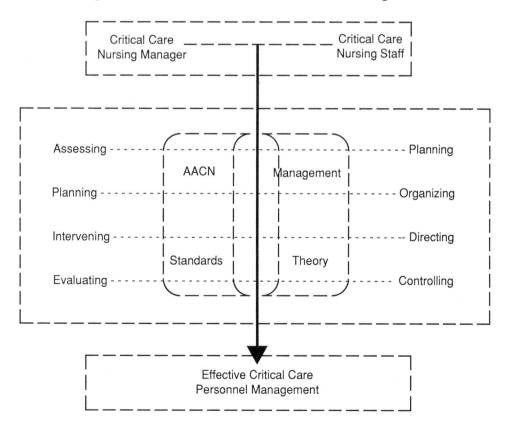

The art of personnel management evolves through the mastery of theoretical content as well as practical application and experience. This book incorporates both techniques by stressing management theory and its application in real situations in critical care nursing.

Part I addresses content applicable to the assessing or data gathering phase of the nursing management process. Characteristics of the ideal nurse manager are described and related to effective personnel management. This gives the reader a foundation from which to begin, stimulates questions for the nurse manager to ask about self-possessed traits, provides the nursing administrator with criteria for selection of the ideal personnel manager, and enables the critical care nurse who is considering pursuing a management career to determine whether these characteristics are present or worth developing. Assessing the very competitive marketplace for critical care staff is also presented as are methods of attracting critical care nurses and ancillary personnel to the institution. Techniques of interviewing, including questions to ask, characteristics to look for, and appropriate critical care nurses to hire, are also included as important steps in shaping the critical care staff into the mold most desirable for effective personnel management.

Part II presents the planning and organizing principles of the nursing management process. A decentralized organizational structure and nursing care delivery system is introduced as a prerequisite for other planning activities. A participatory approach to decision making is viewed as a fundamental necessity for successful personnel management at both the unit and divisional levels in critical care. The importance of nurse managers participating in divisional decisions as well as nursing staff participating in unit-related and direct care decisions is emphasized. Staffing critical care units by a decentralized approach is advocated and creative staffing mechanisms are proposed.

Planning for the professional development of staff is a key component of personnel management, and this chapter outlines steps the nurse manager takes to promote professional development among critical care nurses. Examples of cre-

ative clinical ladders and techniques for increasing staff participation in unit and professional activities are offered. Organizing differences between rural and urban institutions and the impacts of these differences on personnel management are also addressed.

Part III describes the crucial components of intervening with and directing staff in a positive manner. Communication, a pervasive concept essential in personnel management, is explicated here as it applies to critical care nursing and includes current research in this area. Tactics for retaining qualified staff are delineated, and the effect of management style on turnover rates is emphasized. Other directing functions of the personnel manager covered in individual chapters in this book include the arts of mentoring, motivating, and negotiating. Specific situations and case examples guide the reader in the "how-to" of these artful techniques.

Part IV highlights evaluating and controlling desired outcomes in personnel management. One chapter is devoted to conducting periodic performance appraisals and successful techniques to employ in staff evaluations. Other specific forms of evaluations thought to be important include appraising clinical judgment of critical care nurses as well as the inevitable necessity of assessing staff for chemical dependency. Counseling and disciplinary procedures are outlined as compulsory controlling functions the nurse manager performs. The final chapter provides the nurse manager with the rules of labor law and its application in critical care.

The principal belief in a professional approach to personnel management is evident throughout this book with the implementation of the proposed model. Specific instructions for the personnel manager to achieve desired outcomes include sample interview questions, counseling sessions, and written performance appraisals. With these proven strategies the nurse manager will acquire the skills of successful critical care personnel management and ultimately provision of the most effective critical care.

Suzette Cardin, RN, MS, CCRN
Cathy Ward, RN, MS, CCRN

# Acknowledgments

The publication of *Personnel Management in Critical Care Nursing* marks the beginning of a series of four management books sponsored by AACN. We are grateful to our distinguished contributors for their expertise and enthusiasm that have made this premier text possible. Special thanks is graciously extended to our colleagues who tirelessly assisted in the review and critique of the manuscripts: Janice Hanc, Sheri Monsein, Carol Pifer, and Maryle Olivier. Laurel Torczon and Cheryl Riley were invaluable in the preparation of the manuscripts and in their editorial assistance. Working collaboratively in a joint venture with AACN has been professionally rewarding, and we would like to acknowledge Linda Searle for her support of this project as well as Ellen French who has proven to be a loyal liaison throughout the entire process. The AACN Management Special Interest Group and the Communications Committee deserve recognition for the conception of the management book series idea. The staff of Williams & Wilkins have been outstanding in their guidance and facilitation of this text and our gratitude is offered to Susan Glover, Marjorie Keating, and Raymond Reter. We are indebted to nursing administrators and professors who have inspired our managerial paths, with distinct appreciation to Vera Cardin, Carol Mandle, and the late Drucilla Mantle for their visionary approach to nursing.

# Contributors

Rita M. Barden, RN, MSN, CCRN
Nurse Manager, Intensive Care Unit
Coronado Hospital
San Diego, California

Donna L. Bertram, RN, MBA, CNA
Vice President, Nursing
Penrose—St. Francis Healthcare System
Colorado Springs, Colorado

Chris Breu, RN, MN
Assistant Director of Nursing
Humana Hospital Surburban
Louisville, Kentucky

Suzette Cardin, RN, MS, CCRN
Nurse Manager
Coronary Care Unit/Coronary Observation Unit
UCLA Medical Center
Assistant Clinical Professor
UCLA School of Nursing
Los Angeles, California

Susan L. Chamberlain, RN, MSN
Director, Surgical/Psychiatric Nursing
Beth Israel Hospital
Boston, Massachusetts

John M. Clochesy, RN, MS, CS
Instructor
Frances Payne Bolton School of Nursing
Case Western Reserve University
Cleveland, Ohio

Rosemary Dale, RN, EdD, CNAA
Vice President, Nursing and Patient Services
Medical Center Hospital of Vermont
Dean, School of Nursing
University of Vermont
Burlington, Vermont

Dolores Gomez, RN, MN
Director of Critical Care
Desert Hospital
Palm Springs, California

Mary Ellen Guy, PhD
Associate Professor
University of Alabama
Birmingham, Alabama

Lynnette M. Holder, RN, MSN, CNAA
Assistant General Director
Albert Einstein Medical Center
Philadelphia, Pennsylvania

Patricia Kallweit Kaldor, RN, MSN
Vice President, Patient Services
St. Mary's Medical Center
Racine, Wisconsin

Rebecca Katz, RN, MA, CCRN
Clinical Nurse Specialist
Grant Medical Center
Columbus, Ohio

Donna Kemp, RN, MN, CCRN
Neonatal Consultant
San Diego, California

Shirley Koczan, RN, MS, CCRN
Clinical Nurse, Respiratory-Surgical
  Intensive Care Unit
Beth Israel Hospital
Boston, Massachusetts

Elizabeth A. Levson, RN, MSN, CCRN
Clinical Reviewer
Veterans Administration Medical Center
Birmingham, Alabama

Mary Blichfeldt O'Brien, RN, MS, CCRN
Nurse Consultant, Private Practice
Terre Haute, Indiana

Susan G. Osguthorpe, RN, MS, CCRN
Clinical Director, Critical Care
Virginia Mason Hospital
Seattle, Washington

Annette M. Pingry, BSN, RN
Clinical Nurse III, Respiratory-Surgical
  Intensive Care Unit
Beth Israel Hospital
Boston, Massachusetts

Wanda L. Roberts, RN, MN
Nursing Management Consultant
Taipai, Taiwan

**Jane Ruzanski, BSN, RN**
Nurse Manager, Respiratory-Surgical
  Intensive Care Unit
Beth Israel Hospital
Boston, Massachusetts

**Cheryl A. Sirois, BSN, RN**
CN III, Clinical Research Nurse,
  Cardiothoracic Surgery
Beth Israel Hospital
Boston, Massachusetts

**Cathy Rodgers Ward, RN, MS, CCRN**
Nurse Manager
Cardiothoracic Intensive Care Unit/Intermediate-
  Care Unit
UCLA Medical Center
Assistant Clinical Professor
UCLA School of Nursing
Los Angeles, California

# Contents

Foreword ......................................... vii
Preface .......................................... ix
Acknowledgments .............................. xi
Contributors ................................... xiii

## PART I: ASSESSING AND PLANNING

1 Identifying Competent Critical Care Nurse Managers .................... 2
   *Cathy Rodgers Ward, RN, MS, CCRN*
   *Suzette Cardin, RN, MS, CCRN*
2 Recruiting Critical Care Personnel .................................. 11
   *Dolores Gomez, RN, MN*
3 Identifying Competent Critical Care Staff ............................. 19
   *Donna L. Bertram, RN, MBA, CNA*

## PART II: PLANNING AND ORGANIZING

4 Decentralized Managing ............................................. 30
   *Rosemary Dale, RN, EdD, CNAA*
5 Self-Governing ..................................................... 37
   *Wanda L. Roberts, RN, MN*
6 Creative Staffing .................................................. 47
   *Patricia Kallweit Kaldor, RN, MSN*
7 Promoting the Professional Development of Staff ...................... 59
   *Chris Breu, RN, MN*
8 Planning for Various Settings in Critical Care ....................... 71
   *John M. Clochesy, RN, MS, CS*

## PART III: INTERVENING AND DIRECTING

9 Communicating ..................................................... 78
   *Elizabeth A. Levson, RN, MSN, CCRN*
   *Mary Ellen Guy, PhD*
10 Retaining Qualified Staff .......................................... 92
   *Susan L. Chamberlain, RN, MSN*
   *Shirley Koczan, RN, MS, CCRN*
   *Annette M. Pingry, BSN, RN*
   *Jane Ruzanski, BSN, RN*
   *Cheryl A. Sirois, BSN, RN*
11 Mentoring ........................................................ 107
   *Mary Blichfeldt O'Brien, RN, MS, CCRN*
12 Motivating ....................................................... 124
   *Susan G. Osguthorpe, RN, MS, CCRN*
13 Negotiating ...................................................... 138
   *Cathy Rodgers Ward, RN, MS, CCRN*

## PART IV: EVALUATING AND CONTROLLING

14 Evaluating Performance: Assessing and Developing Critical
   Care Staff ....................................................... 146
   *Rita M. Barden, RN, MSN, CCRN*

**15** Competency-based Managing ....................................... 160
  *Rebecca Katz, RN, MA, CCRN*
**16** Evaluating Chemical Dependency in Critical Care Nurses ............ 176
  *Donna Kemp, RN, MN, CCRN*
**17** Counseling and Disciplining Staff .................................... 189
  *Lynnette M. Holder, RN, MSN, CNAA*
**18** Applying Labor Relations in Critical Care Nursing .................... 208
  *Suzette Cardin, RN, MS, CCRN*

Index ............................................................... 221

# Part I

# ASSESSING
AND
# PLANNING

# Chapter 1

# Selecting Competent Critical Care Nurse Managers

CATHY RODGERS WARD
SUZETTE CARDIN

The scope and responsibility of the nurse manager role in today's health care organization is highly valued. The nurse manager if successful can improve patient care outcomes, influence professional nursing practice, and improve nurse-physician relationships (1, 2). Today's nurse manager in critical care needs to move from a controlling and directing role to one that integrates, facilitates, and coordinates management activities with the clinical activities of the nursing unit (3).

The purpose of this chapter is to focus on the evolution of the nurse manager role, identify the characteristics of a nurse manager in critical care nursing, and discuss the selection and evaluation process for critical care nurse managers.

## EVOLUTION OF THE NURSE MANAGER ROLE

The history of nursing management can be traced to nursing's roots. Florence Nightingale believed that: "To be in charge is certainly not only to carry out the proper measures yourself but to see that everyone else does so too; it is neither to do everything yourself nor to appoint a number of people to each duty, but to ensure that each does that duty to which he is appointed" (4). To be in charge has traditionally been the focus of the nurse who was appointed to manage the unit. Throughout the history of nursing this has usually been the nurse with the most clinical experience or expertise. The nurse who is selected on this basis is likely to have justifiable pride in her self-concept as a clinician. At times there may be great difficulty in reconciling the two roles and if her committment to the clinical self-concept is an overriding one, she may minimize the importance of the management role (5).

The title "head nurse" is still used interchangeably with the title "nurse manager" to designate the person who is responsible for managing the unit. The title "head nurse" still carries the traditional connotations for nurses, patients, and physicians that indicate a set of expectations that are no longer totally effective. It has been suggested in the literature that the title should suggest both role and behavioral expectations, and a title such as "nurse manager" generates better role understanding and identification for all concerned (6).

The head nurse usually functions according to what has been defined as "old age skills." This position is characterized by a style that is very defined, deals with only the issues at hand, and can be conceptualized as nonvisionary in scope. The tools that are utilized in this type of management style are: analysis of the problem, organization, setting of goals, policy setting, and reorganizing. The vision is on daily problem solving and a leadership style that is usually autocratic or laissez-faire.

The nurse manager of today needs to acquire new age skills and attributes in order to be successful. The style is receptive and expressive with an emphasis on being visionary in scope. New age skills include the following: creative insight, sensitivity, versatility, patience, and a focus on what the needs are now and in the future. The leadership style is participative in nature. The functional characteristics of a successful nurse manager should include the following:

1. facilitation of teamwork;
2. establishment of good working relationships;
3. accountability;
4. sense of humor;

5. generation of glue for cohesiveness;
6. positive nurse identity;
7. positive role understanding (7).

Sherman in 1975 established the fact that the head nurse is a manager. This study utilized the seven major functional areas of management that theorists generally agree upon: planning, organizing, staffing, leading, communicating, decision making, and controlling and compared these functions to the head nurse role. Within these functional areas 101 core tasks or specific activities were identified. The study revealed that 77.2% of the management core tasks were performed regularly by the head nurse (8).

The American Association of Critical-Care Nurses (AACN) Scope of Practice (Fig. 1.1) advocates that the role of the manager is to provide a supportive environment for nurses and patients (9). The nurse manager needs to utilize the AACN Scope of Practice as a framework for monitoring of unit activities. Monitoring includes legal, regulatory, social, economic, and political trends to identify potential implications for critical care nursing (10). The position statement on "Role Expectations of the Critical Care Nurse Manager" (Fig. 1.2) is a composite of the functions and attributes of today's critical care nurse manager (11). All components of the role are listed in the position statement with a major emphasis on clinical practice, personnel, fiscal, and environmental management. The position statement supports the nurse manager as the key person in today's health care environment. The nurse manager is seen as the link between the patient, the nurse, and the environment. The AACN Demonstration Project is one arena in which the components of the Position Statement on Role Expectations for the Critical Care manager are being evaluated. In an environment where nurse and physician collaboration is high and nurse empowerment is fostered through participative management, the results have been encouraging. In the Demonstration Project the results indicate that the quality of care is high, mortality is lower than predicted, and costs are minimal (see Chapter 5) (12).

## SELECTING THE "RIGHT" NURSE MANAGER

The nurse manager position at the unit level is recognized as the most important position in accomplishing organizational goals (13). This recognition of the importance and power of the nurse

manager within the organization is not only evolving from the profession of nursing but is also emerging from the health policy and hospital organizational development literature (13, 14). Given the magnitude of responsibility of this role and its impact on the success of the organization, the process of selecting the person to fill this position is a crucial one. The ability of the candidate to potentially implement this role must be carefully scrutinized as the "organizational fit" for this person must be suitable.

The nurse manager role has also been known to have an impact on staff nurse job satisfaction and ultimately retention and attraction of nurses. A study of powerlessness in nurses found that hospital nurses have higher powerlessness scores than nonhospital nurses (15). Of hospital nurses 60% report lack of perceived adequate support from nursing administrators (15). Those nurses who indicate this lack of administrative support demonstrate a significantly higher powerlessness score than those nurses who perceive adequate support (15). Previous nursing studies have shown a correlation between feelings of powerlessness and lack of autonomy and input into decision making (16, 17).

The critical care nurse manager must be able to instill a sense of support in the staff he or she supervises through a participative management style, shared governance (see Chapter 5), and promotion of staff nurse autonomy. Hospitals must heed the key to the success of Japanese companies, which is their focus on style of management and quality of leadership within the organization that improves employee morale and promotes long-term retention (18).

One survey of nearly 17,000 nurses has shown that most job complaints revolve around nursing leadership and management skills of supervisors and their failure to follow through on problems, isolation, and overuse of authority (19). Other studies have noted an inverse relationship between a nurse manager's positive leadership style and staff nurse burnout (20, 21). Another study reports that staff nurse job satisfaction is related to the ranking by the staff of the nurse manager's consideration and concern for staff members (22). Vincent and Billings (2) found that critical care nurses rank unit management as the most stressful factor in intensive care unit (ICU) nursing and that this stress is significantly related to burnout and emotional exhaustion (2).

Clearly the impact of the nurse manager on the staff nurse is powerful and incompetent and misfit managers cannot be tolerated. In today's arena of

# Scope of Critical Care Nursing Practice

### Introduction

AACN builds on the ANA definition of nursing[2] and defines critical care nursing as that specialty within nursing which deals with human responses to life threatening problems[1]. The scope of critical care nursing is defined by the dynamic interaction of the critically ill patient, the critical care nurse, and the critical care environment.

The goal of critical care nursing is to ensure effective interaction of these three requisite elements to effect competent nursing practice and optimal patient outcomes within an environment supportive of both. The framework within which critical care nursing is practiced is based on a scientific body of knowledge, the nursing process, and multidisciplinary collaboration in the care of patients.

Although a distinct specialty, critical care nursing is inseparable from the profession of nursing as a whole. As members of the profession, critical care nurses hold the same commitment to protect, maintain, and restore health as well as to embrace the *Code for Nurses*[3].

### The Critically Ill Patient

Central to the scope of critical care nursing is the critically ill patient who is characterized by the presence of, or being at high risk for developing, life threatening problems. The critically ill patient requires constant intensive, multidisciplinary assessment and intervention in order to restore stability, prevent complications, and achieve and maintain optimal responses.

In recognition of the critically ill patients' primary need for restoration of physiologic stability, the critical care nurse coordinates interventions directed at resolving life-threatening problems. Nursing activities also focus on support of patient adaptation, restoration of health, and preservation of patient rights, including the right to refuse treatment or to die. Inherent in the patients' response to critical illness is the need to maintain psychological, emotional, and social integrity. The familiarity, comfort, and support provided by social relationships can enhance effective coping. Therefore, the concept of the critically ill patient includes the interaction and impact of the patients' family and/or significant other(s).

### The Critical Care Nurse

The critical care nurse is a licensed professional who is responsible for ensuring that all critically ill patients receive optimal care. Basic to accomplishment of this goal is individual professional accountability through adherence to standards of nursing care of the critically ill and through a commitment to act in accordance with ethical principles.

Critical care nursing practice encompasses the diagnosis and treatment of patient responses to life threatening health problems. The critical care nurse is the one constant in the critical care environment. As such, coordination of the care delivered by various health care providers is an intrinsic responsibility of the critical care nurse. With the nursing process as a framework, the critical care nurse uses independent, dependent, and interdependent interventions to restore stability, prevent complications, and achieve and maintain optimal patient responses. Independent nursing interventions are those actions which are in the unique realm of nursing and include manipulation of the environment, teaching, counseling, and initiating referrals. Dependent nursing interventions are those actions prescribed by medicine. Interdependent nursing interventions are actions determined through multidisciplinary collaboration. Underlying the application of these interventions is a holistic approach that expresses human warmth and caring. This art, in conjunction with the science of critical care nursing, is essential to the interaction between the critical care nurse and critically ill patient in attaining optimal outcomes.

The critical care environment is constantly changing. The critical care nurse must respond effectively to the demands created by this environment for the broad application of knowledge. Realization of this goal is accomplished through entry preparation into professional nursing practice at a baccalaureate level and a commitment to maintaining competency in critical care nursing through ongoing education concurrent with an expanding base of experience.

### The Critical Care Environment

The critical care environment can be viewed from three perspectives. On one level the critical care environment is defined by those conditions and circumstances surrounding the direct interaction between the critical care nurse and the critically ill patient. The immediate environment must constantly support this interaction in order to effect desired patient outcomes. Adequate resources, in the form of readily available emergency equipment, needed supplies, effective support systems for managing emergent patient situations, and measures for ensuring patient safety are requisites. The framework for nursing practice in this setting is provided by standards of nursing care of the critically ill.

The institution or setting within which critically ill patients receive care represents another perspective of the critical care environment. At this level, the critical care management and administrative structure ensures effective care delivery systems for various populations of critically ill patients through provision of adequate human, material, and financial resources, through required quality systems, and through maintenance of standards of nursing care of the critically ill.

Additional elements contributing to effective care delivery include:
° Participatory decision-making which ensures that the critical care nurse provides input into decisions affecting the nurse-patient interaction.
° A collaborative practice model that facilitates multi-

**Figure 1.1.**   AACN Position Statement: Scope of Critical Care Nursing Practice (adopted by AACN Board of Directors, November 1986).

disciplinary problem-solving and ethical decision-making.

° Education of critical care nurses consistent with standards for critical care nursing education and practice.

The broadest perspective of the environment encompasses a global view of those factors that impact the provision of care to the critically ill patient. Monitoring of legal, regulatory, social, economic, and political trends is necessary to promote early recognition of the potential implications for critical care nursing and to provide a basis for a timely response.

References:
¹ AACN, "Definition of Critical Care Nursing" AACN Position Statement, February, 1984.
² ANA, *Nursing: A Social Policy Statement*, ANA, Kansas City, Missouri, 1980.
³ ANA, *Code for Nurses*, ANA, Kansas City, Missouri, 1985.

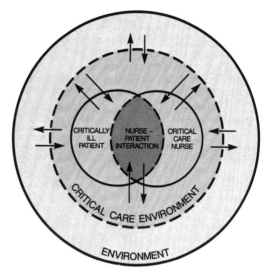

**Figure 1.1** *continued.*

recognizing the critical care staff nurse as a scarce resource, the nursing profession can no longer afford an insensitive, negative, and autocratic nurse manager.

## DESIRED CHARACTERISTICS OF THE NURSE MANAGER

Given the power of the nurse manager within the institution, what characteristics should be sought in the individual to fulfill this position? If a clinical nurse is employing the idea of seeking a nurse manager position, what self-traits should be assessed? To answer these questions, four groups of nurses were surveyed at a major university-affiliated medical center. Critical care nurses, nurse managers, graduate students in Nursing Administration, and senior undergraduate nursing students were included. Each group was asked to list the desired characteristics of a nurse manager in an open-ended questionnaire approach.

Table 1.1 displays the results of the most frequently cited desired characteristics of the nurse manager as suggested by these groups of nurses. All four groups (63 nurses) indicated good communication skills and an attitude supportive of nursing staff as essential traits for the nurse manager to possess. Accessibility, fairness, consistency, approachability, flexibility, professionalism, and knowledge in the clinical area were also considered to be important. Being organized, demonstrating good listening skills, having a positive attitude, and instilling motivation were noted to be positive attributes of a nurse manager. Frequently listed characteristics by critical care staff nurses that were not frequently named by nurse managers included: promotes staff education and development, responds to staff in a timely manner, and frequently gives positive feedback. Staff nurses have a need to be recognized by their nurse manager, and a savvy critical care nurse manager will assess these needs and realize the importance of attention to them. The critical care nurse manager may want to survey the staff on an annual basis as to their perceived desired characteristics of a nurse manager and then have the staff evaluate the nurse manager on these attributes. This type of feedback assists the manager in keeping in touch with the staff nurse's perceptions and gives the staff nurse a chance for input into the manager's performance.

Personality characteristics of a critical care nurse have been identified as aggressiveness, assertiveness, competitiveness, perseverance, moralistic orientation, resourcefulness, and mechanical ability (23). The critical care nurse manager usually has a critical care nurse background and may also exhibit this personality profile but must realize the implications of these traits in the staff he or she manages.

# Role Expectations for the Critical Care Manager

IN *NURSING, A SOCIAL POLICY STATEMENT*, the American Nurses' Association defines nursing as "the diagnosis and treatment of human responses to actual or potential health problems." Critical care nursing is that specialty within nursing which deals specifically with human responses to life threatening problems *(AACN, 1984)*.

Nurse managers "coordinate available resources to efficiently and effectively provide professional nursing care of a quality consistent with nursing care standards and at a cost compatible with the fiscal and other resources of the health care organization" *(ANA, 1978)*. Management of a critical care environment presents a particular challenge because of the magnitude of resources utilized, the timeliness of nursing intervention that is required, the sophisticated technological and clinical interventions that are used, the depth of the data base necessary for decision making and the degree of collaboration needed among disciplines.

WHEREAS, the role of the critical care manager is defined as the coordination and integration of human and material resources necessary to care for a population of critically ill patients

WHEREAS, the trend in administration of patient care units is decentralization, with concurrent increased expectation and responsibilities of the nurse manager

WHEREAS, in response to environmental changes, nursing decisions must also reflect a business orientation

WHEREAS, the vital link between institutional goals and implementation at the unit level is the critical care manager,

THEREFORE, BE IT RESOLVED THAT the manager of a critical care area is a baccalaureate prepared professional nurse who is clinically experienced in the areas of administrative responsibility and competent in the application of management principles,

AND the critical care nurse manager formally participates in institutional planning and decision making that have an impact on the scope of critical care nursing practice and the critical care environment,

AND the critical care nurse manager has responsibility, authority, and accountability for implementation and maintenance of critical care nursing standards.

## Implementation

The critical care manager is the leader and role model for professional nursing practice. The management of critical care also requires a knowledge base, skills, and competencies in clinical nursing and administration. It is the shared responsibility of the nurse manager and the institution to develop and maintain administrative accountabilities that include but are not limited to:

*Clinical Practice Management*
* Implementation of a valid and reliable patient classification system
* Implementation and maintenance of critical care nursing standards
* Direction and coordination of a selected delivery system of patient care
* Provision of support for critically ill patients and their families
* Incorporation of regulatory mandates into critical care practice
* Demonstration of sensitivity to ethical and legal ramifications of nursing practice in the critical care setting
* Delineation of needed knowledge, skills, and competencies of nursing staff and provision of staff development
* Incorporation of current research, new interventions, and technological advances into nursing practice
* Implementation of ongoing quality assurance activities

*Personnel Management*
* Interviewing applicants and hiring qualified critical care staff
* Staffing unit(s) to ensure 24-hour nursing coverage appropriate to patient care needs
* Facilitating staff input into decisions affecting nurse practice
* Identifying and planning for developmental needs of the staff
* Providing appropriate and timely information to staff as a basis for sound decision making
* Conducting timely and periodic performance appraisals based on pre-established standards, and following up appropriately
* Disciplining individual staff as delineated in institutional policy and procedure
* Demonstrating knowledge of labor law applicable to the institution

*Fiscal Management*
* Establishment of a valid statistical data base for budgetary decision making
* Facilitation of the development of realistic annual budget which may include revenue, personnel, supplies and capital equipment
* Establishment of accurate nursing productivity measures
* Regular review of budgetary variances to assure appropriate use of resources
* Promotion of cost effective unit operations
* Anticipation of the impact of institutional financial status on unit operations

**Figure 1.2.** AACN Position Statement: Role Expectations for the Critical Care Manager (adopted by AACN Board of Directors, June 1986).

*Environmental Management*
* Development, implementation, and evaluation of unit goals in concert with departmental and institutional goals
* Implementation and maintenance of structure standards for critical care nursing
* Establishment of effective communication channels to assure coordinated nursing care
* Promotion of a collaborative practice with other health care disciplines to assure an integrated approach to care of the patient
* Implementation of a risk management program to prevent, minimize, or correct risks to patients and staff based on institutional policy and procedure

With the unique combination of clinical, fiscal, and management expertise, the critical care nurse manager is in a key position to promote effective and cost efficient care of patients in the critical care environment.

**References**

American Association of Critical-Care Nurses. *Definition of Critical Care Nursing,* Newport Beach, CA: American Association of Critical-Care Nurses, 1984.

American Nurses' Association. *Roles, Responsibilities, and Qualifications for Nurse Administrators,* Kansas City, KS: American Nurses' Association, 1978.

**Figure 1.2**    *continued.*

Today's critical care nurse manager needs to be visionary. A visionary nurse manager can see beyond the daily tasks of the role and is future oriented. A plan for moving the intensive care unit (ICU) forward should be foremost in the nurse manager's mind with a dream of where that destination will be. A visionary manager constantly asks why things are done and questions habitual nursing practices without foundation. The response "because that's the way we've always done it" is an unacceptable one for the visionary nurse manager. Generation of creative new ideas for critical care nursing practice and striving to have the best ICU that can possibly exist are marks of an open-minded, visionary nurse manager.

A visionary nurse manager should be able to articulate a philosophy for the intensive care unit(s) for which he or she is responsible. When interviewing staff nurses a visionary nurse manager is comfortable in answering astute questions from the applicant such as "What is the philosophy of nursing specific to this critical care unit?" and "What creative plans have you implemented in this past year for this unit?"

Necessary skills for a nurse manager have been described in the nursing literature. Basic survival skills for nurse managers are similar to those in the business world and are listed in Table 1.2 (24). Other qualities predictive of a successful manager include maturity (not age-related), a sense of humor, and an ability to adapt to ever-changing job demands (8, 25).

Tom Peters addresses this desire to be responsive to rapid change in his book *Thriving on Chaos* (26). Peters describes a revolution in the corporate world that refutes previously stable and predictive business markets and promotes the realization of chaotic organizations. These organizations are those that are not only able to respond quickly to shifting circumstances but to proactively take advantage of them.

A successful nurse manager in today's unstable health care environment will recognize the advantages of remaining flexible and learning to love change. The nurse manager must also begin to evaluate staff nurses based on their receptivity to change and to continually ask "What have you changed in our unit?" as well as performing a self-assessment of this question, a common practice throughout all levels of the successful IBM corporation (26).

## SELECTION PROCESS

Including the critical care nursing staff in the interviewing process to hire a nurse manager for the ICU facilitates the staff's feelings of having input into the decision and will ultimately benefit the candidate selected, even if the candidate selected was not the staff's first choice. Identifying the new ICU nurse manager without input from the staff sets the manager up for failure and promotes hostility. The medical director of the ICU, other pertinent physicians, and other supervisory members of the health care team should also be involved in the interviews. Other nurse managers will want to screen potential applicants to ensure the presence of those desired characteristics previously described.

The interview to select the nurse manager should proceed in a systematic fashion and an objective scoring tool should be utilized for each candidate (27). Describing real scenarios and asking the applicant to respond assists in the identification of those desirable or undesirable traits described above.

**Table 1.1.** Identified Desired Characteristics of Nurse Managers

| N | Group | Desired Characteristics |
|---|---|---|
| 20 | Critical care nurses | Good communicator<br>Gives positive feedback<br>Promotes staff education and development<br>Supportive and respectful of nursing staff<br>Approachable and open<br>Knowledgeable in clinical area<br>Good listener<br>Accessible<br>Responds to staff in a timely manner<br>Professional<br>Positive<br>Consistent |
| 11 | Nurse managers | Good communicator<br>Supportive<br>Flexible<br>Consistent<br>Organized<br>Good listener<br>Clinical expertise<br>Honest<br>Professional<br>Fair |
| 23 | Undergraduates | Flexible<br>Supportive of staff<br>Approachable<br>Good communicator<br>Organized<br>Accessible<br>Knowledgeable<br>Open<br>Motivator<br>Promotes staff education<br>Positive |
| 9 | Nursing administration<br>graduate students | Good communicator<br>Positive<br>Supportive of staff<br>Good listener<br>Consistent |

## EDUCATIONAL PREPARATION

What should be the required educational level for the nurse manager role? In light of the need for a theory base in leadership and management content, a baccalaureate degree would seem to be the minimal educational level for the nurse manager. The AACN recommends that a nurse manager should be a baccalaureate-prepared professional nurse who is clinically experienced in the area of administrative responsibility and competent in the application of management principles (11).

In a sample of 288 hospitals surveyed, 49% required a minimum of a baccalaureate degree for the nurse manager role, 43% required a diploma or associate degree, and 3% require a master's-prepared

manager (13). When the chief nurse executives of these hospitals were asked if they believed master's-prepared nurse managers were cost effective, 87% responded affirmatively. In addition, 95% indicated they would hire master's-prepared nurse managers if they were available.

The question of whether master's-prepared clinical nurse specialists should pursue nurse manager positions has come to the forefront in nursing in the past 10 years. Chaska (28) predicted that the traditional nurse manager role may be replaced or redefined by clinical nurse specialists with management expertise (28). Chief nurse executives with experience in hiring clinical nurse specialists into the nurse manager position were asked how effec-

**Table 1.2.**   Basic Survival Skills for Nurse Managers[a]

Well-developed sense of self-awareness
Ability to manage work and personal and family life
Multiple interests and well-rounded experiences
Interpersonal sensitivity
Courage to take risks
Development of competent assistants
Method for self-criticism and self-discipline
Great curiosity
Experiential attitude
Tolerance for sustained work
Sense of calling or mission

[a]Adapted from Moore RC. A pragmatic view of nursing management. In: Sullivan EJ, Decker PJ, eds. Effective management in nursing. Menlo Park, California: Addison-Wesley Publishing Co, 1988, 571–590.

tive these nurses were in implementing the role. Seventy per cent reported that most or all clinical nurse specialists were effective in the role, while 30% reported only some or none were effective (13).

The lack of emphasis on management content in most clinical nurse specialist programs impedes this transition between these roles and points to the need for graduate programs to prepare clinical nurse managers at the master's level. Although traditionally most graduate nursing administration programs have focused on assistant director, director, or vice president level preparation, more recently the importance of the clinical nurse manager role has emerged as evidenced by incorporation of unit level management content into some graduate administration programs. Combining the master's degree in nursing with a master's degree in business administration has also received much attention as nursing turns to business experience for application in nursing management.

Educational preparation of the nurse manager has not been demonstrated to be significantly related to staff job satisfaction or turnover rates, although one study did show that master's-prepared nurse managers tended to have better scores in these areas in their units (29). As the percentage of master's-prepared nurse managers increases further studies should be conducted to detect any significant influences advanced management knowledge may demonstrate in this role.

## EXPERIENCE REQUIRED

Clinical and management experience are desirable for the ideal nurse manager candidate. A minimum of 3 years of experience has been reported as the mean number of years of experience to fulfill this position with a range of 0 to 5 years (13). The

debate over whether nursing experience is necessary at all or if nonnurse managers could be as effective has arisen in the nursing literature (30). In a survey of 216 hospital and nursing administrators, 7% indicated they currently employed a nonnurse in a nursing management position (30). Approximately one-third of hospital administrators and one-fourth of nursing administrators indicated they would be in favor of hiring nonnurses for nursing management positions. Nonnurses are disadvantaged by the lack of clinical experience. Sound critical care clinical experience and knowledge are valuable assets for the critical care nurse manager and assist in understanding the needs of the critical care nurse and patient. Identified advantages of clinical experience in the nurse manager role include: understanding of professional nursing, clinical credibility, and shorter orientation time (30). Further studies are necessary to determine the impact of clinical experience on the success of the nurse manager role.

## UNDESIRABLE CHARACTERISTICS

The Queen Bee syndrome has been identified within nursing and is known to increase with rising levels of management (31). This is a highly undesirable syndrome for a manager to acquire as it connotes a state most opposite of those traits previously described as positive for this role. The Queen Bee identifies with those in positions above her, is aligned with the establishment, resists change, holds antifeminist beliefs that she projects onto others, has a desire to run the show at the expense of others, and avoids group work or group solutions (31). Although the nurse manager role has demonstrated less of a tendency toward the Queen Bee syndrome than higher levels of nursing management, it is possible that this tendency could increase as this role becomes increasingly decentralized and important within the organization (31). It is essential that caution is exercised by the nurse manager entering the role to avoid this pitfall that can be very detrimental to the development of nursing as a profession (31).

Other undesirable characteristics for the critical care nurse manager are opposite of those previously described and include poor communication skills and an unsupportive attitude toward the nursing staff. "Paralysis through analysis" or lack of action has also been cited as a negative factor for nursing managers (32). Staff nurses appreciate a "bias for action" wherein approval does not need to be obtained at multiple levels before action commences (32). The critical care nurse manager must strive to decentralize unit decisions as much as possible and implement them rapidly.

## CONCLUSION

The role of the nurse manager has evolved to one of 24-hour accountability and total responsibility for patient care, patient outcomes, nursing productivity, and the fiscal bottom line of a given department or nursing unit. Nurse managers are now being recognized as department heads and pivotal within the health care organization. Despite this increased responsibility, salaries for this group remain low at a median annual level of $27,500 and there is a reported lower job satisfaction than that expressed by nursing staff (13, 33). Integrating the "right" managers into critical care nurse manager positions or developing those positive attributes identified in this chapter will not only enhance patient outcomes and nursing retention but will also assist in the promotion of the nurse manager role as the key to successful health care administration.

REFERENCES

1. Weeks L, Schneider L. Professional practice: the head nurse set the climate. Nurs Management 1987;*18*(6):48A–48G.
2. Vincent P, Billings C. Unit management as a factor in intensive care nursing personnel. Focus Crit Care 1988;*15*(3):45–49.
3. Porter-O'Grady T. Participatory management: the critical care nurse's role in the 21st century. Dimensions Crit Care Nurs 1987;*6*(3):131–133.
4. Nightingale F. Notes on nursing. Philadelphia: JB Lippincott, 1946.
5. Stevens B. The head nurse as manager. J Nurs Admin 1974;*4*(1):36–40.
6. Mohr M. Developing the first line manager. Nurs Management 1988;*19*(1):59–60.
7. Cardin S. Visionary nurse manager: key for survival. Pacesetter, AACN Los Angeles Chapter, 1987.
8. Fralic M. Developing the head nurse role: a key to survival in nursing service administration. In: Chaska N, ed. A time to speak. New York: McGraw-Hill, 1983:659–670.
9. American Association of Critical-Care Nurses. Scope of critical care nursing practice. Newport Beach, California: AACN, 1986.
10. Hartshorn J. President's message. Focus Crit C. 1987;*14*(3):73–75.
11. American Association of Critical-Care Nurses. Role expectations for the critical care manager. Newport Beach, California: AACN, 1986.
12. Searle L. Of legends and values. Heart & Lung 1988;*17*(4):28A–33A.
13. Hodges LC, Knapp R, Cooper J. Head nurses: their practice and education. J Nurs Admin 1987;*17*(12):39–44.
14. Kaluzny AD, Shortell SM. Creating and managing the future. In: Shortell SM, Kaluzny AD, eds. Health care management: a text in organization theory and behavior. New York: John Wiley & Sons, 1988, 492–522.
15. Sands D, Ismeurt R. Role alienation: staff nurses and powerlessness. Nurs Management 1986;*17*(5):42J–42P.
16. Pearlin L. Alienation from work: a study of nursing personnel. Am Sociolog Rev 1962;*27*:314–326.
17. Hall R. Professionalization and bureaucratization. Am Sociolog Rev 1968;*33*:92–104.
18. Flynn R. The nurse manager and the art of Japanese management. Nurs Management 1987;*18*(10):57–59.
19. Godfrey MA. Job satisfaction—or should it be dissatisfaction? Part 1. Nursing 1978;*8*(4):89–100.
20. Duxbury ML, Henly GA, Armstrong GD. Measurement of the organizational climate of the neonatal intensive care unit. Nurs Res 1982;*31*:83–87.
21. Everly GS, Falcione RL. Perceived dimensions of job satisfaction for staff registered nurses. Nurs Res 1976;*25*:346–348.
22. Duxbury M, Armstrong G, Drew D, et al. Henly S. Head nurse leadership style with staff nurse burnout and job satisfaction in neonatal intensive care units. Nurs Res 1984;*33*:97–101.
23. Levine CD, Wilson SF, Guido GW. Personality factors of critical care nurses. Heart & Lung 1988;*17*(4):392–398.
24. Moore RC. A pragmatic view of nursing management. In: Sullivan EJ, Decker PJ, eds. Effective management in nursing. Menlo Park, California: Addison-Wesley, 1988, 571–590.
25. Warihey PD. First-line managers: training on the cutting edge. Nurs Management 1986;*17*(10):69–72.
26. Peters T. Thriving on chaos: handbook for a management revolution. New York: Alfred A Knopf, Inc, 1987.
27. Urtel J, Runtz S. Eight steps to recruiting the right manager. Nurs Management 1987;*18*(1):28–33.
28. Chaska NL. The nursing profession: a time to speak. New York: McGraw-Hill, 1983.
29. Avent S, Beggerly KB. Head nurse education vs. staff nurse turnover: report of a formal study. Nurs Management 1988;*19*(3):116.
30. Giddens JF, Homan KP, Towns-Culton B. Nursing management positions—for non-nurses? Nurs Management 1988;*19*(12):62–64.
31. Halsey S. The queen bee syndrome: one solution to role conflict for nurse managers. In: Hardy ME, Conway M. (eds.) Role theory perspectives for health professionals. New York: Appleton-Century-Crofts, 1978, 231–249.
32. Kramer M, Schmalenburg C. Magnet hospitals. Part 1. Institutions of excellence. J Nurs Admin 1988; *18*(1):13–24.
33. Baird JE. Changes in nurse attitudes: management strategies for today's environment. J Nurs Admin 1987;*17*(9):38–43.

# Chapter 2

# Recruiting Critical Care Personnel

DOLORES GOMEZ

Hospitals are fast becoming large intensive care facilities. Patients admitted to hospitals are more acutely ill, and length of stay has shortened. Technological advances have skyrocketed and will continue at an accelerating pace. The need for critical care practitioners has never been greater.

## FACTORS INFLUENCING THE CURRENT MARKETPLACE

The health care system in the United States has entered into an era of change. This new health care environment is both highly competitive and regulated. Prospective payment, capitation, managed care, Health Maintenance Organizations (HMOs) and ''discount packages'' have emerged in recent years to combat the rising costs of health care. Added to this turbulent environment is the manpower shortages that currently plague the labor-intensive hospital industry. Successful organizations must develop and implement sound strategies to remain economically sound and maintain quality patient care.

Nursing shortages have been an ongoing reality. According to the United States Department of Labor, registered nurses have been in a shortage condition since 1937, aside from the early 1970s and 1982–1985. However, the current nursing shortage has been heralded to be the most severe to hit the inpatient hospital industry. The American Hospital Association claims the vacancy rate for registered nurses more than doubled, from 6.3 to 13.6% between December 1985 and December 1986 (1).

Reasons for the shortage are numerous. The rapid shift in career goals among working women that occurred in the 1970s is reshaping the labor force. As young women reject low-pay, low-status careers in favor of other professional degrees, colleges produce fewer nurses and more physicians, lawyers, business women, and engineers (2). Between 1983 and 1986 enrollment in baccalaureate degree programs in nursing (BSNs) dropped 19%, enrollment in associate degree programs in nursing (ADNs) dropped 29%, and graduate enrollment was down by 6.2% (3). According to an annual survey sponsored by the Cooperative Institutional Research Program (CIRP) of the University of California at Los Angeles (UCLA) and the American Council on Education (ACE), there was a 50% decline in the proportion of freshman women who plan to pursue a nursing career between 1974 and 1986. This decline was most dramatic between 1983 and 1986 when nursing as a career choice fell from 8.3 to 5.1% (1, 2).

Decreased interest in nursing as a career rests on economic as well as societal factors. Salary compensation and career mobility are major considerations when a student decides a particular avenue of study. Nursing falls drastically short when measured against these economic incentives.

Maximal salaries for experienced registered nurses are less than 40% more than starting salaries. The average base nursing salary in 1987 was 21,127. The average top salary was $29,350 (4, 5). In contrast, physicians, lawyers, and engineers usually realize a three-fold increase in base salary over the course of their career.

The image of nursing in American society has been detrimental to the ability to recruit into professional nursing. Depiction of nurses as hand maidens, sex objects, or ''battle-axes'' by the media has done little to enhance nursing's image. It is clear that society does not value nursing for what nursing accomplishes. Recruitment into nursing is difficult when a poor image and inadequate financial compensation are reality. Consequently, a current college-bound student is less likely to pursue a career in nursing (6).

The shortage of nurses will not easily be resolved. Factors that will continue to accentuate the shortage of in-patient hospital nursing include:

(*a*) competition by alternative delivery systems, businesses, insurance companies, and consulting firms that dilute qualified staff; (*b*) increased patient acuity coupled with advances in technology resulting in increased demand; (*c*) a decreasing pool of nursing graduates as workforce demographics change and societal issues influence career choice; and (*d*) lack of effective retention programs and career mobility within the hospital setting.

## CRITICAL CARE NURSING: SUPPLY VERSUS DEMAND

Hardest hit by the recent registered nurse shortage are the critical care units of hospitals. It is in these units that the complex, acutely ill patient requires the expert knowledge and skills of the critical care registered nurse. The highest concentration of registered nurses are employed in critical care units where the ratio of nurse to patient is 1:2 or 1:1, depending on the patient's acuity status.

The number of beds devoted to intensive care has increased significantly since the 1960s when the first coronary care units (CCUs) were established. Intensive care units (ICUs) have become larger, specialty ICUs have emerged (i.e., Neuro ICU, Trauma ICU, CCU, Surgical ICU, etc.), and technological developments have been concentrated in these areas. The shift to more intensive hospital care has resulted in an increased manpower demand at a time when a severe shortage of registered nurses has drastically reduced the supply.

The effects of the registered nurse (RN) shortage has widespread implications and consequences for nurses, hospital administrators, and the health care industry. The shortage is affecting quality of patient care, the work environment for RNs, and access to health services according to the Secretary's Commission on Nursing (6). Identified factors include: (*a*) increased work stress due to increased patient severity of illness and decreased support services; (*b*) increased workload resulting in prioritized care—that which is absolutely essential is provided; (*c*) decreased morale; (*d*) agency nurse utilization that affects work environment and quality of patient care; and (*e*) closure of intensive care unit beds and emergency rooms due to lack of critical care RNs thereby compromising access to health services.

According to a recent study by the American Association of Critical-Care Nurses (AACN) (7) as many as 125,000 critical care nurses are needed now to fill existing vacancies in hospitals nationwide. Despite the employment of 194,000 critical care nurses in hospitals today, a 13.8% critical care nurse vacancy rate still exists. The study also predicts that by 1990 a 42% to 90% increase in the number of critical care nurses will be needed to care for the critically ill.

Two supply issues emerge in the discussion of critical care nursing. Not only must there be an adequate supply of registered nurses to care for these acutely ill patients, but they must also be educated and certified in critical care nursing beyond basic nursing education. The addition of this lag time (6 months–1 year) to develop competence in critical care nursing has been devastating and has compounded the problem of inadequate numbers of qualified critical care nurses.

The supply of critical care practitioners is not only affected by the number of nurses entering the profession, but also by the number who stay in nursing. Annual turnover rates for critical care nurses average approximately 25% and may be as high as 50% (7). Staff satisfaction and emphasis on retention are therefore imperative to ensure availability of potential critical care nurses. As stated by the past president of the American Association of Critical-Care Nurses, Jeanette Hartshorn, "The major challenge in critical care today is to get the kind of nurses needed, and to keep them once you get them" (8).

Few nurses enter critical care units immediately after graduation. More commonly, nurses will work on an acute care unit for a period of time to sharpen basic nursing skills before applying to work in a critical care unit. Once hired, development of specialty skills involves an additional time commitment or lag time before these nurses are able to assume a full patient load.

Recruitment of new graduates into intensive care has increased as the supply of experienced RNs has decreased. The development of critical care internship programs, extensive critical care courses, traineeships, and postgraduate fellowships in critical care are aimed primarily at attracting new nurses into intensive care. Critical care content has also been incorporated into the undergraduate curriculum in many accredited nursing schools across the United States. In 1985 approximately 40% of accredited schools included a structured critical care course (9). An expansion to include critical care in all undergraduate nursing curricula is needed as a learning experience for hospital-bound nurses as well as a possible feeder mechanism into critical care as a future practice setting.

## SUCCESSFUL RECRUITMENT STRATEGIES

Successful recruitment of critical care nurses encompasses a variety of strategies. Hospitals should utilize a combination of strategies that address both supply and demand in their recruitment program. Recruitment strategies include advertising, marketing, financial incentives, feeder mechanisms, and demand (see Table 2.1).

A well thought-out and planned recruitment program is necessary to ensure an adequate supply of critical care nurses. It is vital that the critical care nurse manager who is responsible for ensuring "appropriately qualified staff to provide care on a 24-hour basis" (AACN Structure Comprehensive Standard VII) (10) be actively involved in all aspects of the recruitment plan. Components of the recruitment plan include: (*a*) data collection, e.g., recruitment needs, marketplace, and turnover statistics; (*b*) analysis of the data; (*c*) methodology of recruitment strategies; (*d*) evaluation of results; and (*e*) feedback to determine adjustments to the plan. Additional input from all levels of the organization should be solicited in the development and implementation of the recruitment plan (11).

### Advertising/Marketing

Advertisement is the primary recruitment mechanism that informs the nursing community of available positions within the institution. Methods include exhibiting at job fairs, career days, and conventions; advertising in local and nonlocal newspapers, specialty area journals, and career directories; hosting open-house activities; and participating in various activities associated with recruiting nursing students. Style and presentation are important components of the advertising campaign. These should be consistent with the image and philosophy of the institution as well as that of professional critical care nursing.

Participation of the nurse manager in advertisement activities is crucial for a successful campaign. Active involvement at job fairs, conventions, and career days provides the prospective hire with the opportunity to meet the nurse manager and get questions about the critical care unit answered immediately. On the spot interviews can take place accelerating the hiring process. Open house activities should also be attended by the nurse manager of the critical care unit. One-on-one contact can

**Table 2.1.** Recruitment Strategies

Advertising
  Newspapers
  Professional magazines
  Schools of nursing
  Career days/fairs
  Professional meetings/conferences
  Open house

Marketing
  Image of nursing
  Unique programs
  Public relations
  Involvement in local clubs
  Senior/junior high affiliation

Financial incentives
  Specialty differential
  Sign-on bonus
  Recruitment bonus
  Creative benefits programs
  Shift/weekend incentives
  Tuition reimbursement
  Nursing scholarship
  Relocation
  Competitive wages

Feeder mechanisms
  Student work-study programs
  Student financial assistance
  LVN to RN incentive
  Recruitment from within
  Critical care course
  Specialty courses
  Student rotations
  In-house registry

Demand
  Practice environment
  Authority/autonomy over practice
  Clinical ladder
  Participative management
  Nursing leaders
  Shared governance
  Flexible hours
  Orientation program
  Professional practice model
  Continuing education
  Clinical nurse specialist
  Nursing school affiliation

be made, interviews conducted, and tours of the unit provided by the individual most knowledgeable of the area.

Content of the advertisements submitted for publication in newspapers, journals, and career directories should also be determined by the nurse manager. A particular focus, specialty, or aspect of care delivery may enhance and/or direct the advertisement to a particular market niche. The unit manager is also ensured that the advertisement adequately describes the critical care environment and needs at the appropriate time.

Marketing involves advertisement as well as professional and public relations activities. Informing the professional and lay community about critical care nursing is an important component of a successful recruitment program. Methods may include advertising critical care nursing in the newspaper or on local radio, marketing and involvement with local clubs and charities, community education activities sponsored through the hospital utilizing critical care personnel [i.e., cardiopulmonary resuscitation (CPR) classes, health education], program sponsorship of junior and senior high school training programs, and information sharing within the critical care nursing community regarding unique programs and specialties within the hospital organization (12, 13).

## Financial Incentives

Within the current competitive marketplace for critical care nurses, the utilization of financial incentives is useful in attracting some nurses to one institution over another. Relocation monies and sign-on bonuses are short-range attempts to recruit nurses on the front end (14). Higher salaries that do more than keep up with inflation and are competitive within the recruiting market should be maintained. A specialty differential for critical care nurses or certification in critical care nursing (CCRN) is particularly useful in targeting this population (15). Differentials for night, evening, and weekend shifts at a significant rate are necessary to attract nurses to these difficult-to-fill positions.

Creative benefit programs that are flexible to meet the needs of the individual nurse are effective recruitment strategies in today's marketplace. An analysis of the demographics of the nursing population within the institution can determine benefit options to be provided. These flexible benefits may include child care, tuition reimbursement, increased pay/no benefits option, reimbursement accounts, benefits to part-time employees, retirement programs, and other insurance and benefit options (16, 17).

Another recruitment strategy is the implementation of financial compensation to employed personnel for the recruitment of critical care nurses. Involvement and utilization of critical care nurses in the recruitment program can produce favorable results from both a recruitment and retention standpoint. Strategies may include monetary reward through a recruitment bonus, sending nurses on recruitment trips to conventions and job fairs, and returning nurses to their schools of nursing to recruit students.

## Feeder Mechanisms

The development of "feeder mechanisms," i.e., the ability to pull into the institution potential future critical care personnel, is an essential component of the recruitment program. There are many types of feeder mechanisms that can be utilized. Variation exists regarding the methods instituted by particular hospitals in their implementation of this recruitment strategy. The larger number of feeder mechanisms used, the greater is the potential for successful recruitment of critical care personnel.

Affiliation with schools of nursing that offer critical care rotations should be sought and maintained. It is important that the student's experience is a positive one, therefore critical care staff involvement is crucial. Critical care nurses need to become student advocates, student preceptorships should be developed, and positive feedback mechanisms must be maintained with both the instructor and student (14). In addition, encouragement of joint appointments of critical care nurse managers, clinical nurse specialists, and qualified critical care personnel with schools of nursing can enhance the attraction of nursing students into critical care practice in a hospital.

Student nurse financial assistance programs are offered by many hospitals as a contractual agreement to assure employment after graduation. The student nurse is assisted monetarily through a loan program that is "pardoned" after an agreed-upon tenure of postgraduation employment. This recruitment strategy is a generic one aimed at attracting new nurses into the hospital. Such a program will, however, increase the available pool of registered nurses for potential employment in the intensive care setting.

Work-study programs aimed at employment of student nurses during the school year and summer months comprise another potent feeder mechanism. Students can be employed in the critical care unit as secretaries, nurse aides, technicians, or ancillary personnel. Internship or externship programs developed specifically for the training of student nurses for these ancillary functions are useful to promote a smooth transition and positive experience for the student nurse. Nurse manager input and participation in program design and responsibility for unit-specific implementation are crucial elements of internship and externship programs. Recruitment of these student nurses after graduation has been highly successful in a number of institutions.

Incentives aimed at encouraging existing non-professional staff to pursue RN licensure through educational assistance programs is a widely utilized feeder strategy. Although use of Licensed Vocational Nurses (LVNs) within intensive care units is not advocated by most hospitals and professional nursing organizations, many organizations do employ LVNs in ICUs. Financial and employment incentives for these individuals to return to school should be developed. Experience factors for postlicensure salary can be instituted to retain these staff after graduation.

Recruitment of nurses from within the hospital to work in intensive care may meet with some resistance from other nursing areas. Shortages have been realized in all areas of hospital nursing. However, intensive care nursing has been hardest hit and is the most difficult to recruit. Development of a critical care course aimed at in-house nurses, traineeships for particular specialty intensive care units, or a stepladder career program (i.e., telemetry unit, subacute coronary care, acute coronary care) may serve to enhance this recruitment strategy. Programs developed that offer critical care training and education for interested staff nurses have been successful in filling critical care vacancies (18, 19).

Critical care courses offered to the community provide yet another avenue for recruitment. Visibility as a center for critical care education can serve to attract nurses to the hospital. Participation by nurse managers, clinical nurse specialists, and qualified critical care staff in the delivery of course content establishes contact with potential future employees. A tour of the intensive care facility by the critical care nurse manager for interested course participants should be considered. Other specialty courses can be developed for presentation to the critical care nursing community.

In-house nurse registries or "pools" can be another area from which to tap future critical care personnel. Nurses may join a pool to gain experience within different areas of the hospital before deciding on permanent employment on a particular unit or in a certain specialty. The benefits of recruiting pool nurses into intensive care are the strong

nursing skills and experience these nurses have generally acquired.

## Demand Strategies

Demand strategies focus upon creation of organizational conditions within the hospital that will attract and retain qualified critical care nurses. These strategies include designing and testing nursing service delivery systems that incorporate improved practice environments, authority and autonomy in nursing practice, involvement in hospital management decisions regarding standards of practice and support services, and adequate compensation linked to competence and performance (20–22).

Results of the Magnet Hospital Study (23) conducted by the American Nurses Association (ANA), which focused on hospitals that attract and retain professional nurses, provide direction for demand strategy development. The major elements identified by the Magnet Hospital Study to have contributed to the magnetism of these 41 hospitals are: a participatory management style; strong, supportive quality leadership; decentralized organizational structure with nursing involvement in hospital committees; ample, qualified nursing staff; competitive salaries and benefits; flexible work schedules; presence of career ladders; high quality care standards; professional practice models that incorporate autonomy and peer support; high value placed on education and teaching; professional image that is valued and respected; emphasis on professional growth and development; and continuous efforts toward improvement of the practice environment.

The magnet study results emphasize the importance of these elements throughout the hospital organization. The crucial link or key is the nurse manager who operationalizes these elements within the critical care setting. The critical care nurse manager should be a role model, participate in specialty nursing organization activities, engage in education and teaching activities, emphasize professional growth and development of the critical care staff, and pursue high quality standards and expectations. It is the nurse manager who ultimately determines the demand strategy for the critical care unit.

The AACN Demonstration Project (24), aimed at the improvement of the practice environment through value identification and subsequent implementation of strategies to uphold the values believed to be essential for effective critical care nursing practice, provides additional information for demand strategy development. Identified fundamental values of critical care nursing practice are: (*a*) an all RN staff, (*b*) nurses with expertise in critical care, (*c*) nurse-physician collaboration, (*d*) use of critical care standards, and (*e*) participative management. Results of Phase I of the AACN Demonstration Project include high nursing expertise, low turnover (8%), increased morale, positive patient outcomes, increased job satisfaction, and a high degree of nurse-physician collaboration. The critical care nurse manager is responsible for upholding the fundamental values of critical care nursing practice within the intensive care environment.

Strategies that focus on demand are long term in nature and involve an in-depth analysis of the state of affairs of an institution. Determinations of staff satisfaction, identification of critical care retention issues, and analysis of exit interview information are necessary to ascertain the current practice environment. A comparison of like elements to the Magnet hospitals and the AACN Demonstration Project can provide additional information and direction.

## REDUCING DEMAND

Demand-reducing strategies are self-limiting within the critical care environment. Patient acuity and severity of illness require an adequate number of professional critical care nurses to delivery quality care. Therefore, strategies employed to reduce the demand of critical care nurses should be instituted with caution. Job restructuring and delegation of tasks to ancillary personnel and support departments must be carefully implemented with the focus on patient outcome indicators.

Improvement of staff productivity to reduce demand provides additional strategy options. These include automated patient care systems, bedside computer terminals, productivity incentives, improved support services, and reduction and/or ease of staff nurse administrative responsibilities and paperwork. Operationalizing these strategy options may, however, be cost prohibitive.

## UTILIZING ANCILLARY PERSONNEL

Cost-cutting strategies employed by hospitals to survive the changes in the health care environment included decreasing "nonessential" staff personnel (25). In the intensive care unit reintrenchment often meant the loss of ancillary personnel such as secretaries, monitor technicians, nurse aides,

and supply technicians. Support departments such as housekeeping and dietary were also affected by cost cuts, resulting in a leaner staff and decreased service. Consequently, professional registered nurses in the intensive care units were held responsible for performing nonnursing duties as well as the delivery of high quality direct patient care.

The pendulum is now forced to swing in the opposite direction. A decrease in the number of available critical care nurses to provide bedside care demands that ancillary personnel be hired to perform nonnursing duties to support professional nursing. Ancillary personnel should therefore be used in the intensive care unit for the provision of nonnursing functions and as a support service to nursing.

Utilization of ancillary personnel in critical care for nonpatient care activities should be specifically defined. Job descriptions and task lists should be developed that clearly delineate scope of job responsibility and function. Nonnursing tasks in critical care include secretarial duties; computer data input and retrieval (nursing station); supply ordering, acquisition, and disposal; equipment setup and maintenance; transport and errands; and monitor surveillance.

Use of ancillary personnel for nurse aide activities in intensive care is controversial at this time (25). The American Association of Critical-Care Nurses position states "use of non-nursing personnel in patient care situations is not the answer to the nursing shortage. The multidimensional needs of critically ill patients can only be met by critical care nurses" (26). However, many hospitals are utilizing ICU technicians or aides to assist nurses in the provision of care. Care tasks may include assisting with a bath, assisting in turning patients, emptying urinary bags, sitting with an agitated patient to prevent injury, and being a second hand when needed (see Table 2.2).

Delivery of quality critical care at the bedside is nursing's responsibility. The critical care nurse makes decisions regarding the care to be provided and techniques used for its delivery. Critical care managers and administrators must carefully analyze and determine the impact of utilizing ancillary personnel in these practice settings. Workload analysis, quality assurance indicators, patient outcome measures, staff satisfaction, and turnover statistics will aid the nurse manager in this analysis.

Job restructuring to support the delivery of bed-

**Table 2.2.**   Ancillary Task Responsibilities

Secretarial/clerical
 Telephone
 Transcription
 Computer entry
 Paperwork duties
 Desk management

Technological
 Electrocardiogram monitor technician
 Setup of bedside equipment
 Equipment maintenance
 Supply-equipment inventory

Support
 Transport activities
  Miscellaneous (lab, x-ray)
  Assistance with patient

Care activities
 Assist RN
  Bed bath
  Turning
  Feeding
  Patient amenities
  Sitter for agitated patient
  Linen changes

side nursing is not synonymous with replacement with less qualified care technicians. The 1988 American Medical Association (AMA) proposal to develop a nonnurse, bedside technician called a Registered Care Technologist (RCT) as a solution to the shortage of bedside personnel will have a negative impact on patient care if implemented (27). Nursing administrators must take the forefront in the development of job design for ancillary personnel in the critical care units.

Critical care nurse managers are responsible for the development and implementation of a thorough orientation program for ancillary personnel in the critical care unit. The critical nature of the intensive care unit, the high degree of technology, and fast pace necessitate specialty training for all personnel employed in the setting. Training should include specific task education with return demonstration. Various techniques for the delivery of content can be utilized such as classroom lecture, videotaped information, checklists, and preceptor assignment. Scope and boundary delineation of the role must also be communicated during the orientation program.

Selection of appropriate and qualified individuals to work as support personnel in the critical care environment is vitally important. The person chosen should be bright and energetic, have the

capacity and interest to learn new tasks, possess good interpersonal and communication skills and the ability to follow directions. Past experience as a ward secretary, monitor technician, or hospital employee may be considered as qualifications. Nursing students make excellent candidates, however availability may be problematic due to school schedule commitments. Students pursuing other careers within the health care field may also prove to be good candidates for these positions. Ultimately, the bottom line decision by the nurse manager rests on the ability of the applicant to meet the job requirements of the position. Selection of the right individual will ensure adequate support for nursing within the intensive care unit.

## FUTURE TRENDS FOR NURSE RECRUITMENT

Recruitment for critical care personnel will continue to be the primary focus and concern of hospital human resource and recruitment programs. This will be particularly true for tertiary, public, and teaching hospitals where the number of intensive care beds continues to expand. Changing demographics to that of an older patient population with multiple medical and nursing care requirements will increase the demand side of the equation (demand>supply). Utilization of short-term, quick-fix strategies to fill immediate vacancies is likely to continue.

Likewise, the critical care nurse manager will see a continuing expansion of her/his role in recruitment activities. These will include activities aimed at both short-term (advertisement) and long-term (student program development) recruitment strategies. Successful nurse managers must excel in this aspect of role development.

Foreign nurse recruitment is on the rise once again as the shortage becomes more acute. Targeted countries are primarily the Philippines, Australia, Canada, and the British Isles. This recruitment strategy is very costly and can take a great deal of time in immigration approvals. In addition, the actual pool of available foreign nurses willing to relocate is self-limiting (6).

The future trend of nurse recruitment will be an emphasis on long-term strategies aimed at marketing nursing as a career option. Provision of more scholarships, traineeships, loans, and other means of financial assistance are essential so nursing can compete with other career choices. Active lobbying and involvement with the legislature to gain maximal financial assistance for schools of nursing, new clinical training programs, and students are needed.

Strategies that target primary and secondary schools are emerging. Examples of collaborative activities between hospital organizations and schools include planned field trips to hospitals to observe staff nurses in practice; jointly sponsored work-study programs for high school students; development of a speaker bureau to address nursing as a career to PTA groups, counselor organizations, and students; health education classes for student clubs and organizations; and sponsorship of tutoring programs. Availability of volunteer and "candystriper" programs should be publicized.

Hospitals will be forced to expand increasing amounts of resources on recruitment and retention activities. Strategic planning with senior management involvement will be essential in the development of a plan to deal with ongoing manpower shortages. Development of recruitment-retention programs with long-term commitment and support of hospital administrators is key to resolving nursing shortages within the hospital organization now and for the future (22, 28).

REFERENCES

1. American Hospital Association. The nursing shortage: you can't afford to lose this nurse. Teleconference Proceedings, April 21, 1988.
2. Green K. Who wants to be a nurse? Am Demographics 1988;10(1):46–61.
3. American Hospital Association. Protecting an endangered species. Program Notes: November, 1987.
4. Powills S. Nurses: a sound investment for financial stability. Hospitals 1988;62(9):46–50.
5. American Nurses' Association. ANA Campaign to Recruit and Retain RNs. Am Nurse 1988;20(3):15–16, 22.
6. Secretary's Commission on Nursing. Executive summary. Interim Rep July, 1988.
7. Levine and Associates. Summary analysis of critical care nurse supply and requirements. American Association of Critical-Care Nurses, Newport Beach, California: 1988.
8. Hartshorn J. Nobody does it better. Heart & Lung 1987;16(5):24A–25.
9. Jeffries P. Undergraduates need critical care, too. Focus Crit Care. 1988;15(2):73–75.
10. American Association of Critical-Care Nurses. Standards for the nursing care of the critically ill. Reston, Virginia: Reston Publishing Co, Inc, 1981.
11. Wall L. Plan development for a nurse recruitment-retention program. J Nurs Admin 1988;18(2):20–26.
12. Connelly J, Strauser J. Managing recruitment and retention problems: an application of the marketing process. J Nurs Admin 1983;3(10):17–22.
13. Leadership Institute AACN Task Force. Attract nursing students into critical care practice. Newport Beach, California: AACN, 1987.
14. Vestal K, ed. Bonus programs ease staff shortage. Aspen's advisor for nurse executives. 1987;2(8):1,7.
15. Dunbar S. Should CCRN nurses receive a salary differential? Dimensions Crit Care Nurs 1985;4(6):361–367.
16. McDonagh K, Sorensen M. Restructuring nursing salaries: a mandate for the future. Nurs Management 1988;19(2):39–41.
17. Curtin L. A shortage of nurses: traditional approaches won't work this time. Nurs Management. 1987;18(9):7–8.
18. Monaghan J, Perro K, Haran M. Critical care staff shortages. Nurs Management 1983;14(1):38–39.
19. Wickes M, Mandak B. New beginning: ICU nursing shortage eliminated internally. Nurs Management 1987;18(7):72A–72H.
20. Spero J. American Association of Colleges of Nursing statement on the nursing shortage. Washington DC: National Center for Higher Education, 1988.
21. Scherer P. Hospitals that attract (and keep) nurses. Am J Nurs 1988;88(1):34–40.
22. American Hospital Association. Final report of the special committee on nursing. Executive summary. Presented at American Hospital Association Convention, New Orleans, 1988.
23. McClure M, Poulin M, Sovie M, et al. Magnet hospitals: attraction and retention of professional nurses. Kansas City: American Nurses Association, 1982:83–98.
24. Mitchell P. American Association of Critical-Care Nurses Demonstration Project Phase I Report. Newport Beach, California: AACN, 1988.
25. Will G. The dignity of nursing. Newsweek 1988; May 23:80.
26. American Association of Critical-Care Nurses. Technician issue addressed by AACN. Focus Crit Care 1988;15(4):73–74.
27. American Medical Association. Registered care technologist proposal. June, 1988.
28. Mowry M, Korpman R. Hospitals, nursing, and medicine: the years ahead. J Nurs Admin 1987;(17)11:16–22.

# Chapter 3

# Identifying Competent Critical Care Staff

DONNA L. BERTRAM

Patients in critical care units may present with various physiological problems, psychosocial issues, and educational needs that require the expertise of a competent registered nurse. With the focus on effectiveness and efficiency in critical care units, the nurse manager must hire and develop a competent critical care staff. The staff members represent the best asset in any unit. They work with patients, families, physicians, and others representing both the facility and the nursing profession. Each staff member utilizes time, money, and human resources in carrying out the nursing process with critically ill patients. Identifying desired characteristics and selecting competent critical care staff encompass the most important roles of the manager. Competence along with caring and professional behaviors leads to a successful unit. Choosing the right type of staff may create a unit that promotes professionalism, lengthens retention, maintains efficiency, and decreases hassles.

## COMPETENCE

Critical care managers desire to choose staff who are dedicated, enthusiastic, knowedgeable, and competent. Competence refers to being adequate, suitable, and properly qualified for the position. Definitions of competent performance may vary with technological changes, geographic areas, institutional desires, and nursing practices. The area of competence in critical care requires both knowing and doing nursing practice. In critical care this includes technical competence, patient outcome achievement, professional and personal contributions, personal behavior, intellectual ability, and work methods.

Measurement of competence in critical care nursing has not yet been derived from thorough research (1). Many techniques for measurement have been identified, but not one technique has been widely used (2). In fact, nursing educators and nursing administrators have not yet achieved consensus on appropriate competencies for beginning practitioners or on the differentiation of competencies between educational levels. More research remains to be done in outlining necessary clinical competency requirements. Some authors have developed helpful materials. Toth and Ritchey describe the use of the Basic Knowledge Assessment Tool (BKAT) for critical care nursing that can assist in-service educators in preparing staff for critical care (3). Internal credentialing as a means of identifying staff competency has been described by Scrima who developed a program to document proficiencies in certain clinical areas (4).

Many nursing organizations offer certification programs as measures of competence. The American Association of Critical-Care Nurses (AACN) Certification Corporation tests for competence in critical care. The CCRN credential is awarded to those who successfully pass the examination. The AACN validated the test structure and knowledge base through the Role Delineation Study. The use of CCRNs offers the value of clinical expertise important to the caring of the critically ill. The AACN Demonstration Project reflected that the high use of an all registered nurse staff with 39% CCRNs positively affected retention, quality, and patient satisfaction (5).

The understanding, implementation, and evaluation of standards of practice offer a framework for the manager in determining competence. Standards for nursing care of critically ill patients have been identified by the AACN in "AACN Standards for Nursing Care of the Critically Ill" (6). These standards serve as a guide for providing quality care from a structure, process, and outcome approach. The Joint Commission on Accreditation of Hospitals Organization provides standards for special care units that assist the manager in identifying various characteristics necessary for nursing staff (7).

Before the critical care manager can choose competent staff, the essentials of the performance required must be identified. The job description offers the main activities involved in the work required. Each of the identified performance requirements may be comprised of many skills and tasks. The manager who clearly knows what the staff are expected to do in meeting patient outcomes has a basis for choosing desirable employees. A check list that includes important and expected skills and tasks necessary for the patient population helps in clarifying expectations for both the new employee and the manager. Basic curriculum content for critical care nurse education has been outlined by Alspach (8). Basic content for critical care needs to cover arrhythmia interpretation, body fluid monitoring, cardiopulmonary resuscitation, hemodynamic monitoring, and mechanical ventilator management (9). Specific content unique to each unit determines necessary skills for competence in practice.

In reviewing the job description, each expected performance requirement needs to be observable, measurable, and specific. Failure to highlight key expectations may lead to disappointment after the employee has been hired. The employee may be unsure of how to implement an activity or perform a certain task in the new setting. The job description and skills check list can be given to the applicant for discussion at the interview. Key responsibilities and specifications for the job may be highlighted and explained. Prerequisites such as rotating shifts, working evenings, nights, or weekends also need to be reviewed in light of expectations of performance.

## ASSESSMENT OF DESIRED CHARACTERISTICS

Eight major characteristics provide the identification of a competent critical care nurse. These characteristics include knowledge, experience, intellectual factors, motivation, personality, human relationships, communication skills, and professional involvement (10–13). Assessing each candidate in these areas helps the manager choose the right person who can meet the expectations. Suggested questions for each area are identified in the implementation of the selection process.

Knowledge focuses on what the candidate knows about the aspects and requirements for the job. The basis for this comes predominantly from their educational experience, continuing education, self-study, and certification (14). Knowledge alone can be powerful but the interviewer needs to differentiate the knowledge base from the application and implementation of that knowledge. The unit manager may need to determine the use of a new graduate versus a nurse with 3 years of medical nursing knowledge. The manager must assess what knowledge will best fit unit needs. Factors include the type of nursing education offered by the candidate, the acuity demands of the patient, any previous critical care content, and grade point averages. Key elements in seeking more information include exploration of physical assessment knowledge and application, scientific principles, school references, awards and achievements, pertinent papers, or research projects. Simulation models have been used to test problem solving, decision making, and creative abilities (15). Educational requirements need to be relevant to the job position. Knowledge can be assessed by state board scores or the evidence of completion of certification examinations. The AACN Demonstration Project revealed that with a high level of CCRNs, the unit had a low attrition rate, lower than predicated mortality, and effective unit functioning (5).

Experience refers to work history. Often on the application, the candidate fills out the last three to five jobs. The unit manager determines the appropriateness of the experience for the current job being sought. Experience may include clinical time in critical care and non-critical care areas, working in nonnursing jobs, full or part-time work, and the types of job duties that were done. The unit manager looks at the type, length and recentness of previous jobs and any outstanding achievements. New graduates and experienced nurses bring different backgrounds to the unit. When both types of practitioners are hired, the manager needs to develop specific orientation programs appropriate for the different levels of practice. The American Association of Critical-Care Nurses' position statement on the "Integration of New Graduates into Critical Care" developed strategies to assist a manager in successfully using new graduates (16). These strategies focus on clinical, personnel, fiscal, and environmental management. Areas of emphasis include the manager's commitment, utilization of standards, developmental areas for the new graduate, orientation programs, use of preceptorships, and quality assurance activities. Personnel management strategies include choosing candidates who are most likely to be successful, providing adequate staffing during orientation, and offering student clinical experiences in critical care. Budgeting for recruitment activities, cost of preceptorships and orientation programs, and materials are important strategies in fiscal management. The environmental strategies outline the need to review unit goals, promote collaborative practice, and provide stress management.

Intellectual factors represent a desired characteristic in critical care. This area incorporates the use of a decision making process and the capacity for understanding concepts and facts. Critical thinking skills become a priority in a rapidly changing environment such as an intensive care unit. The early detection of problems followed by the right interventions become the patient's link to successful outcomes. Critical thinking involves proactive and reactive actions. Preparing for problems and responding to them requires judgment and logical thinking. Often the educational preparation provides the nurse with the necessary knowledge for basic care. As the nurse gains more experience, the ability to problem solve and make sound judgments strengthens. One study on diagnostic reasoning strategies of nurses revealed that with more knowledge and experience, nurses were more accurate in diagnosis and tended toward using a more systematic method of acquiring data (17). The unit manager can assess critical thinking skills by how well the candidate uses the problem solving process, analyzing the ability to make certain decisions, the type of planning the candidate may use, the listening ability, and how well the candidate organizes thoughts. The use of scenarios or fictitious problems will give the manager clues to critical thinking ability (15). The manager may present a clinical situation involving a patient care problem that may affect quality outcome or present a situation with two possible solutions. Asking the applicant to solve or think out loud helps the unit manager assess the critical thinking skill.

Motivation plays an integral part in the evaluation of the applicant. Motivation by an individual determines how much they can accomplish in the position. The unit manager may not motivate an employee but can manage the environment and understand work behavior. Employees have reasons for doing what they do in the job and make choices to meet their own objectives. Their choice represents a value to them. The value or reward may be internal or external. Internal rewards represent satisfaction, achievement, self-esteem, or ambition. External rewards focus on promotion, recognition, money, or benefits. Employees' choices allow them to gain the rewards they seek, which can reinforce their behavior. The manager creates and maintains a motivating climate that allows the staff to seek attainable personal goals. The unit manager needs to understand the motivational elements when selecting staff (11). These factors cover the quality of work, security, advancement, fair play, pay and benefits, supervision, and work surroundings. Morale of the team plays a unique role in motivation. The unit manager looks for candidates who can maintain the esprit de corps in the group. Information needs to be obtained about applicants' affiliative and achievement needs. Assessing new members for their enthusiasm, creativity, optimism, and health adds to the dimension of the unit. Some of these areas may be picked up by the impression the applicant makes and certain clues in the conversation. The amount and type of individual motivation present in the applicant assists the unit manager in developing a partnership relationship.

Personality factors can be gathered throughout the interview. Making a good first impression starts the process. The first 5 minutes can tell much about the person (10). Personality factors include a sense of humor, caring, ability to cope with stress and frustration, creativity, friendliness, honesty, self-confidence, conscientiousness, and distinctiveness. Exploring outside interests and hobbies help determine clues to personality traits. Looking at the type of dress and style offers further tips of the individual. Listening ability, speech patterns, and conversation disclose much about a person.

Human relationship skills involve assertiveness, approachability, and ability to collaborate. Seeking information about friendships and mentors may uncover skills. The applicant with affiliative needs may be more interested in the type of people in the unit and the morale rather than in productivity or financial considerations. They have a high desire to belong to a group. Some people have power needs that direct them to be in charge or have some influence over others. Making an impact and seeing the results can affect relations with others if not handled properly. Other applicants may have high achievement needs and are interested in solving problems and overcoming obstacles or challenges. All of these factors can result in team harmony and create a cohesive unit. Because many units are physically constrained by lack of space, the importance of a good fit by the new person with the rest of the staff cannot be underestimated.

Communication skills represent a key element in choosing staff. Both verbal and nonverbal skills play important roles in selecting staff. Self-expression, listening, and relaying appropriate information give evidence of effective verbal skills. Nonverbal communication includes writing ability, posture, facial expression, and body language. Picking up discrepancies between the nonverbal and verbal communication provides clues to feelings and attitudes. For example, when questioning about possible conflicts with families or physicians, watching for clues of facial expression, tone of voice, body position, as well as what is being said may reveal a problem. The nurse who says, "I enjoy talking with families" but maintains closed arms, shows no emotion, fails to make eye contact, or shows extreme nervousness or forced voice hostility reflects this discrepancy.

Establishing rapport with patients, families, employees, and others facilitates an effective climate in the critical care unit. The ability to positively confront and seek win-win solutions requires good communication skills. Presenting a scenario on negotiation of visiting time may help the interviewer to assess these skills.

The last desired characteristic of an applicant comprises professional and community involvement. Professional involvement can focus on the amount and type of continuing education, achievement of certification, publication, research, and organizational activity. Commitment to nursing as a profession can enhance both the work and the work place. Community involvement shows the interest of the applicant in seeking new experiences as well as offering service. Teaching cardiopulmonary resuscitation, checking blood pressures, teaching classes, or volunteering for civic activities show interest and represent nursing to others.

The unit manager determines the type of desired characteristics needed for the patients and the unit. Focusing on these eight characteristics and assessing the strengths, weaknesses, and opportunities of each candidate develops a process that leads to a good decision. The unit manager specifies key desires in an applicant by clearly looking for those aspects that support the milieu of the unit. Prospective employees also assess whether or not they can do the job required and meet the expectations. When employees sense that personal and professional goals can be met in an environment with appropriate rewards, then management energies can be directed toward outcome achievement.

## UNDESIRABLE CHARACTERISTICS

Although each individual applicant brings unique traits to the critical care environment, some characteristics may not be desirable. The unit manager must consider patient care needs, team rapport, and time involvement in working with a marginal applicant. Some characteristics for the unit manager to consider include the number of jobs held in a short time period or job hopping, absence of credibility, extreme nervousness, frequent interruptions in conversation, poor or inappropriate speech patterns such as foul language, focus on money and benefits over nursing care, criticism of former employers, rudeness, and poor appearance in dress or grooming. Some applicants may start the interview with nervousness or shyness. The unit manager who controls the interview can use personal interest statements or select questions to help overcome the hurdle of these initial reactions. Some applicants may relate a problem of drug dependence and how rehabilitation is working for them. In this instance, the manager needs to assess state board status as well as consider the willingness to work with this problem. (See Chapter 16) Working through how this may affect the unit staff and identifying strategies will help. Strategies include the use of random drug screening of blood and urine specimens, continuance of written counseling, selecting the shift to be worked, determining how narcotics will be handled, and how absences will be addressed. Often a written contract will help identify these parameters. Many state boards of nursing have impaired nurse programs that serve as a resource to the manager and the employee. The importance of education and support of both the individual employee and the staff can also be very helpful.

## PLANNING FOR THE SELECTION PROCESS

Before the selection process occurs, a mechanism for effectively and efficiently processing each candidate needs to be developed. Normally this starts in the personnel department. The application process must be completed. A screening interview may occur in personnel or with the nurse recruiter. A general tour of the hospital may be given. Preemployment health testing or other screening mechanisms will need to occur. Some facilities give a medication test before employment. Personnel may verify state licensure and check references. The unit manager prearranges with personnel for interview preferences and available times. Often candidates will arrive with no appointment. The unit manager must decide if sufficient time is available to conduct an in-depth interview. Other arrangements may need to be made. Sometimes the department director will fill in for the unit manager. In choosing competent care givers, the selection process can be rigorous and involved. Time allocated to the process at the beginning by the nurse manager pays off in the end by choosing the right candidate.

The manager reviews the application for type of education, experience, job being sought, work history, and salary requested. The reference checks and license need to be reviewed. The manager looks for interruptions in work history, reasons for leaving a position, results from any testing, outstanding accomplishments, and any other information that is provided. Often candidates will attach a resume to the application.

Staff involvement in the selection process plays an important role for building team cohesiveness. A team interview by select staff may offer new insights about the candidate. The team may be composed of nursing staff from the same shift or another, clinical nurse specialist, manager, and/or the director. In some cases physicians and others may comprise the team. If a team interview is planned, the candidate should be informed during the application process. Often the unit manager may interview first, screen the applicants, and then schedule a team interview when all can participate. The staff need to receive information about the candidate ahead of time. When a team interview is not possible, a staff nurse can show the applicant around the unit and conduct an interview. The staff nurse can then provide feedback to the manager about the applicant. The staff nurse becomes a part of the decision making process and feels involved. This can build the team.

Using a score sheet may help in differentiating among candidates as well as help the staff who participate in the process. Each desired characteristic can be identified and scored. The score sheet is shown in Figure 3.1 and outlines a three-point

system: 1 = highly qualified, meets or exceeds expectations; 2 = qualified, meets most expectations; 3 = not qualified. The lowest score reflects the best choice if a score sheet is used. The job description may be attached along with any critical tasks specific for this unit. A place for comments is provided on the score sheet for identification of other information about the applicant. The candidate's resume needs to be distributed ahead of time and may be attached to the score sheet.

The interview process requires a room or office where interruptions can be avoided. If the team is large, a conference room may need to be scheduled. The team should not overwhelm the applicant so numbers should be kept to five or less. A schedule of the time and place needs to be distributed so that all members may arrive on time. Before the interview, the manager gives a brief overview of who will be there to the candidate. Sometimes it is helpful when both the staff and the candidate write down questions they plan on asking.

## IMPLEMENTATION OF THE SELECTION PROCESS

The goal of a face-to-face interview is to ensure selection of the best possible employee. The interview structure is outlined in Figure 3.2. During the process, the best results can be elicited by using open-ended questions and those that do not generate a "yes," "no," or "maybe" response. The interviewer can plan to use some basic questions. Listening carefully to each answer generates new insights and further questions. It is important for the interviewer to allow the applicant to talk. Seeking clarity, use of pauses, and reflecting back on statements facilitate a good interview (10). The interviewer should not read each question to the applicant as this makes the process very stiff, uncomfortable, and regimented. The interviewer needs to consider how the applicant may feel during the process.

Each manager can experiment with various questions to develop a style that is most comfortable and effective. Note taking during the interview may help to explore further items as well as provide information to be reviewed later. The interviewer needs to be aware of the clock and adjust questions as needed to meet the time allowed.

Position _____ Qualifications _____

Candidate _____ Date _____ Interviewer _____

| Area | Score | Comments |
|------|-------|----------|
| Education | | |
| Experience | | |
| Intellectual ability | | |
| Motivation | | |
| Personality | | |
| Communication | | |
| Job knowledge | | |
| Nursing knowledge | | |
| Professional involvement | | |
| Community involvement | | |
| Human relationships | | |
| First impression | | |
| Test results | | |
| Certifications | | |
| Other characteristics | | |
| Miscellaneous | | |

_____

_____

Score: 1 = Highly qualified, meets or exceeds expectations, very positive.
      2 = Qualified, meets most expectations, some concerns.
      3 = Not qualified.

**Figure 3.1** Candidate Scoring Sheet

## INTERVIEW

### Brief Introduction

Call the candidate by name and ask if he or she prefers using another. Tell the candidate your name. Show the applicant where to sit. Close the door and request the secretary to stop interruptions.

Introduce a general statement to put the candidate at ease. This may include statements of where the candidate is from, school attended, or mutual acquaintances. Engage in a few moments of small talk if this seems to put the person at ease. This may include discussing the directions to the hospital, parking, traffic, or even the weather! These help serve as ice breakers.

### Explanation of the Process

#### One Interviewer

Explain the format of the interview and what the candidate can expect. Outline the amount of time it may take. A script would be:

> I would like to get to know more about you so I will be asking questions about your education, experience, knowledge areas, and aspects of you as a person. Feel free to ask me questions. I'll tell you about the position and some of my expecta-

tions. This should take us about 1 hour. I may take a few notes during the process.

#### Team Interview

Introduce the candidate and have each team member introduce his- or herself and area. Explain the format of the interview, the expectations, and the time involved. A script would be: "The process will involve each member asking you questions and exploring areas of interest. Feel free to ask questions or seek more information. This process will take about an hour". Sometimes the unit manager may want to leave the interview to allow the new applicant an opportunity to question the staff about management style. If this option is chosen, the explanation needs to be included. "I will leave for about 10 minutes to give you an opportunity to ask the staff some questions about my management style." During the team interview, the manager can observe verbal and nonverbal communication and pick up valuable information.

### Resume Review

#### Education

> What prompted you to choose nursing?
> What attracts you to critical care?

Brief Introduction
    Social Amenities
    General Comments

Explanation of the Process
    Interview Scope
    Time Allotment
    Outcome

Resume Review
    Education
    Experience

Job Knowledge
    Clinical
    Management

Nursing Profession
Motivation
Personality
Human Relationships
Communication Skills
Professional and Community Involvement
Other Characteristics
Elements of the Job
Question Exchange
Conclusion
    Assessment Completion
    Orientation

**Figure 3.2**   Interview Structure

What were your favorite subjects? Why?

What subjects did you not do so well in?

If you could take your college (school) years over, what would you do differently?

If I called one of the faculty, what may the person say about your abilities?

What elective courses did you take?

Tell me about critical care experiences you may have had while in school.

What kinds of grades did you make? (Review transcript if provided).

Tell me about one learning experience that was particularly meaningful to you.

In what areas do you feel the need for more education?

Why did you choose this school?

Tell me about any future school plans.

What kind of school activities did you enjoy?

How involved were you in extracurricular events?

How do you learn concepts and skills best?

Did you receive any awards or recognition?

If I called a fellow student, how would you be described?

How did you finance your education?

What continuing education have you done?

*Experience*

Tell me about the positive aspects of your current or most recent job.

What are (were) some of the minuses?

In your career, what has been your greatest accomplishment?

If I called your immediate supervisor, what would be said about you?

What aspects of your job are particularly difficult for you?

How do you feel about the way you were managed in your last job?

What gives you a sense of satisfaction in your work?

What causes frustration and what do you do about it?

Why are you seeking this job?

What one experience have you had that has been the most meaningful to you?

What type of people do you like to work with?

What are some things you would like to avoid in a job?

What made you successful in your last job?

What skills did you learn in your last job?

If I called a peer, what would be said about you?

I notice that you interrupted your work pattern. What did you do during this gap?

What kinds of patients do you enjoy caring for?

Which kinds of patients do you not like to take care of?

What kinds of emergencies have you been involved in at work?

I notice that you have had many jobs in a short time frame. Tell me why this occurred.

**Job Knowledge**

*Clinical*

What skills do you do best? Not as well?

What types of patients have you cared for?

In looking at the nursing process, what aspect do you do best? What needs improvement?

What types of clinical courses have you attended and when were they?

What level do you consider yourself: novice, intermediate, advanced?

How do you maintain your skills and knowledge?

Tell me what you would do with an intubated patient with deteriorating blood gases who is fighting the respirator (or ask applicable question).

Tell me about one emergency situation that had a different outcome than you expected.

How do you proceed in new situations?

How do you determine whether a nurse cares?

What has been your most difficult clinical situation? How did you handle it?

Tell me about certifications you possess. Why did you seek certification?

What gives you satisfaction in working?

What gives you frustrations?

What would a nurse who works after you say about your care?

What have physicians, patients, and families said about your care?

What type of orientation do you need?

Have you made any errors? Tell me about one that you are willing to share?

What shifts have you worked?

How many patients do you normally care for?

Tell me how I would know that you are competent?

*Management*

What is the manager's role in critical care?

How do you interface with management?

Have you had any management courses?

Tell me how you feel about the statement, ''Every nurse is a manager.''

Tell me what you like about your current boss?

How do you make decisions?

How do you see the role of the clinical nurse specialist in critical care?

How do you handle your performance review if you don't agree with it?

What was your last performance review like?

How has your career helped you take on more responsibilities?

What do you expect from your boss (peers)?

What is your view of administration?

When faced with a decision from administration that you disagree with, what do you do?

## Nursing Profession

Where is nursing headed?

What unique opportunities do you see for the profession?

Would you encourage your son or daughter to be a nurse? Why or why not?

Why are you a nurse?

What do you think about entry into practice?

What are the strengths of the nursing profession?

If you could do one thing in nursing, what would you do?

What would you change in nursing?

How do you see nurses' role in the health system?

What role does the nurse play in the critical care unit?

## Motivation

Where would you like to be in 5 years?

What will make you successful?

What kinds of things would you avoid in future jobs? Why?

Who is your role model? Why?

What career objectives do you have?

What makes you satisfied on a job?

How do you receive criticism?

What kind of people do you enjoy working with?

Tell me about your autonomy.

How do you like to be recognized?

What keeps you in a position?

How would you describe your attitude?

What motivates you?

What keeps you in critical care?

Is there anything that would prevent you from doing this job?

What makes you satisfied?

## Personality

What are some of your good qualities or traits?

What is a growth area for you?

What kinds of things increase your confidence?

Tell me about your sense of humor.

How have you changed in the last few years?

What frustrates you?

What do you do to relieve stress?

Tell me about some things away from work that you enjoy.

Do you consider yourself aggressive, assertive, or a mix? Describe yourself.

What would a close friend say about you?

What do you do when in a conflict with someone else?

Among these three aspects—belonging to a group, making things happen, or overcoming obstacles—which one describes you best?

## Communication

What communication style do you use?

How do you know when someone understands what you have said?

How much do you talk? Listen?

When in a group how do you communicate?

What do you do when you need more information?

How do you use nonverbal communication?

What type of writer are you?

How would you communicate with someone who is angry?

How do you communicate with families?

How do you communicate with a difficult or demanding patient?

How do you establish rapport?

Tell me how you like to receive feedback.

What are the elements of good communication?

## Professional and Community Involvement

What organizations do you belong to?
What kinds of activities have you participated in?
Tell me about publications or research you have done (focus on one or two).
How active are you in the nursing organizations?
What community activities do you participate in?
What role do you see for nursing in the community?
Why are you interested (or not interested) in these activities?

## Other Characteristics Observed

Appearance. Neat? Clean? Makeup? Hairstyle? Jewelry?
Dress and Grooming. Neat? Clean? Appropriate?
Posture. Slouched? Relaxed? Attentive?
Timeliness. Late? Early?
Listening ability. Repeated questions frequently? Answered a different question?
Speech patterns. Clear? Sentence structure?
Focus of conversation. Too much on peripheral items? Display of job interest?
Eye contact. Maintained? Appropriate? Shifted?
Nervous mannerisms. Tapped feet or legs? Played with hair or jewelry? Overtalkative? Too loud?
Language. Word choices? Foul language used?
Criticisms of others. Constructive? Derogatory?
Legibility. Application readable? Neat? Resume typed?

## Elements of the Job

If the candidate has not received all of the information about the job, the interviewer provides what is lacking. This may include: reporting mechanisms, delivery system, performance review, critical tasks, quality indicators, nursing activities, historical perspective, patient population, physician practices, research activities, educational opportunities, and other expectations.

## Question Exchange

The candidate uses this opportunity to ask questions, seek clarity, or provide commitment to the position. Normally aspects of the job that will be questioned will include hours, salary, benefits, type of nursing, patient care load, overtime requirements, and orientation specifics.

## Conclusion

### Assessment completion

Ask final questions. Seek any other questions from candidate. Explain the completion of the process. Outline the time frame for decision making. Explain the follow up process. Discuss salary and benefits if not done previously. Seek interest and/or commitment. Tour the unit if not already done. Introduce the applicant to the director or others if not done. Thank the candidate.

### Orientation

Explain the date, time, and place. Identify any other specific information such as where to park, what to wear, what to bring. Send a follow-up letter welcoming the candidate as an employee.

## EVALUATION OF THE PROCESS

There are several ways of evaluating the selection of competent critical care staff. Unfortunately even though the interview process may be rigorous and involved, some people interview well but do not perform as well as hoped. Input from the staff, performance reviews, patient and family feedback, observation, and input from other team members will provide the necessary information as time goes by. By utilizing a good and thorough interview process the expected outcome of having a competent care giver can be hoped for. Some managers in addition to the interview process described ask the candidate to spend a day in the unit with a nurse preceptor. This provides additional input and feedback.

The unit manager evaluates the success of appropriate selection by reviewing the process. Looking at the strengths and weaknesses of the interview helps improve the next selection process. The following series of questions may assist in the refinement of the selection process.

Was there sufficient time to interview?
How well did the staff participate?
What were their feelings about the process?
What were the overall tone and body language?
Was the room adequate?
What put the applicant at ease?
How did the interview begin and end?
Were all the key points covered?
What could be done differently the next time?
What were some sensitive areas?
How did the process flow?

The unit manager reviews the score sheet, resume, reference checks, job description, applicant reactions, and other information in assessing candidates (13). Taking all of the information coupled with the needs of the unit and the intuitive and intellectual sense of the unit manager, the selection of competent critical care staff is achieved. Giving both the staff and the candidate feedback is important. Articulating competence is different from demonstrating it but through a comprehensive process, the person hired will be the right one for the job. The impression of a thorough and thoughtful interview shows a value and commitment to the new staff member.

Choosing competent critical care staff can avoid future problems of poor morale, turnover, excessive absenteeism, and poor productivity. The decision to hire the right person for the right job is one of the most important roles of the critical care nurse manager. The patients, staff, and institution all benefit when the right candidate is chosen. The selection process that objectively identifies clinical and management knowledge, experience, intellect, motivation, personality, human relationships, communication skills, professional involvement, and other characteristics result in a good job fit. The new person chosen under such a method may have increased job satisfaction knowing that he or she is the right person. The unit manager and the staff also feel good due to the preparation, process, and selection. After the orientation process, the new employee can verify with the unit manager the accuracy of information received during the interview and any thoughts about the process. This ongoing evaluation assists in the next selection process.

Choosing competent critical care staff requires assessment, planning, implementation, and evaluation. The time and attention given to the process pays off for all with the right person in the right job doing the right thing. Ensuring competence in the staff leads to job satisfaction, allows for professional growth, maintains quality outcomes, and supports the unit being the best that it can be in all areas. The role of the critical care nurse manager in this process becomes crucial for the efficiency and effectiveness of a smooth running unit.

REFERENCES

1. Canfield A. Controversy over clinical competencies. Heart & Lung 1982;11(3):197–199.
2. Scott B. Competency based learning: a literature review. Int J Nurs Stud 1982;19(3):119–124.
3. Toth JC, Ritchey KA. New from nursing research: the basic knowledge assessment tool for critical care nursing. Heart & Lung 1984;13(3):272–279.
4. Scrima DA. Assessing staff competency. J N Admin 1987;17(2):41–45.
5. AACN Demonstration Project Information. July, 1988:1–19.
6. American Association of Critical-Care Nurses. Standards for nursing care of the critically ill. AACN Reston, Virginia: Reston Publishing Company, 1981.
7. Accreditation Manual for Hospitals 1988. Chicago, Illinois: Joint Commission on Accreditation of Hospitals. 1987:269–286.
8. Alspach J. The education process in critical care nursing. St Louis: CV Mosby, 1982.
9. Roberts W, Alspach J, Canobbio M., et al. Critical care nursing education: an overview. Heart & Lung 1986;15(2):115–126.
10. Arthur D. Recruiting, interviewing, selecting, and orienting new employees. New York: Amacom. American Management Association. 1986:1–18.
11. Veninga RL. The human side of health administration. Englewood Cliffs, New Jersey: Prentice Hall Inc, 1982:105–152.
12. King N. The first five minutes. New York: Prentice Hall Press, 1987:105–120.
13. Fear RA. The evaluation interview. New York: McGraw-Hill Book Co, 1984:47–82.
14. Benner P, Tanner C. How expert nurses use intuition. Am J Nurs, 1987;87:23–31.
15. Walters JA. An innovative method of job interviewing. J Nurs Admin 1987;17(5):25–29.
16. AACN Management Special Interest Group. Integration of new graduates into critical care. Newport Beach, California: AACN, 1988.
17. Tanner C, Padrick K, Westfall U, Putzier D. Diagnostic reasoning strategies of nurses and nursing students. Nurs Res 1987;36(6):358–362.

# Part II

# PLANNING
AND
# ORGANIZING

# Chapter 4

# Decentralized Managing

ROSEMARY DALE

Decentralization is an organizational style of management consisting of a selective sharing of planning and decision making at all levels of the occupational system. A reversal from complete control of organization by top level management to involvement of employees at the operational level can have a positive effect on all aspects of an operation of business. This approach was initially formulated in industry to increase productivity. In the 1920s, the General Motors Company was restructured to a decentralized model. The purpose for the decentralization was to allow the company to respond more rapidly to market demands and technology (1).

## DEFINITION

The definition for decentralization is not an explicit or absolute term but has a variety of meanings and applications. It can, for example, refer to decentralization of geography or authority. Geographical decentralization consists of the spreading out of the physical environment. Organizational decentralization refers to the spreading out of authority, responsibility, and decision making to all members of an organization rather than to dominant executives only (2).

Life in today's society can be characterized as a series of organizational memberships. Organizations are portrayed as systematic arrangements or individual interactions. This involves the act or power of regulating or directing with authority. The policy of an organization for management functioning could be democratic versus autocratic or centralized versus decentralized.

This chapter will address the philosophy of decentralization as a key element for improving health care systems, factors motivating a transition to a decentralized model, approaches for structuring decentralized nursing, the evaluation of the process, and the outcome of promoting parrticipative staff decision making.

## MOTIVATING FACTORS

Major health care issues today address the high level of health care costs and the nursing shortage. The extent to which these factors affect nurses is an important consideration for nursing management.

A prime factor that would result in a greater retention of nurses in the health care environment would be to improve job satisfaction. The improved morale and positive feelings expressed could also influence potential candidates for nursing and increase recruitment resources.

Nurse managers need to be aware of staff members' professional needs and utilize all members to their highest extent. A more organized, effective use of all resources will also affect health care finances. Consequently, nursing administrators have the potential to bring the state of health care to a more desirable level by improving nurses' satisfaction with their role.

What would promote job satisfaction? Many studies have assessed the causes and highlighted nurses' frustrations. Issues have included: salaries, flexibility of time, professional growth and development needs, workload stress, and lack of involvement in planning and decision making (3–5).

Decentralization is a mechanism by which job satisfaction can materialize. Professional nurses with years of education and experience are most capable of decision making and want to be so recognized. Nurse executive utilization of a decentralized system for management enhances job satisfaction (6).

## APPROACHES TO STRUCTURING DECENTRALIZATION

### Agreement

The first step in converting to a decentralized system is for the top level nursing management team to assess the environment and reach agreement that decentralization is a desirable management approach. There is a level of organizational maturity that must be built before moving to decentralization. Implementation of a management style that vests considerable responsibility and authority at various levels in an organization requires planning. Incumbents, at some levels, may have had limited experiential or didactic exposure to the management or principles of decentralized decision making. When the decision has been made to implement a decentralized management style, the process of educating the individuals involved must begin and a specific plan to accomplish decentralization should be prepared.

## Plan

The second step in establishing a decentralized system is to formulate a clear plan. This plan should be reviewed and accepted by senior nursing management and senior hospital management. The implementation of a decentralized management style for the nursing department, a unit or shift, can have significant ramifications for individuals and services that interact.

Communication and operational decision making needs to be approached differently in a decentralized environment. Therefore, communication within the unit to be decentralized as well as communication with interacting departments or services is a high priority. For any system to succeed, it must be understood and supported by the maximal number of people.

### Formulating the Plan

The nursing administrative group, i.e., vice presidents/directors or directors/nurse managers, can draft the plan. The plan should determine issues to be handled at various levels of the department or cost center. The choice of who will actually make the decision at the department or cost center level will depend upon the subject. Adequate time should be built in to allow multiple drafts to be shared and to receive input from staff.

As is true in any organization, the levels or strata of management will depend upon the size and complexity of the institution and services. In formulating a plan to decentralize, the entire organization must be considered. For instance, the surgical intensive care unit (SICU) that decides to take a decentralized approach to the management of that unit must understand the organizational perogatives that unit has for decision making. In most organizations it would not be reasonable for the

**Table 4.1.** Examples of Decentralized Organizational Systems

| |
|---|
| Director |
|   Supervisors |
|     Nurse managers |
| Director |
|   Associate directors |
|     Supervisors |
|       Nurse managers |
|         Assistant nurse managers |
| Vice President |
|   Associate vice president |
|     Directors |
|       Supervisors |
|         Nurse managers |
|           Assistant nurse managers |

SICU to make decisions on third party billing and contracting or on loan amortization. On the other hand, it is more appropriate for the SICU to make decisions about the selection of equipment and supplies for the unit, staff scheduling, policies and procedures, and the standards for patient care. It is therefore important to understand the levels of management within the organization and where the perogatives for decision making currently lay within the organization.

## Understanding Traditional Levels of Management

Levels of nursing management will depend upon the size of the institution and the volume of the services. These could include various levels of vice presidents, directors, supervisors, nurse managers or assistant nurse managers (Table 4.1).

### First Level Administrator

The first level administrator, (vice president, director of nursing) is the principal source for determining the prime responsibilities of the nursing department. Based on the interaction with other hospital administrators, the top executive's skills and knowledge are at a greater level for decision making in regard to the direction the organization must take (7).

The first level administrator traditionally has a reporting line to the chief executive officer in the organization or in a large and complex organization, to the chief operating officer.

### Second Level Administrator

Second level administrators, (i.e., directors/clinical coordinators), manage specified nursing units, supervise all aspects of unit goals, act as a resource and consultant for the unit nurse manager.

### Supervisors

The supervisors' administrative responsibilities may vary. The supervisor, a resource person for unit staff, may be assigned to specific units to act administratively and/or may function as a clinical expert in the absence of the nurse manager.

### First Line Managers

The nurse manager or individual immediately responsible for a given cost center is a first-line manager. Shoemaker and El-Ahraf, in a 1983 survey, revealed that the majority of nursing respondents viewed the nurse manager role as the most important nursing position (2). The nurse manager role is critical for the achievement of organizational goals. The ultimate goal of any health care agency is high quality patient care. The nurse manager is the manager directly involved with staff who give actual patient care. The nurse manager is responsible for managing and motivating staff, staying within the budget, and assuring that hospital and unit goals are met.

In a decentralization system the nurse manager is also involved with the planning of the budget, policies, procedures, and the hiring or firing of staff. The nurse manager coordinates his or her activities with unit support personnel or the assistant nurse manager. The assistant nurse manager may have specific staff-related responsibilities such as orienting, clinical problem solving, or working with staff on unit projects. The nurse manager and assistant nurse managers are role models for staff and strongly influence productivity and the quality of patient care.

In a decentralized management system these individuals have a key role in assuring staff nurse involvement in the program. The nurse manager and assistant nurse manager will delegate projects and practices to appropriate staff nurses and involve them in decision making such as the formation and revision of policies, procedures, and other practices relating to direct care decisions and unit-related management issues.

Decentralized staffing (see Chapter 6) is an example of staff input into unit-related management issues. For example in one medical intensive care unit (MICU) the staff restructured their weekend scheduling so as to achieve the goal of more weekends off. Staff nurses worked 12-hour shifts on weekends and 8-hour shifts during the week. This allowed the MICU staff to work every third weekend and has proven to be a positive retention strategy.

The staff in one SICU collaborated with pharmacy and cardiac surgery to develop a cardiac surgical pain protocol. The staff nursing caring for the patient determines the amount of pain medication that will be given. The decision that is based on a protocol is made at the lowest level in the organization, which has the greatest impact on the patient and on the decision making ability of the nurse.

### Education to Effect the Change

The process of implementing a decentralized management style will take time for manager and staff adjustment. It is imperative that the plan for decentralization be clearly articulated to all members of the staff. Orientation sessions related to decentralized management, decision making, and budgeting should be provided before the conversion to decentralization (8). Understanding the reasons for the change and the essence of the change will foster receptivity to the change. Similarly, professional nurses, usually chosen for management positions because of their high level of clinical competence, may not be experienced in regard to management responsibilities. Significant orientation is essential for anyone involved in the process. In the orientation packet for new staff to the ICU there should be a rationale for decision making in the unit. It is here that the nurse manager can have a significant impact. When the philosophy is clearly articulated and expectations are delineated, the orientees will feel a part of the unit and begin to feel that they do make a difference and that their input is welcomed.

Changes in the system need to be included in relevant departmental systems such as job descriptions, performance standards, policies, and procedures. Stevens (9) reports that such changes, well planned and executed, will be quickly accepted (9).

### Evaluation

Manager involvement and commitment toward meeting personal and departmental goals have a major influence on the success of the plans for promoting decentralized management.

When a facility or cost center embarks on a plan to decentralize, there are specific goals or objectives to be accomplished. Measurement of the accomplishment of the goals and objectives occurs as an evaluation.

Adequate evaluation points should be built into the process of implementation. The reality is that the process of decentralization can be accomplished within weeks or can span years. The major factors influencing the time are: (*a*) the size and complexity of the organization, and (*b*) the organizational and individual preparedness for the change.

Processes for intermittent measurement and accomplishment of goals and objectives should be formulated. This process is best monitored through a committee structure. A single purpose ad hoc committee can be formulated or a standing committee can monitor the process as a special project. Standing committees to be considered are the quality assurance committee, the staff governance committee, and the staff advisory committee.

The processes to measure staff reaction can include staff attitude surveys, quality of care indices, recruitment, attendance and turnover data, to name only a few.

## OUTCOME

The effects of decentralization should be increased staff involvement and staff control relating to patient care decisions. Innovative approaches to patient care should expand. As the perception of the effects of decentralization evolves, managers and staff will begin to increase productivity levels. The outcome should be higher quality of patient care, increased job satisfaction, better relationships between coworkers, feelings of professional recognition, greater trust between the various nursing levels, less absenteeism, increased nursing retention (resulting in a decreased nursing shortage), and an improvement in financial economics because of increased productivity and innovative ideas of the nursing staff. All of these areas lend themselves to analysis. Some areas such as absenteeism, staff retention, and economic benefits can be described quantitatively. Areas such as trust, professional recognition, and job satisfaction can be qualitatively described and compared.

## CASE STUDY

In 1981 the nursing service at the Medical Center Hospital of Vermont (MCHV), Burlington, Vermont, decided to take a decentralized approach

to managing. MCHV is a 500-bed tertiary care facility. It is a community controlled, nonprofit facility located adjacent to the University of Vermont (UVM). The MCHV complex is categorized as an academic health center.

At MCHV, the nursing department was moved from a highly centralized, and in many ways autocratic organization of the 1970s, to a decentralized system with a high component of shared governance in the eighties. The motivation for effecting the change grew from expressed staff nurse desire to have more control over practice issues. Centrally vested authority for clinical decision making was clearly becoming unfeasible as clinical specialization and technology grew.

Another significant influence for decentralization was the evolution of the role of the chief nurse executive. As the health care environment became increasingly complex, hospital administrators came to place increasing value on the opinion and decisions of the chief nurse executive. This caused a cascade effect on responsibilities as the chief nurse executive altered her traditional responsibilities.

The vice president for nursing and patient services as the chief nurse executive is ultimately responsible for patient care. The vice president is a member of the executive policy-making body of the hospital and the medical executive board. As the prime sources of leadership of the decentralized nursing system, the vice president initiates the delegation of authority and responsibility necessary for accomplishing nursing functions and assuring that nursing care standards are maintained.

In 1987 the vice president for patient services role was merged with the role of the dean of the school of nursing at the University of Vermont. The combined role of vice president and dean of the UVM School of Nursing has increased collaboration between the two areas and consequently has been of benefit to professional growth and role satisfaction for both nursing students and staff.

### Medical Center Structure

The Medical Center Hospital of Vermont has been broken into major divisions, each division headed by a director reporting directly to the chief nurse executive. Divisions are set along clinical lines (i.e., maternal, child, critical care). Each division has approximately 160 full-time employees (FTEs) and may have as many as 300 employees.

The director is supported by a unit specialist and an inservice instructor. These positions are defined as:

Unit Specialist—Senior unit secretary, responsible for orientation and management of unit secretaries within the division. Provides clerical support for the director and assists in the financial monitoring of the division.

Inservice Instructor—Master's-prepared practitioner responsible for orientation and education in the division. Monitors quality assurance activities, is a clinical resource and role model for staff.

The directors are responsible for the delivery system in the division and are resources and consultants to the nurse manager. The director assesses and resolves administrative and clinical problems with the nurse managers, plans the budget with the nurse manager, fosters professional development and utilization of staff, and participates in the planning process for future program development within the respective clinical division.

Nursing supervisors are the primary resource people for nursing and for administrative staff issues on the evening, night, and on weekends shifts. These individuals, although while clearly managerial, have no direct line authority to the nursing staff.

Nurse managers, primary role models, are the direct resource for the nursing staff on a given unit. They are responsible for the administration of a patient care unit and nursing service personnel on a 24-hour basis.

The nurse managers work with the staff and other managers associated with their individual units to plan systems of care. Budget planning is the responsibility of the nurse manager in collaboration with the director. Budget maintenance is the responsibility of the nurse manager. Clinically, the nurse manager is an advanced practitioner who serves as a role model for staff. He or she promotes staff to utilize their skills and become involved in revising standards and procedures. Unit-based quality assurance and research studies also fall within the scope of the nurse manager.

In the MICU the nurse manager collaborates with the unit-based quality assurance nurse. This nurse who is master's prepared works part-time as a staff nurse and part-time as the nurse for quality assurance. She has a working knowledge of the unit and is able to actively assist the nurse manager in monitoring and implementing a unit-based quality assurance program. The staff in the SICU revised their emergency cart to provide an easier mechanism to ensure compliance with the Joint Commission on Accreditation of Healthcare Organizations. The nurse manager was a consultant to staff in this area of practice.

Staff nurses progress in a career ladder through three levels, I–III (see Chapters 14 and 15). Inexperienced nurses begin at Level I and provide patient care while focusing on developing nursing abilities. The staff nurse I is supported by a preceptor and works through an orientation program tailored to the unit by the unit staff, nurse manager, and inservice instructor. Level II staff are fully functional practitioners who can direct the work of others. Level III staff are those who demonstrate a high level of competence in decision making revolving around the process of assessment, prescription for action, and evaluation of outcomes of patient problems. They also provide a depth of knowledge and skill in the areas of administration, clinical practice, education, and research.

The classification of nurses according to their level of practice also provides a source of recognition. This promotes job satisfaction and motivates staff to increase their level of expertise. The level III staff nurse position is a promotional position. Staff in each unit with consultation from the nurse manager have developed specific guidelines for implementation. Specific criteria for promotion include: ability to be an effective charge nurse, certification program in critical care nursing offered by the American Association of Critical-Care Nurses Certification Corporation (CCRN credential), and advanced nursing practice judgment. Another aspect of recognition is an increase in salary for each level. The nurse manager on the unit, along with staff, create the criteria for each performance level. Directors remain involved as advisors and maintain an equanimity among units and divisions.

All staff members are encouraged to be involved in decision making regarding patient care practices relating to areas in which they have shown expertise. Staff and nurse managers in the division chair the nursing policy and procedure committees. These committees are segregated according to specialty areas. Policies and procedures are reviewed yearly

**Table 4.2.**  Interactive Groups

| | |
|---|---|
| Group: | Administrative staff |
| Members: | Nurse managers, clinicians, instructors |
| Time: | Every 3 months |
| Group: | Administrative group |
| Members: | Vice president, directors, supervisors |
| Time: | Monthly |
| Group: | Vice president/directors |
| Members: | Same |
| Time: | Monthly |
| Group: | Nurse advisory council |
| Members: | Vice president/staff nurses |
| Time: | Monthly (days) |
| Group: | Evening forum |
| Members: | Supervisor/unit staff representative |
| Time: | Monthly (evenings) |

by committees composed of staff representatives. The procedure is then reviewed by the nurse manager and the director.

The committee was asked to review the drug verapamil for intravenous usage in the critical care areas and the emergency department (ED) (10). Clinical research was done at the staff nurse level on the use of verapamil in the clinical setting. The committee recommended that nurses in the ICU could push intravenous verapamil while nurses in the ED were not permitted to push the drug. The decision was based on the constant observation of the patient in the ICU versus the limited, one-time exposure to the patient in the ED.

Other committees that include all levels of nursing are: quality assurance, research, and computer development in nursing.

A variety of meetings (Table 4.2) are held regularly to provide communication and interaction between managers and/or staff nurses. Such group interactions are valuable for: providing recognition of staff, receiving input in relation to scheduled topics or issues raised and sharing of current or planned unit activities. Ultimately they produce a useful means for motivating the group members.

The Nurse Advisory Council provides a direct link between the staff nurse and the vice president for nursing. Each unit selects its own representative who in turn relates the unit issues and concerns to the advisory council. Topics include salary and benefits, floating, holiday time, and parking. The issues at this level are related to the operational organization of the nursing department. The evening forum is another avenue for dialogue. Issues that directly relate to a specific shift are discussed.

Clinical issues such as scope of practice on the off shifts, the role of the practical nurse, and nurse-physician concerns are issues that the unit representative could bring to this meeting.

Decentralization at MCHV has proven to be a positive advantage. A considerable number of nurses on all units have displayed innovative ideas relating to nursing practice and patient care, utilizing their expertise to the fullest. In the SICU the unit instructor suggested that senior nursing students be utilized as nurse aides/nurse helpers. Staff have actively supported this innovation. They feel that the student functioning in this capacity has had a positive impact on their workload and this has also been a recruitment tool for the ICU. The students feel that it has demystified the ICU experience for them. Six students have been successfully recruited into the ICU setting at MCHV.

Another innovative idea resulted in a grant for a surgical unit. The unit began to care for acquired immune deficiency syndrome (AIDS) patients and developed an AIDS task force. It was at this level that the idea for a grant was developed on caring for the AIDS patient.

Relating to a 1987 study (11) that resulted in support of the belief that decentralized structures help retain nursing staff, the 1988 3% nursing shortage of MCHV, compared to the national average of 11%, would support the advantage of decentralized system.

The transition to a decentralized model has not been without problems. Two areas of difficulty have been selected for this illustration:

## COMMUNICATION AND INTERACTION WITH ANCILLARY DEPARTMENTS

### Communication

In a decentralized model information dissemination becomes the responsiblity of a chain of individuals. Over time the staff mix has changed. Currently in both ICUs (surgical and medical) there is a large staff to support a combined total of 32 ICU beds. The physical layout lends itself to isolation. Many of the staff are part-timers and communication is a problem at times. The ability to communicate to every level of the organization and to each staff member is as strong as the weakest individual within the chain of communication.

The experience at MCHV was that communication related to institutional goals and activities was not uniformly distributed to the staff in a timely fashion. In response to this the organization has:

1. instituted a monthly newsletter for the nursing service. Ideas are generated from the nurse advisory council.
2. provided communication workshops for staff and managers;
3. conducted round-the-clock staff meetings with staff.

### Interaction with Ancillaries

Decentralization can be a frustrating experience for departments interacting with a decentralized service. For instance, food services attempting to synchronize tray delivery hours, security attempting to negotiate a policy to safeguard patient valuables, and the morgue trying to implement a postmortem care system found that there was no key person to work with in the nursing service. Each nurse manager could speak for his or her own area. The chief nurse executive, director and nurse manager in today's health care system have neither the time nor inclination to participate in these types of decisions.

To resolve this problem, the MCHV employed a nurse, referred to as an administrative supervisor. This individual dealt with many of the issues for which the traditional day supervisor had been responsible. The administrative supervisor is staff to the directors and negotiates those issues not related to clinical practice. The nurse manager has benefited a great deal from this position. The administrative supervisor worked with the laboratory in clarifying how laboratory tests were to be ordered in the ICUs. She was the link between the clinical laboratory department and data processing. Every nurse manager has encountered problems with missing patient belongings especially at the time of a patient's death. The administrative supervisor has actively worked out a system with the morgue and the department of nursing to correct this ongoing dilemma.

### CONCLUSION

Decentralization is one approach to structuring an organization. The experience of this author has been positive with the decentralized model. It should be emphasized that careful organizational analysis and discussion are necessary to identify the style or model that will yield the greatest satisfaction and productivity in a critical care environment.

REFERENCES

1. Greenwood RG. Managerial decentralization. Lexington, Massachusetts: DC Heath and Company, 1974, p 1.
2. Shoemaker MA, El-Ahraf A. Decentralization of nursing service management and its impact on job satisfaction. Nurs Admin Q 1983;7(2):69–76.
3. Editors. Nursing shortage poll report. Nursing 88 1988;18:33–41.
4. Scherer P. When every day is Saturday: the shortage. Am J Nurs 1987;87(10)1284–1289.
5. Huey FL, Hartley S. What keeps nurses in nursing. Am J Nurs 1987;88(2):181–188.
6. Przestrzelski D. Decentralization: are nurses satisfied? J Nurs Admin 1987;17(10):23–28.
7. Callahan CB, Wall LL. Participative management: a contingency approach. J Nurs Admin 1987;17(9):9–15.
8. Wellington M. Decentralization: how it affects nurses. Nurs Outlook 1986;34(1):36–39.
9. Stevens B. The nurse as executive. 2nd ed. Wakefield, Massachussets: Nursing Resources, Inc, 1980; p 178.
10. Cardin S. Nursing considerations in the administration of verapamil. J Cardiovas Nurs 1988;2(2):73–75.
11. Barkyte DY, Counte MD, Christman LP. The effects of decentralization on nurses' job attendance behaviors. Nurs Admin Q 1987;11:37–46.

# Chapter 5

# Self-Governing

WANDA L. ROBERTS

Shared governance has recently been identified as a "strategy for transforming organizations (1)," a "treatment for an unhealthy nursing culture" (2), and a "giant step forward" (3) for institutional nursing practice. The curiosity generated by these statements can quickly revert to genuine excitement when organizations with more mature shared governance programs reveal signs of their success—high job satisfaction and staff morale, low annual attrition rates, and significant 5-year retention rates. An illustration of these outcomes can be seen in the results of the American Association of Critical-Care Nurses (AACN) Demonstration project conducted in the critical care unit at Overlake Hospital Medical Center, where a shared governance system was in operation for several years. The findings (4) included the following:

- The annual turnover rate of critical care nurses was 3.3%.
- There was a mortality rate 50% below predictions in the population of critical care patients studied.
- Nurses had significantly higher morale than that found in other groups of critical care nurses.
- Nurses enjoyed their work and did not want to work anywhere else, and they perceived their jobs as less stressful than nurses in other critical care units.
- Nurses perceived they had significant power to make decisions about patient care.
- Nurses perceived they had a high degree of influence over how they do their work and how they acquired what they needed to do their work.
- Nurses perceived a high degree of collaboration with physicians in the care of patients.
- Patient satisfaction with care was very high.

Indeed, these results deserve attention in light of the fact that nearly every critical care unit in the nation's hospitals have now felt, in some way, the impact of an acute nationwide shortage of nurses. Threats of future, more constant, and critical short-

ages loom overhead with reports of steadily declining enrollments in nursing schools and ever greater demands for nursing services. Nurses who are working in hospitals are not silent about their frustration, stress, and dissatisfaction with current working conditions, compensation, and lack of opportunities for advancement. Few nursing managers or administrators would disagree—"the climate, the culture of nursing, must change" (2).

The working conditions and constraints that exist in traditional, authoritarian health care organizations are no longer acceptable to today's professional nurse. Nurses now want a voice and an active role in decisions that affect their practice and the environment in which they work. They want fair and adequate compensation. They want challenging and satisfying work. They want reasonable working schedules, ones that do not decrease the quality or quantity of their personal or recreational time. They want to make a worthwhile contribution to the overall service delivered to patients. They also want to be recognized and rewarded for a job well done. Nurses are not the only group of people who want these things. Workers in general throughout the industrial sector have similar needs and desires.

Peterson and Allen described six societal changes they believed accounted for the alteration in values and attitudes of workers toward institutions and authority. First, there is a general lack of confidence in organizations, a realization that organizations can be harmful to workers as well as helpful. Widespread layoffs within industries most recently magnified this realization. Second, and compounding this lack of confidence, is a diminishing authority base in organizations. Organizations, like the rest of society, are in a state of flux. They no longer provide stable symbols for the worker. They are no longer "authorities" for defining career advancement and success or for providing job security. When institutions cannot be relied on for stability and security, employees tend to modify their commitment to the organization and develop other reference points. This third factor offers reasons for why balance in one's life, between work and other more personal aspects, becomes more important. Workers expect the work environment to conform to their lifestyles rather than the other way around. Another example of the changing attitudes of workers toward organizations is the observation that more employees are identifying themselves in generic terms rather than with a specific organization. Saying "I am a nursing manager" or "I am a critical care nurse" today expresses what workers see as a more permanent relationship, i.e., one with a generic focus of work. How employees now view leaders within an organization is another dimension of the societal upheaval that is occurring. The leader as the "father figure" is no longer accepted. Workers want identity and contact with the organizational leader, they want someone who provides meaning to their work by being someone worth working for. They seek an organization with expressed values corresponding to their own. Last, the flow of information within organizations has been redefined. Because of technology that has made work more sophisticated and contributed to more rapid information processing and a general knowledge increase among staff members, traditional systems are not as effective. Relationships and communications within organizations consequently tend to be overlapping and multidirectional. Structures that depend on strictly downward and upward flow of information are antiquated. Because of all of these changes, Peterson and Allen concluded that fundamental restructuring of our organizations must occur. We must have organizational transformation (1).

To transform is to change dramatically. The concept implies that old ways are replaced by new ways of thinking and acting. It requires a shift of beliefs and attitudes. It demands new perspectives and new norms. Because transformation deals with a change of some of the most elusive cultural elements—values and beliefs—it does not occur rapidly, directly, or by decree. Rather, transformation takes place over a long period of time, through deliberate and redundant activities (2).

Nursing shared governance is one model for bringing about transformation of nursing organizations. The shared governance concept receives underlying support from participative management theory, a basic premise that decisions should be made closest to where the results will be felt. In

other types of working environments, participative systems have realized a number of favorable effects (5). That the positive effects of participation in other settings could also be experienced within hospital nursing organizations was the belief upon which the shared governance idea was founded. In short, nursing shared governance is a formalized system whereby nurses exercise control over how nursing care is delivered and the manner in which it is delivered within the institutions where they work. Shared governance structures can also provide mechanisms for addressing issues related to the environment in which nurses practice such as scheduling, staffing, recognition and reward systems, professional development, and compensation and benefits.

There is no single shared governance system that will work in every setting. Any model that is implemented has to be tailored to fit the specific environment, group of employees, and their expectations. In order to assist nursing leaders to design, implement, and evaluate the most appropriate shared governance system or participative intervention for their organization, Allen et al. recently published an interesting conceptual model (5). This model, synthesized from a review of over 100 research reports on participative decision making in a variety of settings, depicts the almost universal relationship between decisional participation and satisfaction. The connections among organizational factors that mediate this relationship occupy the remainder of the model.

Basically, two pathways are identified, one termed information and the other action. The information pathway deals with the quantity and type of work-related information one has, and it reinforces the need for a free flow of information in all directions. A crucial element in this pathway is the relationship between performance and reward. The action pathway is concerned with the nature of the work a person does and emphasizes challenge. Productive participation in decision making, as it impacts the organizational variables shown in the model, can be expected to produce positive outcomes for individuals as well as the organization. Employees will become more satisfied when participating in decisions, more involved in their jobs, more internally motivated, and more committed to the organization. Reinforcement over time may likely occur such that people begin to value responsibility and autonomy. Their work may become more important to them, and they may find more challenge in their jobs (5). Further details of the variables and relationships depicted in this shared governance model will be discussed in sections below as they relate to steps in developing a shared governance system.

Implementing a shared governance system is not easy. Managers and staff alike are well aware of the chaos, ambiguity, and grieving that accompanies major change. The energy output required, particularly by first line managers, during the initial developmental phase (which can easily span several years) is tremendous. The desire to hold onto old ways and structures will be strong. However, unless nursing managers transcend this downside of change and take the risk, the organizational transformation will not occur. The culture of nursing will remain unhealthy and unable to respond effectively to changes in the environment and the organization. The care of patients will suffer.

As with any major and complex undertaking, operationalizing a shared governance system can be broken down into a number of steps or tasks. Some tasks obviously precede others. Other tasks can occur simultaneously with prior or subsequent ones. Ordering and pacing the transformation process is beneficial so that individuals and the organization are not overwhelmed. People feel significant loss of control and helplessness during change when they are unprepared for it, when their current skills and fund of knowledge are inadequate to make a successful transition, and when no resources are available to help them (2). Let this knowledge guide your thinking and your actions as you implement the change. The tasks involved in establishing a shared governance program are described below. Some practical examples and suggestions are also provided.

## IDENTIFY AND ADOPT THE VALUES AND BELIEFS

One of the first tasks in developing a shared governance system is to commit to the beliefs behind it (6). Commitment implies fully understanding the beliefs as they relate to the operational philosophy and adopting those beliefs as a foundation for formulating future judgments and making decisions. The principles upon which shared governance was founded address beliefs about: the nature, needs, desires, and responsibilities of people within the organization; who, when, and how

problems are solved; and beliefs about organizational leadership.

Methodist Hospital in Madison, Wisconsin, developed the following belief statements for their leadership group at the onset of their shared governance project.

We can achieve our full potential and will work hard to do so.

People are honest and trustworthy; they want and deserve to be treated with respect and dignity.

We understand the purpose of our work and the goals of this nursing service.

We are accountable and responsible for patient care delivered to individuals interacting with this system.

We are able to identify and correct mistakes and problems before they escalate or are shifted to higher levels of the organization.

Leaders have a responsibility to teach staff how the organization operates.

There is no such thing as an information monopoly; leaders assure that information is shared and that communication is a two-way process.

We have a responsibility to each other, or staffs, and those with whom we interact. This responsibility translates to a sense of empathy, understanding, caring, nurturing, and mutual support (6).

These beliefs were further translated into divisional goals:

Deliver efficient and effective nursing care to all patients and clients of Methodist Health Services, Inc.

Work cooperatively as colleagues with all staff and all disciplines.

Demonstrate caring, understanding, empathy, and support to all patients and staff.

Work within a nursing environment comprised of informed, communicating, positive, and motivated nursing staffs (6).

As another example, Overlake Hospital Medical Center nurses in Bellevue, Washington, united their goal and belief statements in a preamble to the bylaws of their nursing shared governance organization, called nursing congress (7).

The Overlake Hospital Nursing Congress is committed to providing quality patient care in a cost-effective manner. The Nursing Congress supports the mission, philosophy, goals and objectives of the hospital. On an annual basis, nursing participates in the development of the goals and objectives of the hospital.

The Overlake Hospital Nursing Congress supports a decentralized organization that places the responsibility and authority for decision-making at the level closest to the situation, thereby supporting the goal of delivering the highest possible level of quality patient care in a environment conducive to professional practice.

We believe that patient care at Overlake Hospital is a collaborative effort of all health care team members: nurses, physicians and all allied health care professionals. Further, we believe that the effort of all team members should be directed towards resolving illness to the extent possible and promoting wellness of each individual patient.

We believe nursing is a unique profession that relies upon physiological and psychosocial scientific principles to provide advocacy to each individual patient. We believe that the foundation of effective nursing practice is the application of the nursing process. Because the nursing process is dynamic, we believe that learning and professional development must be continuous and pertinent. We believe that we are accountable to the individual patient, the Overlake Hospital community and to each other as professionals.

The Overlake Hospital Nursing Congress is committed to fostering an environment that facilitates professional and personal growth while achieving organizational goals in a manner that develops and utilizes decision-making and accountability of staff at all levels.

Note that similar elements existed in the goals and beliefs elaborated in both of the preceding examples. Although no documentation of beliefs and goals of other shared governance systems could be found, it is likely that similarities will again be seen judging from what is known about the operation of these other participative nursing programs (8).

## GATHER SUPPORT

Every organization has key people, gatekeepers of the organizational culture, whose support is essential for change to occur. In the hospital setting these gatekeepers can be charge nurses, staff nurse leaders, other managers, physicians, or administrators. Gaining universal understanding of the tenets of shared governance among these key individuals may be one of the most difficult tasks to accomplish. No matter how bad current conditions are perceived to be, there remain comfort

and security in old structures and ways of doing things. Giving up control and being willing to take risks, with all of the accompanying vulnerabilities, require trust. Trust between staff, managers, physicians, and administrators is essential for a shared governance system to succeed. Check your trust titer as a critical care nurse manager. For example, do you profess an open door policy with your staff but no one seems to use it? Is the only way you find out about problems is when there is an "explosion"? If so, chances are trust is low. In this case, trust building activities are paramount.

Trust is developed in many ways, some large, many small. Meaningful contact between managers and staff is basic to developing trust. Nurses today want leaders who are visiable, who understand their practice and their individual needs and wants, and with whom they can talk freely without fear of misunderstanding or reprisal. They want to see and "feel" their manager's support. There are endless opportunities for gaining trust and support for a shared governance system, however, the majority of these arise at the point where the practice takes place, at the bedside, on the unit. So, seek them out. Manage by walking around. Lead by example.

An example of how one can operationalize participative beliefs is one in which a staff nurse is exceptionally disgruntled about not receiving immediate approval for a 10-week maternity leave. Six weeks is the policy and the standard. The nurse is criticizing the manager's hesitation in granting the request to "any and all who will listen." Finally, her peers start questioning the manager's motives. The resolution of this problem rests on the belief that everyone "owns" the problem, inasmuch as granting the leave request will affect the schedules and workload of the other staff in the unit in order to provide coverage. A forum, to which affected staff are invited, might be held to resolve the issue. It is exceedingly important to make sure the nurse requesting the leave is not viewed as the "bad guy," for she too has special needs and is a valued member of the group. The request is presented as well as the implications for staffing and patient care during the nurse's absence. Everyone has the information and everyone has an equal voice in resolving the issue. Experience has shown that this type of approach can produce very positive results in terms of staff satisfaction with the outcome and in staff growth.

In addition to living the beliefs and achieving

local successes, education of others about the shared governance philosophy is important. Although there is not a great deal of detail published about successful shared governance programs, information can be acquired through talking, corresponding, or visiting with colleagues experiencing such a system. Learn about their achievements. Discuss the benefits with members of your own organization.

## DEFINE PARTICIPATION IN DECISION MAKING

At some early juncture in developing a shared governance system, decision making should be addressed and defined. Participation can occur in individual jobs or small groups, at the divisional level, or at the corporate level. It can vary in degree from joint consultation, in which management maintains executive control over the final decision, all the way to worker control. The content of participation in decisions can include employment conditions, practice models, productivity, cost and labor reductions, personnel policies, wages, as well as strategic decisions (5). Each organization defines participation according to their own peculiar characteristics and circumstances.

As more people get involved in making decisions, there tends to be a variable loss of efficiency in the decision making process. This is not necessarily bad, particularly in light of the positive effects of participation that can be achieved, however, it does require attention. In some programs the degree of staff participation is decided by the urgency of the decision (6). The more urgent the decision, the fewer the number of people involved in deciding. Staff in this situation may be kept informed and later provided opportunity to discuss the decision and the circumstances dictating urgency. The discussion portion of this process is important and should not be ignored. Staff education on how the organization works and how it influences and is influenced by internal and external forces is crucial in a shared governance system. Good decisions are well-informed decisions.

Another way to define decision making is to clearly outline the types of decisions in which staff may participate. For example, staff may provide input relative to nursing standards, but they may not in the area of employee wages and benefits because of third party involvement in this arena. Care must be taken with the more directive approach such that the reasons for excluding partic-

ipation in some circumstances are sound and made clear to staff. If participation is not feasible and the decision is already final, then do not ask for input. A perception that participation is nothing more than "tokenism" will be highly destructive to a shared governance system.

That virtually any decision that affects the practice of nursing or the environment in which nurses work has a potential for staff involvement is a participative philosophy adopted by some organizations. The nursing management staff triage problems and issues as they arise and decide on the level of staff input needed. Among other factors, triage decisions are based on the urgency of the decision, staff desire for input, the level of professional maturation of the staff, growth opportunities provided by participation, management maturation relative to loss of control, and the negotiability of the issue. This approach works well in organizations in which a reasonable amount of trust exists between staff and management and not a lot of structure is needed.

Communication of the acceptable decision making process to staff may be formal or informal. Published grids or flow charts have been used that depict the route decisions take from problem identification through resolution, implementation, and follow-up communication (6). A description of the actions needed for completion of each step in the decision making process can also be included. For example, the observations, discussions and feedback required for determining when a perceived problem is a real problem may be delineated. More informal communication of the process such as communication forums or role playing examples can also be effective. The key is achieving clarity of process among all participants and minimizing ambiguity.

## ASSURE TWO-WAY COMMUNICATION

A free flow of information in all directions is fundamental to a shared governance system. Allen et al. described how having access to work-related information affects satisfaction in participative systems. Role conflict and role ambiguity, they concluded, can be reduced or eliminated through information. Role conflict occurs when two role expectations are incompatible (e.g., having to answer to two bosses—physicians and administrators). Having an active voice in decisions about one's job helps the employee gain information that will help make conflicting expectations more obvious and provide alternatives for reconciling demands. Role ambiguity occurs when one is unsure of what one is expected to do or how one fits into the organization as a whole. Opportunities for clarifying ambiguities occur through participation. Even when conflict cannot be eliminated, people tend to be less dissatisfied with the results because of the knowledge gained. Participation can give people control over how much energy is spent on ambiguous functions or can give them the ability to redirect rewards away from the conflicting expectations (5).

In a shared governance system nursing leaders have the responsibility for assuring that staff receive and understand available information. Staff have the responsibility for accessing established communication channels to obtain information, to ask questions, and to communicate information to managers. All communication should occur in a timely manner. Newsletters, written reports, forums, staff meetings, communication books, and "walking rounds," are all effectively used mechanisms for communication exchange. The effectiveness of this two-way communication process is again dependent upon trust—trust that information shared with peers, supervisors, or other members of the organization will be handled openly and constructively. The capabilities of an organization in the area of communication can contribute greatly to the success or failure of a shared governance system. Productive participation has a slim chance if there are too many instances in which failure of an innovation is attributable to poor communication, "brick walls" go up between staff and managers because the manner in which information was communicated led to wrong perceptions, or staff resort to "mass revolt" because information was unclear, untimely, or withheld from them. In a mature governance system there should be no information monopolies. Effective participation is informed (6).

A second aspect of communication is giving feedback. Feedback facilitates an employee's awareness of the contribution he or she makes to the delivery of the service or creation of the product of the organization (task identity). An awareness of the importance of an employee's contribution leads to feelings of competence, growth, and increased self-esteem (internal motivation). This in turn leads to greater satisfaction. Participation in decisions enhances feedback. Effective feedback facilities change by reducing the uncertainties associated with attempting and evaluating change. In addition, feedback makes more clear the link between changes and performance, and the relationship of performance to rewards (5).

An openness to feedback should be cultivated in both managers and staff. Skills in giving constructive and sensitive feedback and in receiving criticism without depersonalizing it are not naturally acquired capabilities. Many nurses are paralyzed with fear at the thought of dealing with a conflict situation. Many experience anxiety and self-doubt when required to provide sensitive feedback to their peers. Modeling of desired behaviors by skilled individuals, particularly managers, can be effective in developing skills in staff. Leaders can create an atmosphere of vulnerability to input by being willing to help each other identify and remove barriers that tend to stifle feedback. For example, a person whose first response to every suggestion of change is to describe in detail why it will not work may be assisted to learn how to postpone her judgment and instead first indicate interest in the idea and willingness to explore further the cost and benefits of the suggestion. Individuals responding with emotion—anger, tears, stunned silence—quickly discourage further feedback. Reversal of this approach is essential. Preparing ahead and rehearsing responses can often help mitigate emotional reactions as well as assure the correct message is communicated. Informal discussions about "failure" situations can also be productive. The benefits of admitting responsibility for miscommunication and trying a new approach can be demonstrated. The philosophy here is that a mistake is not synonymous with deliberate disrespect or evil motives.

The shared governance philosophy requires a commitment to a healthy two-way communication process. Training and developmental activities should be considered to assure attainment of this goal. Managers or employees who are unable or unwilling to acquire effective communication skills or who cannot commit to an open atmosphere may choose to seek a position outside the organization.

## IMPLEMENT PARTICIPATIVE STRUCTURES

Providing structures for participation within the organization can occur concurrently with other steps in developing a shared governance system. Participative structures can include forums, staff councils, unit meetings, or standing committees.

One of the pioneering plans, Rose Medical Center in Denver, has a self-governing body called "nursing congress." In close parallel to the medical staff organizational structure, the nursing congress operates under its own bylaws approved by the board of trustees. The bylaws were deemed important to assure continued support for the congress regardless of future changes in the hospital management. Bylaws outline the purposes, goals, and guidelines for conducting business and provide for the congress as the nursing self-governance structure as well as the election of four officers (president, vice president, recording secretary, and corresponding secretary). All employees (nurses, technicians, secretaries) of the nursing division are automatically congress members. The elected officers are members of the executive committee of the congress as are the chairpersons of the eight committees and councils (nursing standards and practice, audit/qaulity assurance, continuing education and research, career ladders, collaborative practice, human resources, rules and regulations, and bylaws). Three elected members at large complete the committee. The congress conducts meetings with the membership on a quarterly and annual basis. The congress, in operation since 1981, has addressed traditional nursing issues (staffing, scheduling, productivity) as well as issues arising from changes brought on by pressures for cost control and the prospective payment system (layoffs, low census schedules) (2, 9). A system very similar to and patterned after the congress of Rose Medical Center exists at Overlake Hospital Medical Center, Bellevue, Washington (7).

Bylaws for a shared governance body, called the "Professional Nursing Organization" (PNO), received approval in 1984 from the hospital executive committee and the board of trustees at the University of Rochester Medical Center Strong Memorial Hospital. A sound participative system was in operation at Strong Memorial several years preceding establishment of the PNO. Elected representatives from each nursing unit served 1-year terms on a staff nurse advisory board. These advisory boards addressed service-specific issues or problems, and met twice monthly with clinical nusing chiefs. In addition, a staff nurse executive committee existed that was composed of the chairpersons of each advisory board. The executive committee met monthly with the associate dean for nursing practice, addressed issues concerning all of nursing, and set the agenda for bimonthly staff forums. The executive committee of the New

Professional Nursing Organization is composed of 40 elected members, nine of whom chair the standing committees. Nurse administrators, faculty, and staff nurses are represented in proportion to the number of FTEs in each respective area. The chairperson of the PNO is also a voting member of the hospital executive committee as is the chairperson of the medical staff organization (3).

Reports of other participative interventions describe similar structures to the Strong and Rose Medical Centers. In several cases participative systems have been implemented on a single nursing unit with staff assuming supervisory and management functions as well as full responsibility and accountability for the care delivered on the unit. In place of traditional line positions staff may elect a staff member and assistants to provide for continuity and overall coordination (8, 10).

Several common structural features emerge as part of these shared governance programs. All have some type of elective system whereby staff representatives are chosen by their peers and colleagues to serve in decision making forums. Representatives, further, have an equal vote in those decisions. Many have self-governance frameworks that derive power and authority from the board of trustees of the organization. This is an important accomplishment in that it recognizes the significance of the contribution nursing makes to the mission of the organization and its protects and promotes nursing's responsibility for clinical self-direction.

Council or committee structures are also seen in the majority of these shared governance plans. Committees research and discuss issues, problems, or suggested innovations and develop a proposal from which decisions can be made. Committees have representation from all nursing constituencies, which assures all perspectives are presented. Committees tend to provide an efficient and practical mechanism for dividing the workload into manageable portions and maximizing staff involvement and input.

## DEFINE COSTS

The strong emphasis on cost containment and efficiency in today's health care institutions is an undeniable reality. In some respects, this emphasis facilitated the shared governance movement in that hospitals came to realize gains in efficiency by decentralizing and shifting more problem-solving responsibility to the unit level. Innovations by nurses that increased productivity, trimmed unnecessary inventory, or reduced use of costly supplies were welcomed and rewarded. Practice patterns that seemed to incorporate a ''more is better'' philosophy were analyzed, challenged, and altered. In other respects, however, the shared governance philosophy has the potential to be undermined by approaches that put too much emphasis on efficiency. On the surface, participative interventions appear costly. Involvement in the meetings, group work sessions, and developmental activities needed for a shared governance system demand staff time, nonproductive time, time away from patient care. A great deal of management time is also required in making the system succeed. However, a cost-benefit analysis will illustrate that the benefits of shared governance system outweigh those costs.

In determining costs, decide which activities will be considered as ''paid time'' versus which will be considered unpaid ''professional obligation'' time. For example, attendance at all official meetings may be reimbursed while work outside committees may be unpaid. Consider staff replacement costs to provide coverage for nurses attending meetings during work time. Costs for brochures, newsletters, and advertisements should also be examined. In addition, receptions or forums aimed at generating staff enthusiasm, support, and involvement may be needed. Consider, overall time demands of participation, even if unpaid, since this has an impact on peoples' rest and personal time. Last, the types and number of educational programs required in developing employee skills will need to be delineated.

The benefits derived from a successful shared governance system are not all as tangible or quantifiable as some of the cost factors. However, some logical arguments can be made. Participation has been shown to lead to increased employee satisfaction and organizational commitment. This in turn leads to reduced employee turnover and increased retention. All one has to do is calculate the tremendous costs associated with replacing *one* staff nurse, current estimates ranging from $10,000 to $80,000, to see the potential cost savings. And then, calculate the costs incurred by *not* being able to replace one nurse because of current shortages. How much can be gained by keeping hospital beds open or by not pushing existing staff to the limits of their endurance? Another factor to consider, although difficult to measure, is the quality of patient care delivered by an experienced, stable, and satisfied nursing staff. Hospitals with mature shared governance structures or similar participative interventions are also noted for their high quality of patient care. Although a cause and effect relationship between these factors has not been established, the coincidence, if you will, offers a convincing course of reasoning. A reputation for delivery of a high quality service is an invaluable asset to any hospital in today's competitive environment. Simply put, it means more business.

## NURTURE THE SYSTEM

Transformation requires a shift in perspectives, attitudes, and beliefs (1). It requires translation of existing skills into assets for the new culture (2). To accomplish this, resources must be made available to assist staff and managers in the transition. A commitment to leadership development is essential. Nurturing includes the activities of guiding, teaching, directing, developing, and rewarding. Although initially very intensive, the energy expended in these activities can be rechanneled into more creative and visionary directions as staff and managers develop proficiency in effecting change within the organization.

The atmosphere developed in a shared governance system must be one that expects and expands the accountability and responsibility of every individual within the organization. Likewise, the service delivered must be seen as the product of the *combined* efforts of all individuals, not one individual, group, or discipline. First line managers have an essential role in developing this environment. Through consistent modeling, coaching, counseling, and supporting, the manager can help staff develop skills for articulating problems or concerns in a clear, factual, and positive manner. Staff can learn to distinguish reliable from unreliable sources of information, to separate personal from professional issues, and to analyze both local and more global implications of proposed changes. In addition, they need to learn how to provide feedback sensitively and in a timely way.

From experience, developing staff comfort and skill with confrontation is one of the most difficult goals to attain. Conflict produces many degrees of tension. To transcend this, conflict has to be seen as a challenge, a mechanism to achieving personal growth through victory over one's fears, or an organizational or professional responsibility. Selecting conflict situations in which staff can experience successful resolution initially is important.

Preparing responses ahead of time, rehearsing these, and role playing potential spontaneous interactions can be beneficial in building confidence and increasing the chances of success. Treating the results of less positive confrontational experiences matter of factly and focusing on the usefulness of the knowledge gained from the situation can further help reduce tension.

Mechanisms for follow-up on issues and projects need to be developed throughout the system. If accountability is the standard, then issues should not be lost and responses to concerns or requests should materialize as expected or promised. In addition, those individuals who avoid participation and those who expend their energy in chronic complaining and griping need special attention. The expectations that participation is the norm and that problem resolution occurs through established routes must be made explicit. Gentle nudging into participative situations by the nurse manager will assist staff to learn from, and be influenced by, their more mature peers.

Developing leadership at all levels is another important aspect of the nurturing process. Peterson and Allen described transformational leaders as those who manage with the head and the heart, are sensitive to individual needs, and understand the connection of the whole. These leaders are not "controllers" and, in fact, realize no organization can be controlled from the top. These people are responsible for creating and holding the vision and for supporting policies and structure. They teach others how the system works and assure that others understand corporate and management values and beliefs. Last, the authors stated, for successful transformation it is essential that leaders operate in a way that promotes the influence and power of the whole, not individuals or structures (1).

A final and crucial area that needs to be addressed as positive changes in performance occur and responsible participation grows is the relationship between performance and rewards. Nurses who believe that rewards correspond to the quality of their performance are more satisfied and tend to value opportunities for participation more than those nurses who do not believe this linkage exists (5). Rewards and recognition systems should become content for participative decision making. This will assist employees to clarify and create connections between the quality of patient care they deliver and the rewards they receive as well as help them understand how their roles contribute to the products of the organization. Participative forums also provide an opportunity for the hospital to discover the types of rewards most desired by staff. Most of the shared governance systems reviewed have some form of career/clinical ladder recognition program in place.

## DEVELOP CRITERIA FOR EVALUATION

Demonstrating organizational progress toward achieving the desired goals of a shared governance system has many benefits. Experiencing progress, in and of itself, is energizing. It provides a form of recompense for the high degree of energy expended in bringing about the change. It also provides justification for continuing. Those who may not be convinced that participation is the ideal may be nudged into supporting the plan by evidence of success.

Some of the most quantifiable criteria by which to evaluate progress are the annual staff turnover rates and staff retention rates. Although these factors may not change early in the program, when they do, the impact can be powerful. Anything that appears to reduce the actual or potential internal nursing shortage generates significant interest and support.

Attitudinal surveys can assist in collecting data about staff perceptions of satisfaction and morale. Important elements of satisfaction may include cohesion with peers, enjoyment of friendly relationships among coworkers, esprit de corps, low stress, and low burnout. Work satisfaction measures may include perceptions of supervisory support, collaboration with peers and physicians, the effectiveness of the unit in providing good care, the challenge provided by one's work, autonomy, and the degree of power and influence one has over how they do their work. Physicians can also be surveyed for perceptions about the quality of care delivered and satisfaction relative to their working relationships with staff and managers. Patient and family perceptions of satisfaction should also be sought. Audits provide a mechanism for analyzing the care delivered by the nursing staff. The percentage of time nurses meet standards, including documentation requirements as well as the number and type of preventable patient incidents (e.g., medication errors, falls) could be examined.

The percentage of total staff actively involved in shared governance structures could be used as a measure of success, although the absolute percentage of participation is a rather weak indicator.

About a 20% staff involvement rate is usual in the more advanced programs (8). What is more important is that there is consistent active involvement and that the nurses involved are dynamic and feel satisified with their accomplishments. One factor found to be of great significance at Rose Medical Center was the increased ability of the nurses to accommodate to change. As an example, when this organization was faced with a forced layoff of 80 employees because of a period of persistent low census, the nurses designed and implemented a voluntary day-off schedule, thereby protecting the nursing units from staff cuts (2). In another institution, when several patient populations had to be relocated throughout various nursing units because of changes in service demands, the nurses successfully executed a plan that preserved current staff positions and schedules and maintained cohesion of work groups. These are not insignificant gains and, although not numerically quantifiable, can be easily seen as marks of success of a participative system.

Last, remember transformation is slow. Success is often measured in inches. If one resistant nurse accepts accountability for one issue, you have made progress. If even one time you are informed of a problem after the staff have satisfactorily solved it, you are on your way to success.

## SUMMARY

The proponents of shared governance systems agree that the positive outcomes of decisional participation attained in other types of organizations can also be achieved in nursing organizations. Indeed, the signs of success of more mature programs are evidence of this and are enviable. Dramatic organizational change is needed today because of the societal changes affecting the attitudes of workers toward organizations and authority. This transformation requires an alteration in values and beliefs as well as development of different standards and norms.

The process of implementing a shared governance system involves a number of tasks. These tasks are discussed throughout the chapter and include suggestions for gaining support for a gov-

ernance system, providing participative structures, defining decisional participation, nurturing the system, defining costs, and developing evaluation criteria. Each organization is different so it must tailor any system to fit its own characteristics and circumstances.

Nursing leaders who desire to implement a shared governance system or similar transformational strategy will need to make a significant commitment to the beliefs behind the system. Major change is slow and can create varying degrees of chaos. Time and energy demands are initially immense. The perceived loss of control over decisions can be frightening. However, over time, as individuals within the organization become more adept in accomplishing change and, accountability and responsibility become the standard, these developmental demands will decrease. Energy can then be channeled toward creating proactive responses to an everchanging environment and directing the future of the profession of nursing.

## REFERENCES

1. Peterson M, Allen D. Shared governance: a strategy for transforming organizations, part I. J Nurs Admin 1986;16(1):9–12.
2. Johnson LM. Self-governance: treatment for an unhealthy nursing culture. Health Prog 1987;4:41–43.
3. Ortiz ME, Gehring P, Sovie MD. Moving to shared governance. Am J Nurs 1987;7:923–926.
4. Mitchell P, Armstrong S, Forshee T, et al. American Association of Critical-Care Nurses demonstration project: phase I report. AACN, Newport Beach, California, 1988, unpublished.
5. Allen D, Calkin J, Peterson M. Making shared governance work, a conceptual model. J Nurs Admin 1988;18(1):37–43.
6. Peterson M, Allen D. Shared governance: a strategy for transforming organizations, part II. J Nurs Admin 1988;16(2):11–16.
7. Nursing congress bylaws. Overlake Hospital Medical Center, Bellevue, Washington, 1983, unpublished.
8. News. By whatever name, the movement to put nurses in charge of their practice is gaining ground. AM J Nurs 1987;87(5):712–726.
9. News. Nurses in Denver adopt self-governance. AORN J 1981;34:778–779.
10. Elpern EH, White PM, Donahue MF. Staff governance: the experience of one nursing unit. J Nurs Admin 1984;6:9–15.

# Chapter 6

# Creative Staffing

PATRICIA KALLWEIT KALDOR

Providing adequate staff to give the nursing care that is required is the ongoing and continual responsibility of every critical care nurse manager. The patient and family are the focus of all care. Staffing revolves around the provision of this care. Staff nurses are a key element to a successful staffing and scheduling program and must be included in its planning and implementation.

Scheduling and staffing are two managerial functions, alike in their results but different in timing. For the purpose of this discussion, *scheduling* is the assignment of individual staff based on forecasted nursing workload. It is based on what we know. The more we know, the better our estimation. Scheduling accommodates the predictable variabilities in workload and in staff availability. On the other hand, *staffing* is the process of adjusting the number of staff working according to the acutal workload. Staffing accommodates the unpredictable variability in workload and staff availability. For each, there must be assessment of the situation and a plan with options and contingencies.

## ASSESSING STAFFING NEEDS

A creative staffing program begins with in-depth assessment of factors both internally and externally that have an impact on the decisions that need to be made in regard to staffing. In addition, the types of patients cared for and the flow of workload within the organization will have an effect. Once the environment is assessed for the amount of staffing needed, it will be necessary to decide how it can best be provided. The type and mix of staff will need to be determined as well as how the work will be organized (nursing care delivery system). Scheduling can then be accomplished in either a centralized or a decentralized fashion based on the needs of the organization. The provision of regular staff as well as staffing contingencies is part of a complete program. Creative staffing alternatives need to continually be explored as the health care

environment and the needs of the employees change. It is essential that the scheduling and staffing program includes a process for evaluating its effectiveness. This feedback will provide information to the nurse manager to make appropriate staffing adjustments.

### Internal Factors

Assessment of staffing needs begins with a review of many internal factors. The organization philosophy of providing care, or the mission statement, as well as the goals of the nursing services should address the desire to provide quality care in a cost-effective manner and in a caring environment. Unit-based staffing guidelines are established based either on past history or on time studies of nursing care activities. From this data, productivity standards are established, budgets prepared, and productivity monitored. Scheduling decisions are made based on the established standards. The physical environment, i.e., size of the unit, private rooms versus wards, location of supplies and equipment, and access to support departments, affects the efficiency of staffing and thus determines scheduling. Nursing and patient care rituals also determine staffing levels and need to be critically assessed on an ongoing basis to determine current relevance to practice. Daily weights, heights on infants, vital signs taken every shift, and head-to-toe assessments every shift are examples of rituals that have been questioned at times because the routine 8-hour shifts have become ten and 12-hour shifts.

### External Factors

Prospective payment, competition, and consumerism are critical components of today's health care environment and are among the many external forces that have an impact on staffing decisions. The Joint Commission on Accreditation of Healthcare Organizations (JCAHO) has established nursing services standards that relate to staffing (1) (Table 6.1).

**Table 6.1.** Joint Commission on Accreditation of Healthcare Organizations (JCAHO) Nursing Services

| | |
|---|---|
| NR.1.1 | The nursing department/service takes all reasonable steps to provide quality nursing care. |
| NR.3 | The nursing department/service is organized to meet the nursing care needs of patients and to maintain established standards of nursing practice. |
| NR.4 | Nursing department/service assignments in the provision of nursing care are commensurate with the qualifications of nursing personnel and are designed to meet the nursing care needs of patients. |
| NR4.1 | A sufficient number of qualified registered nurses are on duty at all times to give patients the nursing care that requires the judgment and specialized skills of a registered nurses. |
| NR.4.2 | Nursing personnel staffing also is sufficient to assure prompt recognition of any untoward change in the patient's condition and to facilitate appropriate intervention by the nursing, medical, or hospital staffs. |
| NR.4.3 | In striving to assure quality nursing care and a safe patient environment, nursing personnel staffing and assignment are based on at least the following: |
| NR.4.3.1 | A registered nurse plans, supervises, and evaluates the nursing care of each patient. |
| NR.4.3.2 | To the extent possible, a registered nurse makes a patient assessment before delegating appropriate aspects of care to other nursing personnel. |
| NR.4.3.3 | The patient care assignment minimizes the risk of the transfer of infection and accidental contamination. |
| NR.4.3.4 | The patient care assignment is commensurate with the qualifications of each nursing staff member, the identified nursing needs of the patient, and the prescribed medical regimen. |
| NR.4.3.5 | Responsibility for nursing care and related duties is retained by the hospital nursing department/service when nursing students and nursing personnel from outside sources are providing care within a patient care unit. |
| NR.4.4 | The nursing department/service defines, implements, and maintains a system for determining patient requirements for nursing care on the basis of demonstrated patient needs, appropriate nursing intervention, and priority for care. |

In addition to JCAHO standards that apply to all hospital nursing services, specialized nursing organizations, such as the American Association of Critical-Care Nurses (AACN), have established standards that can be applied to the staffing of critical care units (2). Comprehensive Standard VII is an example of an AACN staffing standard: The critical care unit shall have appropriately qualified staff to provide care on a 24-hour basis.

The support standards to Comprehensive Standard VII address the issues of staff acquiring a knowledge base and psychomotor skills common to and requisite for the care of critically ill patients and the nurse:patient ratio reflecting recognition of patients' acuity and required nursing care. The support standards also require unit staff participation in development of staffing patterns to assure flexibility, utilization of at least a 50% registered nurse staff, restriction of unlicensed personnel from delivery of direct nursing care, ability of staff to intermittently support other areas, and contingency plans to assure availability of qualified critical care nursing staff.

AACN further delineates its position on specific aspects of critical care in its development of position statements. Since 1983, when AACN published its position on "Use of Technical Personnel in Critical Care Settings," clarification of the registered nurse's role has existed, strengthening the registered nurse's accountability for coordinating and implementing the nursing process and facilitating the delivery of nursing care to the critically ill patient. Technical personnel may assist the professional registered nurse in the data collection phases of the nursing process. Role delineation of the technical position must include a written position description, an available training program, and clear lines of responsibility and accountability as evidenced on the organizational chart (3).

In 1986, AACN described the role of the critical care manager in its position statement entitled, "Role Expectations for the Critical Care Manager," which reinforces staffing concerns as addressed by JCAHO with specific application to critical care units (4). This position statement refers to a statement published by the American Nurses' Association in 1978: Nurse managers "coordinate available resources to efficiently and effectively provide professional nursing care of a quality consistent with nursing care standards and at a cost compatible with the fiscal and other resources of the health care organization'' (5). The position statement, like that of JCAHO, requires implementation of a patient classification system, nursing standards, and a defined nursing care delivery system—all factors affecting staffing. The critical care manager must participate in interviewing and hiring of qualified and needed staff to ensure 24-hour nursing coverage appropriate to patient care needs.

On the legal side, staffing may be more of a concern today than in the past. A staffing problem can be a simple matter of numbers (too few people) or of staff members who are not competent to practice in a particular setting. ''In a negligence case, lack of competency is more frequently raised as a main issue: insufficient staff is usually a collateral issue introduced to emphasize a negligent departure from accepted standards of practice'' (6). Every nurse manager ought to be well versed in the laws in his or her particular state that describe standards of practice for nursing. Authority, definitions of nursing care, supervision and direction of delegated nursing acts, and violations of standards are described in detail.

Basic to any business decision is a cost/benefit analysis. Standards for providing care have been discussed, however, only what can be afforded can be provided. Medicare patients currently represent approximately 50% of all hospital admissions and this percentage is expected to continue to increase as our population becomes increasingly elderly. Medicare, as a prospective payment system, pays not for the actual care that has been provided but what it has determined it should cost to provide the necessary care. Like Medicare, health maintenance organizations (HMOs), preferred provider organizations (PPOs), and self-insured businesses, are imposing capitation costs on providers of care. Care cannot cost more to provide than the organization will receive in reimbursement. This fact imposes serious constraints on the management of critical care units, including what can be afforded to appropriately staff the unit.

### Acuity of Nursing Care Needs

When assessing staffing needs, a review and analysis of unit-specific factors is necessary. The extent of the patients' nursing care needs and the unit activity level should be included in the analysis. The inpatient population will continue to be increasingly more elderly. As a result, patients with an acute health care problem will also have many concomitant and/or chronic health care problems. As described by JCAHO and other professional organizations, a patient classification or nursing dependency system must be implemented that attempts to accurately describe nursing care needs of patients so that can be established (7). Phillips et al. (8) note, that

nursing dependency techniques indicate quantity of care rather than quality. It is difficult to categorize patients accurately, there can be no ''standard'' time for procedures, and studies have difficulty in analyzing crisis or potential crisis situations. In calculating staff requirements, the need for time for senior staff to administer the unit, to orient new staff, to supervise and teach, and to solve problems must be recognized. These issues cannot be excluded in any calculation regarding direct patient care.

Regardless of its difficulty, however, it is recognized that patient acuity/nursing dependency systems do allow a more accurate estimation of nursing staff members required. Ideally, the system should be time based.

There are two common methods for quantifying or estimating nursing resources needed. One of these entails classifying patients with similar requirements for nursing care and assigning an average amount of nursing care hours required. In this system, a level of care or a category is assigned to each patient. This type of system is useful for patients who are homogeneous, such as in cardiac recovery or newborn intensive care, or when changes in status are infrequent or easily predicted as the patient moves from one level to another (9). The second approach involves determining standard times for each major nursing activity and multiplying by the number of times that activity occurs. These are then totaled to determine the nursing resource requirements for patients (10).

The resultant number of care hours can be used in two ways. They can be used to determine staffing shift to shift. If sufficient nursing resources are readily available, this is an excellent way to assure adequate staffing. If, however, contingencies and flexibility of staff have been difficult to establish, these care hours are better used to forecast long-range staffing. In other words, positions can be approved based on trends realized. These scheduling plans are then based on nursing care that has been quantified according to the patient's dependence on the nursing care. It is more important to measure need for nursing resources than to determine how acutely ill the patient is. An example of this is the ventilator-dependent patient in an intensive care unit (ICU) versus a patient on a large intermediate care unit with a Cheyne-Stokes breathing pattern and copious oral secretions. The nursing time to maintain a patent airway may well be doubled for the second patient.

## Unit Activity

The nurse manager needs to carefully analyze unit activity and monitor trends continuously. Unit activity refers to both census history as well as workload within the shift. Fluctuation in census can be trended over time to establish high and low volume times by season, month, day of week, and shift. Within each shift, trends can be established for workload related to activity such as admissions, transfers, discharges, specialized procedures performed in the unit, and expected changes in patient population requiring additional patient monitoring. A decreasing average length of stay for any given patient population may indicate a need for more intense nursing care. There simply is less time to provide the care. Patient populations should be defined for each unit with care needs identified. The more homogeneous the patient population on a unit, the more efficient the unit can be managed. Steps should be taken, of course, to minimize variability in patient census because census variations are a key reason scheduling is difficult. Nursing units should be consolidated when census drops significantly because empty beds cost nearly as much to maintain as beds that are occupied and revenue producing. Patient placement policies should be reviewed so that homogeneous patient populations can be cared for together and, as a result, nursing requirements can be decreased. Program changes should be planned for as well as patient volumes projected. Full attention to unit activity by the nurse manager will support thoughtful scheduling decisions (11).

Assessing staffing needs is the most important step to providing adequate nursing care to patients who require it. Both internal and external factors must be critically reviewed. Nursing intensity must be measured and unit workload evaluated so that patient care needs can be met by the most appropriate number and skill mix of staff (Table 6.2).

## SCHEDULING TO MEET PATIENT CARE NEEDS

Once the assessment phase is completed, the nurse manager proceeds to plan for the provision of 24-hour coverage to meet patient care needs. Well-defined staffing and scheduling policies are needed to attain staffing patterns that recognize patient needs and provide effective work groups. Core or master staffing is needed as well as variable staffing options. Productivity standards are established and must be met. Staff should have input into schedules and may even be able to accomplish self-scheduling. Nurse managers, responsible for 24-hour coverage, who delegate schedule preparation, must maintain close communication with those preparing the schedules. Costs associated with the staff other than the cost of providing direct patient care, such as orientation and housewide response to cardiac arrests housewide, should be quantified and included when planning staffing. Specific factors involved in this planning process include unit workload, skill mix (professional/nonprofessional/clerical), full-time:part-time ratio, nursing care delivery system, and managed care.

When evaluating unit workload to establish a staffing plan, the size and configuration of the unit must be considered. Efficiency of staffing as it relates to the size of the unit will depend on physical layout as well as the acuity and clinical homogeneity of the patient population. In other words, a respiratory ICU can appropriately be larger than a general medical/surgical ICU. A round configuration with excellent visualization of patients and easy access to a central core of supplies can be staffed more efficiently than private rooms on either side of a long corridor. It will require more complex staffing patterns to provide nursing care on a unit with patient mix ranges from intensive care to telemetry care. The better the physical layout and the more homogeneous the patient population, the more efficient the unit can be staffed.

## Unit Workload

Unit workload also relates to various patterns of admissions: scheduled (e.g., surgicals, postcardiac catheterization laboratory procedures) versus unscheduled (e.g., cardiac arrests, other medical emergencies, postanesthesia recovery); emergency versus internal transfers; percentage of patients returning to the unit versus direct admissions. The question that arises and must be answered in each

**Table 6.2.** Scheduling and Staffing Needs Analysis Checklist

| External forces (most difficult to influence) | Unit specific (easiest to control and make a difference) |
|---|---|
| Health maintenance organization (capitation costs)<br>Consumer interest and expectations<br>Computerization<br>Medicare (Prospective Payment System)<br>Aging population<br>Joint Commission on Accreditation of Healthcare Organizations Standards<br>American Association of Critical-Care Nurses Standards of Care<br>American Association of Critical-Care Nurses Position Statements<br>American Nurses' Association Standards<br>Supply of available nurses | Philosophy<br>Productivity standard<br>Fluctuations in census<br>Staffing guidelines<br>Unit activity: workload within shift<br>Nursing care delivery system<br>Preestablished care gudelines<br>Rituals/nursing routines<br>Physical configuration of unit<br>Cross-training; "Buddy" unit<br>Private rooms/wards<br>Location of supplies/equipment<br>Access to support departments<br>Unit goals and objectives<br>Volumes: average daily census, average length of stay, total patient days<br>Full-time/part-time mix<br>Skills mix<br>Patient populations<br>Flexible scheduling patterns<br>Size of unit<br>Nursing versus nonnursing tasks<br>Unit-based (autonomous) staffing |
| **Organizational**<br>Mission statement<br>Goals and objectives<br>Surgery schedule<br>Product evaluation<br>Product standardization<br>Philosophy<br>Compensation structure<br>Control of hiring<br>Inventory control<br>Competitive bidding | |
| **Nursing services**<br>Philosophy<br>Patient acuity system<br>Centralized versus decentralized scheduling<br>Goals and objectives<br>Scheduling guidelines<br>Full-time/part-time mix recommendations<br>Total full-time equivalents/positions | |

of these situations is whether you can plan staffing to be able to prepare for the arrival of the patient. Only the predictable can be included when planning a schedule.

Historically, critical care nurses have been expected to respond to situations outside their assigned units or regularly assigned duties, e.g., cardiac arrests and care of postanesthesia patients. All nonunit staff time must be quantified and addressed separately from the time required to provide care to patients admitted to the unit. Critical care nurses usually accompany patients to procedures provided outside the critical care environment. A system of patient scheduling, implemented by all departments that provide care or diagnostics to patients, can facilitate optimal utilization of nursing time and optimize the time allowed for the patients' hospitalization. A hospital-wide system

of patient scheduling has been implemented in institutions that have automated admission/discharge/transfer information as well as order entry and can readily expand computer applications.

**Skill Mix**

Skill mix and full-time:part-time ratios are determined based on patients' care needs. The more acutely ill the patient, the more intense the need is to employ professional nurses who can manage the scope of care. Advantages of an all registered nurse (RN) staff in critical care include the RNs' versatility to meet patient and family needs in a demanding and highly technological environment. In addition, RNs can readily expand their function and supplement the rehabilitation and treatment programs of other health care professionals. Finally, there is no need for the RN to take the time to supervise the care of patients otherwise assigned to nonprofessionals when care is provided by an all-RN staff. The cumulative result of these advantages is that an RN staff can deliver the required care with fewer total nursing care hours required per patient day (12).

In an era of a nursing shortage it may be difficult to support an all-RN staff. It may be necessary to determine specific RN functions, eliminate nonnursing tasks, and support the RN whenever feasible. A recent study (13) indicated that "the dominant controllable factor affecting nursing staff productivity is the availability of effective support services, especially materials management, dietary, pharmacy, and transport services. Although many departments will resent the assignment of additional functions, nonnursing tasks must be reassigned to keep costs below reimbursement rates." Each institution must analyze its own situation and formulate a position on this issue before determining staffing needs.

Consideration of the nurse's educational and experiential background must be included in the determination of an optimal staffing pattern. First line managers must maintain control of hiring so appropriate decisions can be made and adequate staffing provided. Part of a nurse manager's staffing responsibility is the hiring of new employees based on needs of the patients, needs of the unit, and qualifications of the applicant. In other words, effective staffing is the result of deliberate, careful selection of specific individuals and a prediction of their effect upon patients and patient care. A good staffing program will include identifying the quality of the product (nursing care), predicting the number and type of staff to produce the volume and quality, developing assignment patterns, and evaluating the effectiveness of the overall staffing pattern. Standards of care attained and costs maintained within budget constraints are indicators that the staffing plans are effective and efficient.

As care needs become less technical and patients become more stable, they are moved to units with a lower RN:patient ratio. As a result, other nonprofessional care givers can be added to complement the new staffing pattern requirements. Depending on census trends on weekends and holidays, full:part-time ratios are established. If routine alternate weekend work schedules are used, half of the number of people on the staff will be working each weekend. If all of the staff are full-time, then half of the people will be working the

weekend and the staffing complement is thus half on weekends as compared to Monday through Friday. This works well if census trends decrease significantly on the weekends. As you increase the percentage of part-timers to full-timers, you increase your staffing on the weekend. If census remains at a constant level, then a 60:40 to 50:50 full-time:part-time ratio is appropriate and necessary.

## Managed Care

Two additional factors to be considered in providing 24-hour coverage are the nursing care delivery system utilized and the extent to which managed care has been implemented. The selected nursing care delivery system will reflect the philosophy of nursing care in the institution. Three systems currently utilized are functional, team, and primary nursing. Functional nursing is task oriented and efficient but delivers fractionated care to the patient, i.e., many individuals provide small components of care. This system continues to be used occasionally but is not preferred. Team nursing is care coordinated, delegated, and often provided by professional registered nurses. In intensive care units, this system is generally no longer used because of the all-RN staffing trend and the desire not to use technical personnel to provide direct patient care. Primary nursing is a comprehensive nursing approach that provides continuous coordinated and individualized care from admission to discharge. The primary nurse is a professional nurse who assumes responsibility and 24-hour accountability for the care of a small number of patients. This is the delivery system of choice in critical care in order to provide both the highest quality of care for the patient and the highest degree of job satisfaction for the professional RN. Primary nursing supports the professional RN in the areas of professional status, administration, nurse-physician relationship, and autonomy (14).

There are two myths about primary nursing that must be eliminated for primary nursing to continue as the nursing care delivery system of choice. Myth I is that primary nursing requires an all-RN staff. Although an all-RN staff is not necessary, it is preferred because successful implementation of primary nursing is more complex with a mixed skill level staff. The team building skills required for managers are higher as they must provide greater supervision and support of the nonprofessional caregivers. The essential ingredient of primary nursing is the establishment of a responsible relationship between the nurse and the patient. The primary nurse delivers care to the patient when he or she is present. More importantly, decisions about the care to be delivered are carried out by those who care for the patient in the nurse's absence. Myth II is that primary nursing requires more staff than team nursing. In reality, when nurses are responsible and accountable, they naturally want to do more and be more successful at what they do. They eliminate some steps to providing care because of the improved continuity, coordination, and commitment (15).

The next logical move from primary nursing is to managed care and preestablished multidisciplinary patient care guidelines. The professional RN becomes the case manager and care is managed over the entire event: prehospitalization to posthospitalization when appropriate. Preestablished care guidelines, designed by the most knowledgeable RNs, map the event and all health care professionals' contributions are indicated and coordinated. These plans should be endorsed by medicine as well. Obviously, the nursing care delivery system used and the extent to which managed care is implemented will affect scheduling and staffing patterns.

## EFFECTIVE SCHEDULING AND STAFFING

Effective scheduling and staffing, then, must incorporate the effect internal and external factors have on the environment as well as the assessment of the current situation within the critical care unit. Once these components are assessed, a decision needs to be made as to whether the function of scheduling and staffing will be accomplished in a centralized or a decentralized manner. A consideration of philosophy and economy should indicate which method an organization will choose. These factors are viewed as they relate to the nurse manager's responsibility for staffing and the budget of the unit.

### Centralized Versus Decentralized

Centralized scheduling and staffing is a method in which staffing levels and mix are determined by nursing services and/or by the nurse manager of the unit and shift-to-shift staffing is managed by a central office. The greatest advantage is that a specific individual is responsible to assess staffing and make a decision to provide optimal staffing housewide. Unfortunately, the disadvantages of centralized scheduling are many. First of all, an additional person or persons (staffing coordinator,

shift supervisors and/or scheduling clerks) must be paid to provide a function that can better be done at the unit level. Regardless of the accuracy of a patient classification system, an individual in a centralized scheduling office cannot be as aware of each staffing situation at the unit level as those employees working in that unit. In addition, a centralized scheduling office generally means floating of staff from one unit to another. Floating is a tremendous job dissatisfier and a factor that may not support the philosophy of quality and continuity of care (7).

Decentralized scheduling and staffing, on the other hand, does support quality of care (16). Decentralized scheduling and staffing is a method in which staffing levels and mix are determined by the nursing unit within agreed upon constraints. Scheduling is the responsibility of the nurse manager and staffing is managed shift to shift by the unit RNs. Variations in the nursing hours required are managed by the nurse manager and staff on each unit based on their professional judgment. The only requirement is that the productivity standard be achieved over time.

### Autonomous Staffing

Decentralized scheduling and staffing in its purest sense is *autonomous staffing*. The philosophy of autonomous staffing is that the highest quality of care is best provided by people with appropriate skills assigned and committed to a clinical area. The objectives of autonomous staffing are twofold: to assist the nurse manager in exercising control of staffing to influence patient care and unit expenses and to assist the staff nurse in identifying his or her responsibility for adequate coverage to meet patient needs. Autonomous staffing allows for those who are responsible for worked hours to manage human resources. Autonomy is a quality of being self-directed or self-governing. Autonomous, then, is the right to self-government without outside control. It also means existing or capable of existing independently. Autonomous staffing, then, is self-regulation of a unit regarding staffing policies and scheduling guidelines. This self-regulation of staffing by a unit must include prearranged staffing contingencies.

Autonomous staffing has advantages and disadvantages for both the nurse manager and the staff nurse. The major advantage and job satisfier for the nurse is that floating to other units is not required. Staff may also take requested days off when workload is down in their area regardless of workload elsewhere. Autonomous staffing generates an increased sense of responsibility for patient care on the patient care unit. Staff rely heavily on each other, as well as medical staff and other health care professionals, to provide the patient care required. As a result, staff cohesiveness and morale can be enhanced when autonomous staffing is implemented. The disadvantage for the nurse can include burn-out during prolonged periods of high census if adequate contingencies are not established.

There are many reasons why nurse managers, especially in highly technical critical care units, should consider autonomous staffing. Participative management and shared governance are integrated into practice as staff make decisions on staffing, a key factor affecting their practice. Additionally, staff become more productive (less time is spent directing floats) and accountable for patient care. Collaboration between physicians and nurses is enhanced as physicians are less frustrated when working with the same RNs. Certainly, patient satisfaction is improved. Temporary agency help, although potentially very qualified, decreases the overall efficiency of the unit and is always more costly than in-house staff. There are three major disadvantages of autonomous staffing. First, fewer in-house RNs are available to provide coverage. This can be especially acute in a critical care unit with high staffing requirements. Second, there are budgetary considerations if the staffing contingencies utilized are quite costly, e.g., excessive overtime of unit staff. Additionally, there can potentially be extended periods of low census when the workload is low and staff must be sent home with potential loss of wages.

There are conditions and a climate necessary for autonomous staffing to be successful. Christman (17) writes that

> an autonomous nursing staff must fulfill four basic requirements: 1.) There must be rigorous demands on staff for competence and skills, and accountability for their own decisions in managing patients. 2.) The unit must be organized based on primary nurse/patient relationships. 3.) There must be systematic methods of assessing, credentialling, and maintaining skills of the staff. 4.) Nurses must have the right to obtain consultation on request and the obligation to undergo periodic reviews of clinical consistency and results.

Nursing services must be organized to support decentralization, and the professional staff must be committed to the profession and to their unit. A nurse who believes that being there makes the difference will be there and support the staffing requirements of the unit.

Not all units may desire or be able to implement autonomous staffing. There are units, however, that have implemented self-scheduling, which is another method to increase staff nurses' feelings of autonomy and job satisfaction (18). Self-scheduling is the process by which staff nurses on the unit collectively decide and implement the schedule given the criteria for adequate staffing as determined by the nurse manager. The criteria must indicate number and mix of staff as well as time needed for off-unit activities such as meeting and mandating educational activities. Benefits of self-scheduling include less time spent by the nurse manager in preparing schedules. More important, however, staff nurses gain control of an issue that is key to their satisfaction with the job and the work environment and that is their work schedules (19). There is an increased awareness by the nurses of the unit need for nursing care and methods to establish adequate staffing designed and implemented with a renewed commitment from the staff.

## Establishing Staffing Contingencies

Obviously, if each unit is to be autonomous as it relates to scheduling and staffing, then adequate contingencies for personnel resources must be established. Nursing services may centrally establish and support some of these contingencies, e.g., an internal pool of nurses (per diem) who are able to work as requested but for whom no hours are promised. Hospitals within a corporate system should investigate pools of RNs that can work within the system. Generally, then, costs can be controlled both in salaries and benefits. There may potentially be a group of nurses who are hired as regular employees who are not assigned to a specific unit but who are "float" nurses and are cross-trained for several units to fill in where needed. An attempt should be made to be area specific in order to support the RN's professional growth through experiential and educational opportunities provided in the area. Additionally, the RN will feel an increased commitment to area standards of care. The difficulty utilizing RNs across several units is that RNs with specific skills, e.g., care of the cardiac patient, can be needed on all cardiac care units when busy and then not needed when the census is low in all units. In other words, cross-training should be planned for units with different volume trends. A good example is a general ICU and an emergency room (ER). The ER is generally busiest in the summer, whereas many general medical/surgical and/or cardiac ICUs experience lower volumes in the summer. Cross-training for these two departments is practical and logical and requires a similar RN personality for both. Nurse managers in like areas should consider coordinating vacations, leaves of absence, and other planned staffing changes with one another on a regular basis.

Unit-based contingencies might include restrictive floating (to similar patient populations) or rotation to other shifts. Personnel can be placed "on call" to extend an 8-hour shift to a 12-hour shift to fill a vacancy on a shift. For example, if an RN is not available for the evening shift, a day shift RN would work an additional 4 hours and a night shift RN could come in 4 hours early. An entire staffing pattern could be arranged to all 12-hours shifts, requiring fewer employees to provide the same staffing levels and eliminating the evening shift that may be difficult to staff. Some organizations, in order to provide adequate staffing on weekends, are offering bonuses for extra weekends worked, differentials for any weekend hours worked, or full-time status and pay if an individual works 24 hours every weekend (24 of 40). Incentives vary from area to area, are market driven, and will depend on seriousness of vacancy rates.

### Agency Personnel

Utilization of agency personnel is always an option. Although a hospital can be held liable for the negligence of such personnel, highly skilled and competent RNs are available from outside agencies. The Division of Nursing, Department of Health and Human Services, developed a contract to study the utilization and effects of temporary nursing services. These studies have shown that agency RNs are at least as well prepared educationally and have considerable and variable experience. They are more likely to work weekends, evenings, and nights. Additionally, critical care is the most frequent environment requested, second only to the medical/surgical areas (20). The advantages for an RN to work through an agency are higher hourly wages and control over hours worked. In addition, agency RNs do not get involved in unit politics, allowing them to reportedly spend more time than

regular staff in direct physical care of patients (21, 22). These factors need to be remembered and considered as scheduling options are developed.

The need for and value of utilizing agency help must be critically assessed. The advantages for the organization to utilize outside agency RNs includes financial aspects such as savings realized when benefits and educational time (which is high in critical care) do not need to be paid for these individuals. Agency personnel are available on short notice to fill vacancies or give regular staff needed time off. They are frequently available when regular staff are not available. These RNs can enhance staff morale because the regular staff no longer works short-handed. Frequently these RNs introduce new ideas and/or methods and serve as a transfer of information from one hospital to another. The cost of agency staff may also be a financial disadvantage. These individuals are very expensive. Their hourly cost to the organization can be greater than 200% of the regular employees. In addition, there is a cost associated with the time it takes to screen, schedule, orient, and evaluate agency RNs. Another disadvantage is the inability of individual RNs to work independently and with an assignment equal to a regular employee. The regular employee spends much time throughout the shift teaching (in particular, hospital policy and procedure, physician standing orders, nursing standards of care) and directing when outside agency RNs are utilized. This decreases staff morale. Additionally, the fact that agency RNs frequently receive better schedules and higher remuneration disheartens regular staff. The use of agency help must be carefully controlled and monitored (23).

## EXPLORING CREATIVE STAFFING ALTERNATIVES

### Establish Goals of Staffing

Effective scheduling and staffing can be achieved. Creative staffing alternatives must be explored. Scheduling is never a fixed science but an evolving art. The process begins with the establishment of the goals of scheduling and staffing. Shaheen (24) suggested this definition of the goals for staffing and scheduling nursing personnel:

> Nurses provide responsive human intervention based on scientific knowledge which sustains preventative and curative treatment to biological changes in the human condition of sick persons, regardless of the moment in time these changes occur. Such interventions meet an optimal level

for standardized performance if, and only if, allocation of human resources guarantees persistent, consistent, and predictable quantity and quality of human resource talent per eight hour shift, 100% of the time, to infinity.

Once the goals are established, decisions are made to reflect these goals. The next step is to generate a creative environment, one in which all RNs can participate in achieving the goals. To do this, values should be clarified. The guiding values come from the philosophy of patient care that is established. From these values develops a cohesive culture that naturally supports and generates creativity. Individuals feel free to propose new ideas in a trusting environment. Together the manager and the employees set objectives to staff the unit adequately and fairly. The objectives change motivation into action as there is a commitment to the behaviors that are necessary to accomplish the goals of staffing. The manager needs to build in rewards for improved and good performance so that positive behaviors are reinforced and recognition by peers is achieved. Opportunities for time off, extra weekends off, educational time, and such things as a no-float policy can be offered as rewards for good performance. Of course, the manager must also identify and direct underachievers in this same environment. This process can be translated into productivity that must also be measured on an ongoing basis by the manager. High expectations lead to high productivity.

### Generating a Creative Environment

Creative scheduling ideas will be generated when barriers to innovative approaches are identified and attempts are made to reduce them. Barriers can include nursing inefficiencies—old rituals that no longer meet patient care demands and/or nonnursing tasks better provided by technical/clerical/or other professional staff. Delivery of food trays, emptying of wastebaskets, pick up of blood from blood bank, making of unoccupied beds, and pick up and delivery of medications are all tasks that can be done by nonprofessional staff. Conservative estimates are that nurses spend up to 38% of all patient care availability time in the performance of nonnursing activities, and there are costs associated with this problem: overtime and downtime costs, increased lengths of stay, erosion of the nursing delivery system, inadequate teaching and discharge planning, poor retention of nursing staff, excessive sick days and chronic absenteeism, and

inordinate reliance on agency personnel at the risk of continuity of care (25).

Physicians need to consider how their orders have an impact on nursing needs and how these same orders place demands on available nursing personnel time. Tedious standing orders may no longer be appropriate in a high-acuity, fast-paced health care environment. All current orders need to be reviewed and eliminated if no longer pertinent. It has been shown that when physicians work collaboratively with nurses, care is improved and more is accomplished with no increase in staff (26).

Despite honest attempts to change, nursing documentation continues to be duplicative, narrative, and time consuming. The Division of Nursing of the American Hospital Association (12) reports that "nurses spend up to 40% of their time writing nursing records which describe their patients, document therapy provided to them, and report the outcome of these interventions." Time spent documenting must be dramatically reduced by an increased use of preestablished care guidelines, flowsheets, exception charting, and/or automation of the patient record. Patient and family teaching may no longer be completely accomplished in the inpatient setting. Perhaps other health care professionals must be accountable for components at which they are experts, e.g., dieticians and pharmacists providing nutritional counseling and instruction in medication administration, respectively. All of these tasks can be barriers to optimal utilization of the professional RN staff and must be identified and reduced.

Alternative scheduling options can be explored with staffing goals considered and barriers to staffing reduced. Certainly the RN role must be assessed in light of the RN shortage. However, the role does not need to be compromised, only more clearly defined. When a professional nursing environment is provided, recruitment will continue and professional care will be maintained.

### Various Scheduling Patterns

There are many defined scheduling patterns: 8-hour, 10-hour, 12-hour, 7/70, and 24/40. Some individuals have opted to work every weekend as it works out well with family and/or educational responsibilities. Any pattern can be used as long as it meets the goals of scheduling, is consistent with the nursing philosophy, and recruits professional nurses. Offering a range of working schedules offers the professional nurse a number of opportunities for economic control and social adjustment. The stresses of caring for the ill demand a work-recreation schedule that will assure the nurses are able to maintain the energy and alertness they need to function over the long term. Family responsibility is the most frequent reason for leaving nursing or for not currently being employed in the profession (25). One needs to consider any scheduling option that will meet the demands of the workload and attract and retain RNs.

An important aspect of a successful scheduling plan is the ability to recruit and retain competent nursing staff. One approach is to investigate the local market place and assess the need to implement competitive differentials for shifts or units that are difficult to staff. In other words, if competitor hospitals are paying an ICU differential, you may have to consider it for your hospital, despite perhaps a philosophical belief that this is not "fair." The payroll budget may have to be divided between a broadened salary scale and shift and/or weekend bonuses. The money must be spent (and there is always a limit to that sum of money) where it is most crucially needed. Some employees are looking for a scheduling option that will provide them with more days off (10-hour, 12-hour). Others see a tremendous benefit to a paid critical care nursing course, tuition reimbursement, or continuing education funds. Survey the strengths and weaknesses of the specific geographical location and market place and among your own staff (27). Retention methods will lead to recruitment.

When considering various scheduling options, the effect of any one choice on patient care should remain the primary concern. There will be advantages and disadvantages to any option implemented. Quality of care and continuity, however, must be maintained. Budget limitations, the management of overtime and shift differentials, and the Federal Fair Labor Standards Act must also be considered. Hospitals generally pay on one of two bases: overtime after 40 hours per week or overtime after 8 hours per day or 80 hours in 14 days. It should be remembered, however, that RNs are professionals and can be exempt from these rules if salaried and guaranteed minimum salary for every week worked. This is an important consideration when planning various scheduling options.

## Cyclical Scheduling

One general method of scheduling regardless of length of shift selected is cyclical scheduling. Cyclical scheduling is a technique for assigning work days and time off in a pattern that repeats itself cyclically while paying heed to the need for proper numbers and mixes of personnel, continuity of patient care, and work groups. Advantages of cyclical scheduling include a reduced amount of highly skilled professional time spent on scheduling functions (i.e., less nurse manager time spent); schedules are known by staff in advance resulting in decreased requests for days off; continuity of care is provided by minimizing floating; equitable and consistent staffing is provided ("good" and "bad" days off spread equitably); and work groups develop team synergy by stabilizing scheduled days off. "The schedule also lends itself to staff input—and they should be encouraged to develop their own preferred cycles within a predetermined unit staffing pattern" (28). Disadvantages to cyclical scheduling are that it can be inflexible and impersonal, and often no requests are allowed except for vacations. Depending on the specifics of the situation, cyclical scheduling can be a positive method, providing predictability of schedule for staff, some personal requests granted, and minimal time invested in the scheduling function for the nurse manager. Certainly, if a cyclical schedule can be developed, accepted, and then also automated, an even greater time savings can be achieved.

## Benefits of Flexible Scheduling

There are tremendous benefits to be realized with flexible, variable scheduling. When planned carefully, flexible scheduling meets the criteria of effective scheduling. The workload is managed, it is cost effective, and it provides options for staff to best serve personal needs while maintaining quality and continuity of care. In addition, a decrease in absenteeism, sick time, and overtime is usually experienced. Improved job satisfaction and recruitment with resultant improved morale is realized.

## EVALUATING STAFFING PROGRAM

Evaluating the staffing system is the final step in any staffing program. Methods for evaluating and determining quality of care relative to acceptable standards must be established. Generally, the approaches taken to measure quality of care fall into three categories: structure, process, and outcome. Structure standards incorporate such things as physical facilities and appropriate staffing levels. AACN Standard VII states that the critical care unit shall have appropriately qualified staff to provide care on a 24-hour basis. Process standards emphasize the actual performance of care and will determine how many and what type of staff will be needed to provide care. Outcome standards measure whether goals for patient care have been achieved. The actualization of these goals could, in part, rely on decisions made about staffing.

In summary Aydelotte (29) describes four elements of a staffing program as follows: (*a*) identification of the quality of the product (care to be rendered to the client); (*b*) the application of a specific method to determine number and kinds of staff required to provide the care; (*c*) selection and arrangement of the nursing staff in specific configurations and the development of assignment patterns for the staff required 24 hours per day, seven days per week; and (*d*) an evaluation of the product provided and a judgment reflecting the impact of the staff upon quality of care. The established goals for scheduling, which reflect the overall philosophy of the organization, will direct the decisions made relating to ongoing staffing. The internal and external environment is carefully assessed. The required number of employees will be utilized to provide the nursing care defined by set standards of care. Next, various scheduling options are implemented to meet the needs. The success of the scheduling and staffing program is evaluated through review of the patient outcomes realized (quality assurance) and the productivity levels maintained (required versus actually staffing).

Providing adequate staff to give the nursing care required is a challenge for every nurse manager. When approached realistically and in an organized fashion, it is not an overwhelming task. It can be rewarding for the manager. It can result in a positive work environment and be a job satisfier for the staff nurse.

REFERENCES

1. Joint Commission on Accreditation of Hospitals. AMA/88 accreditation manual for hospitals. 1987:141–150.
2. American Association of Critical-Care Nurses. Standards for nursing care of the critically ill. Reston, Virginia: Reston Publishing Company, Inc., 1981.
3. American Association of Critical-Care Nurses. Position statement: use of technical personnel in critical care settings. November 1983.
4. American Association of Critical-Care Nurses. Position statement: role expectations for the critical care manager. June 1986.
5. American Nurses' Association. Roles, responsibilities, and qualifications for nurse administrators. Kansas City, Kansas: American Nurses' Association, 1978.
6. Cushing M. Staffing: sometimes a no-win situation. Am J Nurs 1986;86(2):131–132.
7. Boston CM, Karzel S. Will the nursing shortage lead to liability suits? Hospitals 1987;6122):64–68.
8. Phillips GD, Chong C, Gordon PJ. Nurse staffing in intensive care units. Anesthesia Intensive Care 1983;11(2):118–124.
9. Billings DM. Patient classification in critical care. Dimensions Crit Care Nurs 1983;2(1):36–43.
10. Gallagher JR. Developing a powerful and acceptable nurse staffing system. Nurs Management 1987;18(3):45–49.
11. Kirby KK, Wiczai LJ. Implementing and monitoring variable staffing. Nurs Economics 1985;3:216–222.
12. Sovie MD. Managing nursing resources in a constrained economic environment. Nurs Economics 1985;3:85–94.
13. Tonges MC. Quality with economy: doing the right thing for less. Nurs Economics 1985;3:205–211.
14. Blenkarn H, D'Amico M, Virtue E. Primary nursing and job satisfaction. Nurs Management 1988;19(4):41–42.
15. Manthey M. Myths that threaten. Nurs Management 1988;19(6):54–55.
16. Althaus JN, Hardyck NM, Pierce PB, et al. Nurse staffing in a decentralized organization: part 1. J Nurs Admin March, 1982, p 34–39.
17. Christman L. The autonomous nursing staff in the hospital. Nurs Admin Q 1987;11(3):37–44.
18. Miller ML. Implementing self-scheduling. J Nurs Admin March, 1984, p 33–36.
19. Cooperrider F. Staff input in scheduling boosts morale. Hospitals, August 1, 1980, p 59–61.
20. Kehrer BH, Deiman PA, Szapiro N. The temporary nursing service RN. Nurs Outlook 1984;32(4):212–217.
21. Prescott PA. Use of nurses from supplemental services: implications for hospitals. Nurs Admin Q 1986;11(1):81–88.
22. Laird DD. Supplemental nursing agencies—a tool for combatting the nursing shortage. HCM Rev 1983;8(3):61–67.
23. Davis SH. The use of registry nurses in critical care: a cost-benefit analysis. Dimensions Crit Care Nurs 1982;1(2):88–96.
24. Shaheen PP. Staffing and scheduling: reconcile practical means with the real goal. Nurs Management 1985;16(10):64–72.
25. Caterinicchio RP. Implementing a DRG-driven acuity system. Hospital Topics 1985; May–June:6–13.
26. Knaus W, Draper E, Wagner D, et al. An evaluation of outcome from intensive care in major medical centers. Ann Intern Med 1986;104(3):410–418.
27. Smith DR. Nursing shortage—some practical response please! Nurs Management 1983;14(11):38–39.
28. Marcchionno PM. Modified cyclical scheduling: a practical approach. Nurs Management 1987;18(10):60–62, 64, 66.
29. Aydelotte MK. Staffing for quality care. J Nur Admin 1973;3(2):33.

# Chapter 7

# Promoting the Professional Development of Critical Care Nurses

CHRIS BREU

Critical care nurses are committed, creative, and deliberate in their clinical practice. This group and nurses in general, often fail to utilize those same characteristics when planning for their professional growth and development. For example, many nurses feel that professional growth generally is a result of experience or educational opportunities (academic or continuing education). In reality there are several avenues for professional development. In addition, professional growth is often not a deliberate planned process but is approached in a more haphazard fashion. Many nurses have not been given specific information on how to plan their own professional development. This topic is not often seen in the literature and is frequently not discussed in academic programs. In fact, the recently published "Summary Analysis of Critical Care Nurse Supply and Requirements" stated that career development programs for critical care nurses seem to be nonexistent (1). Thus many critical care nurses have not been given the tools to plan and develop their professional growth.

The primary responsibility of professional development lies with each critical care nurse. This responsibility includes each nurse continually assessing her individual needs and seeking the resources that will help to meet those needs. Dr. Margretta Styles has said that "our efforts, yours and mine, to attain our professionhood as nurses and thus contribute to the professionalism of nursing, as well as to our own self-actualization, must be our major concern (2)." However, because many nurses have not been provided with information on how to best plan for their development (professional self-actualization), the nurse manager has an essential role in facilitating the professional development of the nursing staff. This role has multiple responsibilities that include mobilizing resources, assisting with assessments, and providing guidance and opportunities that will help the staff reach their professional goals. In order to be successful in meeting these objectives, each nurse manager needs to have a thorough understanding of the professional development continuum and the multistepped process needed to enhance and achieve professional development.

This chapter will describe each of these and will also identify specific actions nurse managers can take to enhance professional growth in critical care nurses.

The chapter uses a modified problem solving model. The content is based on theories described in other chapters within this text, specifically Chapters 4, 12, 14, and 15. These related theories are not repeated here but the process discussed is an application of these theories.

## ADVANTAGES OF PLANNED PROFESSIONAL GROWTH

Because it takes a great deal of energy to promote individual growth in staff members, it is helpful to assess the potential advantages of these efforts by nurse managers. There are several positive outcomes that nurse managers should be able to observe if staff are consistently involved with their own professional growth and development. First, there should be an observable increase in the skills and abilities of individual staff members. This increase in skills and abilities should have a positive effect on patient outcomes, consistent implementation of unit standards, and overall quality of patient care. These observations can be informally observed by the nurse manager as well as formally documented through the processes of performance appraisals and quality assurance.

A second, positive outcome from consistent

professional growth of staff is an increase in job satisfaction. Theories that describe what contributes to job satisfaction and employee motivation are complex and varied, (see Chapter 12). However, many theorists have identified professional growth as a key factor. For example, Herzberg's research indicates that personnel are motivated by opportunities for achievement, recognition, responsibility, and growth (3). Argyris has suggested that managers can motivate employees by working toward a match between personnel and jobs. This can be accomplished by making jobs interesting and helping employees meet their needs for self-actualization (4). Alderfer's theory on motivation includes a component on growth needs, stating that each individual has an intrinsic desire for personal development (3). Each of these theorists, as well as others, suggest positive relationships between professional development of staff, job satisfaction, and employee motivation.

These theories seem applicable to the critical care nurse. As they see the positive results of increased knowledge and skills, professional self-esteem should be enhanced. As they witness the beneficial effects they have on patient care, they should realize the control they can have on patient outcomes within their unit.

Other positive outcomes of professional growth can include an increase in unit pride and esprit de corps. Individual staff contributions often complement and enhance the contributions and knowledge of critical care colleagues. The competetiveness that sometimes exists in critical care units can be decreased as staff members realize that they are each in the active process of learning and that they each reap benefits from the enhanced skills of colleagues. The unit environment can become motivating, stimulating, and challenging not only for each individual but for the collective team of critical care nurses who work in the unit.

## CONTINUUM OF PROFESSIONAL DEVELOPMENT

In order to promote some of the positive outcomes of professional development of critical care staff, it is important for each nurse manager to understand the process of professional development.

Every nurse is functioning on a continuum of professional development that begins as a student and progresses as career experiences accumulate. This continuum has probably been best described by Dr. Patricia Benner who has done significant research in this area. She has described the levels of proficiency that each nurse passes through as she progresses throughout her career. This research was based on the Dreyfus model that includes five levels of proficiency: novice, advanced beginner, competent, proficient, and expert. Benner applied these categories to nursing and described how each level pertains to our profession (5). Each level is described below.

### Novice

Novice is the first stage on the proficiency continuum. At this level, the nurse does not have previous experience within the clinical situation. Principles and theory are understood but the context is missing (5). This stage continues throughout the first year in a new clinical setting (5). The nurse who is new to critical care is at the novice level. This nurse is frequently overwhelmed with the myriad responsibilities in caring for the critically ill, has difficulty setting priorities, and is very task oriented. There is often an understanding of the many things that need to be done but there is little integration of the total picture of patient needs. For example, in caring for the respiratory patient who is fighting the ventilator, this nurse would most likely recognize the need to suction the patient, take vital signs, and draw arterial blood gases but is probably unable to integrate the information to alleviate the problem.

### Advanced Beginner

The second stage is reflective of enough experience for the nurse to be able to put some context and meaning to the clinical situations. The nurse at this level still needs some support and help with setting priorities and continues to be task focused. This stage usually continues from 12 through 24 months (5).

In caring for a recent myocardial infarction patient, for example, this nurse should be able to monitor cardiovascular parameters and give meaning to abnormal physiological data. However, this nurse would probably have difficulty in assessing the many variables that indicate when the patient is ready to learn about his or her disease process.

### Competent

At this stage the nurse can see beyond the task to the longer range plan for the patient. He or she does use abstract, conscious contemplation of problems. Support by more experienced staff is still needed and he or she remains very task oriented, yet organized and efficient. This level usually lasts for 2 to 3 years (5).

For example, this nurse can be assigned a patient who had a recent abdominal aortic aneurysm repair and a patient who is actively bleeding gastrointestinally. One requires frequent vascular and post operative assessments and one requires frequent treatments and interventions. The nurse at this level of experience should be able to identify priorities in both patients and arrange care to meet the needs of both. This nurse should also be able to make adjustments in these priorities as the need arises.

## Proficient

At the fourth stage, the nurse is now able to perceive situations as a whole rather than as separate parts. In problem solving, the nurse considers fewer options than the nurse at the competent level and is able to identify the problem more efficiently. This nurse has had enough experience to be able to automatically analyze what is happening in the clinical situation. His or her experience base is from 3 to 5 years (5).

For example, the nurse at this level who is caring for a patient in congestive heart failure should be able to recognize the subtle changes in facial color, patient anxiety, and skin temperature that could indicate the early stages of cardiogenic shock. It is not the significance of any single sign but the integration of the total picture of the patient that alerts her to this possibility.

## Expert

This is the highest level of continuum. This nurse has extensive background and is no longer guided by rules and principles. He or she has had ample experience that enables him or her to be fluid and flexible in various clinical situations. This nurse does little *conscious* problem solving and is able to handle complex problems efficiently (5).

For example, the nurse at this level should be able to take both her personal experiences and those of colleagues in caring for patients who are respirator dependent and make conclusions about the quality of care this population receives in this critical care unit. This nurse should be able to identify the inconsistencies in care and the areas where the unit standard is not being met with these patients. The conclusions made are usually based on a thorough physiologic, psychosocial, and total team perspective.

If a staff member changes roles or clinical positions so that the patient population changes, he or she would naturally move down the continuum until experience with the new population has been gained. Or a given nurse may be at the proficient level in caring for most patients but if a new complex therapy is introduced to that nurse, he or she may move back a step on the continuum in caring for patients with an unfamiliar complex therapy or diagnosis.

An example is the nurse who has worked for 4 years in a coronary care unit. This nurse would probably be at the proficient level in caring for patients in this unit. However, when tissue plasminogen activator therapy is introduced to the unit, this nurse would probably only be at the competent level in caring for these patients until enough experience was acquired to understand the ramifications and potential patient responses to this therapy.

There are three major threads that are developed along this continuum as the nurse progresses through each stage (see Table 7.1). The first is how the nurse approaches a patient. In earlier stages, the patient is viewed as a set of tasks to be accomplished versus in later stages, the clinical situation and the patient are viewed as a whole with all aspects integrated into a smooth flowing plan of care. The second thread is the cognitive approach used by the nurse. Initially clinical problem solving is done by using rules and principles. As experience increases, this changes to more analytical reasoning that is often automatic and requires less deliberate conscious thinking. Therefore conscious contemplation becomes less and less. The last thread is how a nurse approaches and manages a clinical situation. The newer nurse functions quite rigidly with little flexibility whereas the experienced nurse is able to perform in a more fluid, flexible, and organized manner.

Viewing the nursing unit as a whole and being able to contribute to unit level decisions and directions also seem to increase as the nurse progresses along the continuum. For example, the novice and the advanced beginner focus most of their attention on gaining various experiences and increasing their problem solving ability. The more advanced nurse is able to step back, look at, and evaluate care that is provided to a given population of patients. Advanced, more experienced nurses who are further along the continuum should have enough experience to be able to develop standards

**Table 7.1** Professional Growth Continuum

| Approach | Novice | Advanced Beginner | Competent | Proficient | Expert |
|---|---|---|---|---|---|
| Patient | Focuses on individual tasks to be accomplished | | | →| Views the patient situation as a whole |
| Cognitive | Uses rules and principles, deliberate, conscious thinking | | | →| Uses analytical reasoning, automatic thinking |
| Clinical | Functions quite rigidly, lacks organization and speed | | | →| Has a fluid, flexible manner, is quite organized and efficent |

of care for groups of patients, test nursing diagnoses and appropriate interventions, utilize research findings to improve the care they deliver, and demonstrate increased leadership skills and abilities.

## STEPS FOR SYSTEMATIC PLANNED PROFESSIONAL DEVELOPMENT

It is clear that movement along this continuum occurs through two ways, experience in a given area with a certain population of patients and planned professional development. It is the ''planned'' aspect of professional development that often needs facilitating among staff members. In order to promote planned growth in individual staff members, it is necessary that nurse managers are familiar with the various steps that are needed to achieve optimal and consistent professional growth. Each of these is described in Figure 7.1.

### Step 1: Assessing Professional Needs

The nurse manager needs to be concerned with the holistic development of each staff member. This includes developmental components that address: the needs of the specific patient population (including pathophysiological bases, medical therapies, and nursing interventions); the psychosocial needs of both patients and families; the interpersonal skills needed to function effectively as a member of a team (unit and interdisciplinary teams); leadership skills; and advanced nursing skills (research utilization, standards development and testing, nursing diagnosis development and critique, implementing quality assurance projects).

The needs of staff nurses will obviously vary depending on where they are on their own proficiency continuum. Deciding where on the proficiency continuum a staff member is will help to target the priorities for growth for that individual.

This process is facilitated by asking specific questions related to various components of the continuum. These include:

- How much experience has this staff member had in this particular clinical setting, with this level of acuity, with this type of patients?
- What other clinical opportunities has this member had that have provided applicable experiences?
- What is the cognitive approach used by this staff member to solve clinical problems—an approach guided only by rules and principles, or one that is more rapid and analytical?
- How flexible is this staff nurse in clinical situations? Is there demonstrated rigidity in problem solving or is the clinical performance more fluid and flexible?

Answering these questions in view of specific characteristics of the various stages will enable the nurse manager to place each staff member appropriately on the continuum.

The nurse managers can then use a variety of tools to continue the assessment of their staff member. These include orientation checklists (if a new employee), criteria-based performance appraisals (see Chapter 14), learning needs surveys, and expectations derived from unit-based standards of care, policies, and procedures. Another helpful document is the American Association of Critical-Care Nurses (AACN) Certification Corporations statements on knowledge, skills, and abilities of an experienced critical care nurse (6).

Once this assessment is completed, the nurse manager can use this information to facilitate a self-assessment by each staff member. These data can be shared with the staff member when appropriate, but it is essential that the staff members com-

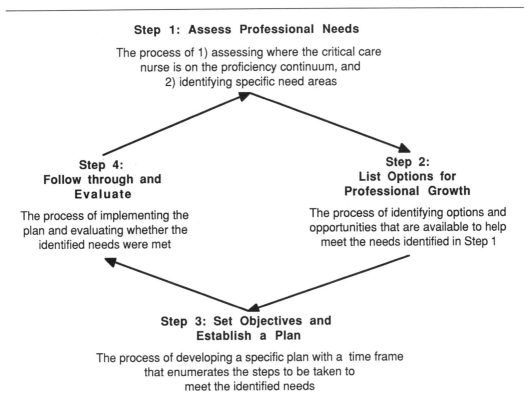

**Figure 7.1.**  Steps for planned professional development.

plete their own assessment. Specific self-assessment questions that would help this process include:

- What special skills and abilities could I acquire that would help me to grow in my current role? Examples include: the ability to manage vasopressor drugs in order to accomplish established therapeutic goals, or the skill to calm an anxious family.
- Of these identified needs what are the most important and have the greatest impact on care?
- What specific *knowledge* could I acquire that would help me to grow in my current role? Examples include: an understanding of the physiology of cardiogenic shock, or an understanding of the psychological responses to illness.
- What professional role do I want 3 years from now? Is it different from my current role? If yes, what skills, abilities, and knowledge do I need to acquire to prepare for this role? For example: to reach the next step on the clinical ladder the skill of teaching new orientees is re-

quired as is the knowledge of the quality assurance process.

This joint assessment by the nurse manager and the staff member should yield specific areas to target for professional growth based on the expectations placed on all staff in the unit, the future goals of the individual staff member, and the current proficiency stage.

**Step 2: Listing Options Available That Match Identified Needs**

The second step in planning for professional growth is to identify options and resources available that can help meet these needs. These include opportunities within the critical care unit, research conduct and/or research utilization activities, in-service and continuing education opportunities, the certification process, lecturing, publishing, and association involvement. Each of these is described below with an emphasis on the nurse manager's role in mobilizing these resources and options.

In this second step the staff member is able to identify the means to have his or her needs met. The nurse manager often has access to and knowledge of many of the available avenues and takes an active role in matching these opportunities with the identified needs of the staff member.

### Step 3: Setting Objectives and Establishing a Plan

This step is often missed. Many of the staff are able to clearly articulate their needs, but they do not carry the process to the next step and develop a formal plan on how to meet those needs. Specificity is key here. The objectives and plan need to be specific and clear with reasonable time frames established. An example follows:

A staff member may state an intention to increase understanding of the psychosocial care of cardiomyopathy patients by preparing an inservice on the topic for colleagues. The individual will review the literature within the next month, develop an outline within 6 weeks, have the outline critiqued by the clinical nurse specialist within 8 weeks, and finalize and present the inservice within 3 months.

The nurse manager plays an essential role at this point, because many staff need guidance in developing clear, reasonable objectives with appropriate time frames. An ideal time to assist with this process is at the annual performance appraisal session.

### Step 4: Following through and Evaluating

As mentioned, it is up to the staff nurse to establish his or her own personal objectives and follow through on the plan. However, the nurse manager is often a source of encouragement and needed resources. Because relatively short-term objectives are more ideal, it is desirable for the nurse manager to assist in evaluating the process more often than on an annual basis. Many nurse managers have found formal semiannual meetings ideal to promote progress toward goals and help with reassessment and identification of new goals as needed.

Considering the usual workload and responsibilities of the nurse manager, this may not seem feasible to some nurse managers. To relieve this time concern, the nurse manager could meet with 3 or 4 staff members at a time. This method would promote peer support in reaching goals and a cross-sharing of developed resources and expertise. An

other option is to delegate follow-up on individual objectives to assistant head nurses or charge nurses. This method would keep the charge nurse aware of the professional goals of the staff he or she most frequently supervises and provide an opportunity to match resources and patient assignments to identified needs. This activity would also foster the development of both leadership and motivational skills in charge nurses. The nurse manager could continue to be a resource for problem solving and identifying resources. The annual appraisal of goal attainment could continue to be done by the nurse manager with input from the charge nurses, or by peer review (see Chapter 14).

Questions the staff member should address at both semiannual meeting times include:

- To what degree did I accomplish each objective?
- Was the process rewarding and satisfying?
- Were there unforeseen barriers that got in the way of accomplishing the goal to the degree desired?
- What frustrations did I experience?
- What would I do differently next time if I chose the same avenue to meet my goal?
- What resources did I develop?
- Were there other professional needs that were unexpectedly met?

Once the objective is met and the evaluation completed, the staff member assesses whether it is appropriate to establish more objectives. If other objectives are being pursued, the answer may be no. If, however, most of the objectives have been accomplished, it may be appropriate to return to step one, do a reassessment, and begin the process over.

It is obvious that this process parallels a simple problem solving model. It is a familiar and easy process to complete. Most staff members, however, are not used to applying this process to their own professional growth and development. In order to assure progress along the proficiency continuum, planned deliberate efforts need to be made. Nurse managers can greatly facilitate staff development by utilizing this process with all staff members and holding them accountable for the objectives they establish.

### PROFESSIONAL GROWTH OPPORTUNITIES

An ongoing challenge for all nurse managers is to match identified needs of the staff with opportunities for professional growth and development.

The major avenues for development of the staff are discussed below.

## Involvement in Unit and Hospital Activities

There are a number of professional development needs that can be met through involvement in unit activities. For example, the need to increase knowledge and understanding of the care of patients with disseminated intravascular coagulaton (DIC) could be accomplished by working with another colleague to develop or update a standard of care for this diagnostic group; the need to develop certain leadership skills could be met by coordinating a unit project; the need to understand how quality can be addressed by unit nurses could be met by having responsibility for aspects of the unit quality assurance program.

Another opportunity within this category is involvement on interdepartmental committees. Many developmental needs can be met by interacting with other departments and disciplines. Examples include: serving on the ethics committee to increase the perspective and the problem solving repertoire of a staff member; serving on other committees and task forces to develop interpersonal skills as well as group communication skills. There is also a secondary gain from increased staff involvement outside the unit. Considering the current dynamic state of the health care industry, it is important that each staff member have an understanding of the pressures affecting their hospital. This is also a crucial time for nurses to have input into decisions that are being made daily that have an impact on the critical care unit. Both of these goals can be accomplished as well as the staff member meeting his or her own identified needs by an increased involvement in hospital-wide activities. All of these examples are reflective of a decentralized management style. In order to provide most of these opportunities for staff members, the nurse manager needs to be comfortable with delegating responsibilities and have a philosophy of promoting unit level decision making.

## Research Conduct or Research Utilization

The second opportunity encompasses all of these activities that are either research conduct or research utilization (RU). The most frequently used method by staff nurses is RU. Nurse managers can support this opportunity for professional development either through individual staff member efforts or unit-wide projects. On an individual basis,

if a staff member has difficulty in a certain area of patient care, he or she can review the literature (including unit level information) and base his or her practice on these new findings. A more advanced clinician can incorporate innovations into practice and also be involved in introducing these concepts to the rest of the staff.

Unit level research utilization projects are excellent ways to promote change within the unit as a whole. Significant change can occur smoothly with full staff support if the process of research utilization is used incorporating a planned change model (7, 8). For example, this process can be used to decrease resistance to having more flexible visiting hours, improving the care of long-term immobilized patients, or changing endotracheal suctioning techniques.

The whole process of research utilization is facilitated if there are pertinent journals and current textbooks available on the unit. Consideration of these ongoing references should be included in the development of the unit budget. In addition, a well-stocked hospital-based library is an essential resource. A computerized literature search system (Medline, Nurse Search, etc.) greatly facilitates the process of research utilization. If there is no access within the facility to a library with pertinent resources, the nurse manager may want to plan a trip each month to the nearest medical library. The staff could generate clinical questions each month, and the nurse manager and a staff member or two could seek pertinent articles related to these topics. This gathering of resources would facilitate research utilization, currency in staff knowledge, and updated standards of care.

Another mechanism that encourages the staff to utilize research findings in their practice is a unit-based journal club. The purpose of the club could be to review and critique applicable clinical articles and review research studies for ways to change or improve practice. The responsibility for coordinating the meetings and the topics can be rotated so that individual as well as group goals can be met. Implementing mechanisms to provide a continuous process of research utilization within the unit will assure ongoing opportunities for professional development of individual staff as well as the critical care unit as a whole.

## Educational Opportunities

Probably the most frequently used avenue to meet professional developmental needs is through formal educational methods, either in-services, continuing education, or academic education. It is a constant challenge for the nurse manager to assess total learning needs within her unit and then try to match those needs with educational opportunities, especially opportunities that will have a direct impact on the quality of care provided in the unit. Using the information gained from staff performance appraisal sessions is an excellent way to identify those needs. However, resources are limited, including the resource of time, and the nurse manager needs to assure that the in-service opportunities that are available to the staff are indeed meeting the priority needs of her staff. Some key questions to ask include:

- Do I utilize results from my unit-based quality assurance (QA) program to develop educational opportunities for my staff? Is this accomplished through a formal feedback system where the link between the QA plan and resulting in-services is clearly identified?
- Is the learning needs survey that I use specific to the unit and the patient population in that unit? Does it reflect the full scope of care and have a balance between medical and nursing models? Is the tool I use sensitive enough to detect the difference between the learning needs related to quality concerns and the interest needs of the staff?
- Do the in-services address the high risk, high volume aspects of the unit?
- Do I have a mechanism for incorporating results from occurrence reports into the unit level in-service plan?
- Do I target certain staff for particular in-service opportunities so that individual needs are assured of being met?
- Do I influence the overall hospital continuing education program to assist in matching the needs within my unit?

Answering these questions will help to assure that the energy and resources that go into the unit in-service program are effective in influencing staff expertise and quality of care.

Many nurse managers find it beneficial to have a departmental-wide in-service program so that the needs of all critical care nurses are being met through a coordinated program. This saves resources but does not eliminate the need to have some in-services specific to individual units. These in-services usually flow from the unit-specific QA program. For example, the intensive care unit staff may be having difficulty doing postoperative vascular assessments that are specific to the surgical procedure that was done. Or the cardiac observation unit staff may not be sure about the priority learning needs for patients after pacemaker implantation.

In addition to in-service education many critical care nurses have returned to school. Because 60% of critical care nurses are prepared at the associate degree or diploma level (1), the most frequent academic educational goal for critical care staff nurses is attainment of a baccalaureate degree in nursing (BSN). The nurse manager can encourage this goal among her staff by providing flexible staffing that accommodates school schedules, and by encouraging a tuition reimbursement program at the hospital level. A formal program should also be in place in the unit that provides encouragement and recognition to staff who are in the process of a BSN completion program. A hospital-wide program that provides recognition for completion is also needed as well as a recognition component incorporated into a clinical ladder if one is being used at the facility.

## Certification

Attainment of CCRN certification has multiple benefits including: professional recognition by peers and patients, personal pride, potential career ladder advancement, and at time monetary compensation (9). In addition, it was one of the identified characteristics that contributed to superior outcomes (e.g., job satisfaction) in the AACN Demonstration Project (10). Finally, the process of CCRN certification is an excellent way to enhance and encourage professional growth. Not only does the process of initial certification promote growth but the process of recertification encompasses a broad array of professional development avenues. These include written care plans, policy and procedure development, committee or local AACN chapter involvement, and publications (9). The CCRN may need assistance with assessing priority development needs, but the recertification process itself will facilitate goal attainment.

Nurse managers should take an active role in influencing the number of certified nurses within their unit. Often staff are hesitant to initially certify without the support of a review course. Collaborative efforts by nurse managers usually have a positive impact on whether there is a review course available to their staff.

Other techniques that promote certification include unit level and hospital-wide recognition of certified nurses, and the incorporation of certification requirements into promotion criteria and career ladders. There is an ongoing controversy as to whether monetary compensation is an appropriate reward for certification attainment (11). However, a number of hospitals do provide some type of monetary reward for successful attainment of CCRN certification.

Considering the significant role certification can have in the professional development of critical care nurses, nurse managers should invest effort into promoting this avenue of professional growth.

## Lecturing and Publishing

Both of these activities can be done on the unit, hospital, community, regional, or national levels. These processes are similar with the result being a sharing of expertise with peers and colleagues. Topics or content areas that are pertinent for a lecture or an article are identified in the assessment process described above.

Often staff need a great deal of support if this is a new professional experience for them. Giving minipresentations to the staff can be a first step for lecturing, progressing to lecturing to staff from other units, and then lecturing in the critical care course or in hospital educational programs. The staff member who is a novice at lecturing will need help with setting expectations and objectives. Pairing this staff member with an experienced member often provides the security and information needed for the first presentation.

Publishing can also begin at the unit level, e.g., writing a small drug informational piece for the staff. Other opportunities include writing for the hospital or local AACN newsletters. Journal publishing is also a realistic goal for many critical care nurse experts, and nurse managers should encourage this activity and provide the needed resources and guidance.

The process involved in both lecturing and publishing is rigorous and usually stimulates tremendous professional growth in a given subject area. Nurse managers do have an influence on how often staff members use these opportunities for professional growth.

## Association Involvement

Involvement in AACN provides many opportunities for professional growth of staff members.

Local chapters provide frequent educational opportunities for their members. Many chapters also provide review programs for attaining CCRN certification. In addition, activities within the chapter system provide collegial and peer support. This network of interfacility communication can significantly broaden the intervention base and problem solving repertoire of staff members.

Other resources are available through the chapter committee structure. Most chapters develop committees and task forces based on community needs and member requests. Many have committees that provide resources on standards, research conduct or utilization, ethical dilemmas, and other common concerns of critical care nurses. Active participation in committee work or in elected positions provides numerous opportunities for professional growth for staff members. Often skills are developed and enhanced in the areas of team communication, group and interpersonal relationships, and program development. All of these skills are transferable to situations within the critical care unit.

Nurse managers can use a variety of techniques that encourage involvement in local AACN chapter activities. Membership brochures, CCRN applications, and information on local and national AACN educational events should be posted throughout the unit. Continuing education events sponsored by the chapter can be incorporated formally into unit events so that attendance is encouraged. The hospital could also host chapter activities.

Individual staff can negotiate some of their personal objectives to include chapter efforts. Active involvement of several staff members in chapter committees will assure that unit priorities are being addressed by the chapter. In addition, each nurse manager should have an active role in the local AACN chapter to further facilitate matching chapter resources with unit needs.

There are also many opportunities available on the national AACN level in both elected and volunteer positions. AACN is continuously seeking the input and involvement of critical care nurses. If any staff members have had experiences that would provide resources at a national level, their involvement should be encouraged. Not only would they be making a worthwhile contribution, but the time donated translates into significant professional growth experiences.

There are several other appropriate organizations that critical care nurses are involved in that provide opportunities for professional growth. These organizations include the: American Nurses' Association, American Heart Association, American Association of Neurosurgical Nurses, Sigma Theta Tau, and others (12). Many of the benefits of involvement with these organizations are similar to those described above.

## CLINICAL LADDERS

For the last couple of decades, it has been important to develop mechanisms that encourage and recognize career development for staff who provide direct patient care. Clinical ladders were introduced into many hospitals in the 1970s and 1980s to provide incentives in the workplace for achieving higher levels of competence from nurses involved in direct patient care (13). The American Academy of Nursing study on magnet hospitals found that staff nurses in "magnet" hospitals "consider a career ladder an essential component of professional development (14)." Within these hospitals, the concept of career ladders is "fast becoming the norm and already an expectation of professional nurses (14). There have also been reports of positive effects of clinical ladders on recruitment and retention (13).

Clinical ladders vary tremendously throughout the nation. Some are two-step ladders, others are multiple-step ladders. Some encompass administrative options, others have only clinical options defined. Some incorporate unit level peer review for promotion, others have facility-wide peer review. Some require validation that expectations continue to be met every few months, others annually, some not at all. It appears that one aspect they all have in common is that it takes a great deal of time, energy, thought, and devotion to the change process to develop and implement a clinical ladder.

If a clinical ladder is not currently available, the nurse manager's role is to work with peers, nursing staff, and the organization to see if this is a beneficial method to use for promoting professional growth within the existing system. If so, it is essential that both nurse managers and staff members become involved in every developmental phase.

Once the ladder is implemented, it is the responsibility of the nurse manager to readily utilize the ladder as a method to promote growth, encourage retention, and keep staff members challenged and stimulated within the critical care unit.

## PITFALLS OF PLANNED PROFESSIONAL GROWTH

There are some precautions to be aware of as nurse managers encourage professional development among their staff. One caution is that most planned professional growth activities occur during the staff members' personal off-duty time. In this environment, with a focus on productivity and costs, it is a rare facility that will be able to support staff professional development sufficiently to meet each staff member's needs. In order for these developmental activities to be consistent and pertinent to individual needs, the staff member must recognize and accept planned professional growth as a *self*-responsibility. This reality makes it necessary for the nurse manager to promote the philosphy of self-responsibility for professional development. Promoting staff responsibility often means utilizing various motivational techniques to encourage staff members to accept this responsibility (see Chapter 12).

In addition, the nurse manager has a responsibility to provide as much hospital support for professional growth as possible. This support can include paid time off for staff to attend educational programs, "released" time during work for staff to develop professional projects, and budgetary allowances for resources. Attaining this kind of support for the staff usually requires the nurse manager to be very skilled at negotiating and very persistent in communicating staff needs to fiscal planners (refer to Chapter 13).

Another caution related to professional growth is that not all of these experiences will be successful. Some will fail due to poor planning, unforeseen events, or other variables. The nurse manager can assist with the evaluative process that identifies the positive aspects about the experience along with what, if anything, could have been done differently to avoid the negative aspects. Encouragement to continue the process may also be necessary at this point.

Professional growth experiences also compete with other priorities in life. Some staff members respond by planning very few developmental experiences due to the other demands in their lives. Other staff members respond by becoming overcommitted in the professional arena and often in other arenas also. For example, some staff members will concurrently be taking academic coursework, active in the local chapter, involved in unit and hos-

and professional g

A final caution is that some nurse managers may fear that as staff develop they may actually be motivated to leave direct patient care. Although there are no research studies available in this area, this author believes that critical care nurses leave the bedside when the frustrations they experience (intershift and/or interdisciplinary conflict, medical mismanagement, inadequate administration support, poor working conditions) outweigh the rewards (professional self-esteem, team spirit, growth opportunities, challenge, nurse/patient/family relationships, control over practice).

This model for professional growth is based on the premise that critical care nurses who are consistently moving to a higher level on their proficiency continuum, in an environment that is supportive and uses participative management techniques, will tend to be motivated and satisfied in their patient care positions. This premise is supported by Porter-O'Grady (15) in his discussions on ways to create a professional environment and establish staff accountability as well as by Peters (16), in his discussions on involving everyone in everything, using self-management teams, and creating an environment that promotes listening, celebrating, and recognizing. Other aspects of participative management are discussed in Chapters 4, 5 and 10.

## PROFESSIONAL GROWTH AND DEVELOPMENT OF THE NURSE MANAGER

Each nurse manager also has the need to plan and implement his or her own professional growth objectives. Using the process described above along with a variety of growth opportunites will help the nurse manager with the accomplishment of objectives. All of the avenues for professional growth previously discussed are appropriate for nurse managers to use depending on their identified needs. It is also important for the nurse manager to have a balance between objectives that address management skills and objectives that address clinical skills. Some nurse managers feel that they need to be clinical *experts* on *all* aspects of patient care. This is unrealistic considering the time, effort, and knowledge needed to maintain this goal and the demands of the nurse manager's role. A more realistic goal is to have staff experts on different aspects of care. The role of the nurse manager then is to facilitate team collaboration and team sharing of expertise resulting in a collectively higher standard of care.

The process of growth of the nurse manager can best be accomplished with the support, input, and encouragement of the nurse manager's supervisor. With all of the components of support visible to the staff, including the nurse manager's commitment to the process, the nurse manager serves as a role model to the staff. This example can translate into a potent motivator for them to achieve their goals.

## SUMMARY

This chapter has identified ways that nurse managers can promote professional development among staff members. Nurse managers are better equipped to facilitate this growth if they have an understanding of both the proficiency continuum and a process for planned professional growth. Several opportunities for professional growth were discussed as well as specific ways nurse managers can encourage use of these opportunities. Advantages and pitfalls of professional development were also discussed.

The nurse manager can have a tremendous impact on the growth and development of staff members. Providing the framework, resources, and encouragement has a positive influence on the degree to which staff members are involved with their own growth and development. It should be noted, however, that the process and methods described above take significant time and energy on the part of the nurse manager. On the other hand, the results from these efforts can also be significant. The potential outcomes include an increase in (a) the quality of care provided, (b) the currency of care provided, (c) staff morale, (d) staff motivation, and (e) staff retention. All of these outcomes make the nurse manager's job easier. In fact, the potential results of these efforts can be so far reaching and have such a positive influence on the critical care unit that this process should be *the priority concern* for every nurse manager.

REFERENCES

1. Summary analysis of critical care nurse supply and requirements. Newport Beach, CA: American Association of Critical-Care Nurses, 1988:11.
2. Styles MM. On nursing: toward a new endowment. St Louis, CV Mosby Company, 1982:8.
3. Luthans F. Organizational behavior. 4th ed. St Louis, McGraw-Hill Book Company, 1985:201.
4. Marriner A. Guide to nursing management. 2nd ed. St Lous, CV Mosby Company, 1984:196.
5. Benner P. From novice to expert: excellence and power in clinical nursing practice. Menlo Park, CA: Addison-Wesley Publishing Company, 1984:13–14.
6. AACN Certification Corporation. Critical care nursing practice statements. Newport Beach, CA: AACN Certification Corporation, 1984.
7. Breu C, Dracup K. Strengthening practice through research utilization. Communicating nursing research. Boulder CO: WICHEN, 1978.
8. Horsely J, Crane J, Reynolds MA. Using nursing research to improve nursing practice. New York: Grune and Stratton, 1981.
9. Coleman B, Stanley M, Chenevey B, et al. CCRN certification: exclusive or expensive? Focus Crit Care 1988;15:23–27.
10. American Association of Critical-Care Nurses. Demonstration project. Newport Beach, CA: AACN, 1988.
11. Dunbar S. Should CCRN nurses receive a salary differential? Dimensions Crit Care 1985;4:361–367.
12. Kelly LY. Other nursing and related organizations in the United States. Dimensions of professional nursing. 4th ed. New York: Macmillan Publishing Co, 1981.
13. Sanford RC. Clinical ladders, do they serve a purpose? J Nurs Admin 1987;17:34.
14. American Nurses' Association Cabinet on Nursing Services. Career ladders: an approach to professional productivity and job satisfaction. Kansas City: American Nurses' Association.
15. Porter-O-Grady T. Creative nursing administration: participative management into the 21st century. Rockville, Maryland: Aspen Publications, 1986;81–130.
16. Peters T. Thriving on chaos: Handbook for a management revolution. New York: Alfred A. Knopf, 1987:284–131.

# Chapter 8

# Planning for Various Settings in Critical Care

JOHN M. CLOCHESY

The "typical" critical care unit in the United States is a mixed medical-surgical intensive care unit (ICU) or coronary care unit (CCU) in a community hospital of fewer than 300 beds (1). Planning for critical care involves identifying and obtaining the resources necessary to provide the desired service(s). This chapter focuses on the human resources needed to provide critical care nursing in a variety of settings. The answers to several questions are necessary for nurse managers to begin the planning process. These questions are:

- What is the nature of the work/task (i.e., what is the product or product line)?
- What kind of staff expertise is needed?
- What are the rules and regulations required by the nature of the work?
- Who makes the decisions about clinical issues?
- Is there task specialization?

The product line will indicate the knowledge and type of technology need. Units with many rules, regulations, procedures, and protocols have a difficult time retaining experienced, well-educated nurses. Such nurses seek control over their practice, "not total independence," but self-determination in practicing according to professional "nursing" standards (2). Once these data are collected, specifics about the hospital setting and type of unit can be explored.

A variety of factors must be considered when planning for critical care personnel. These factors include whether the hospital is rural or urban, whether it is a teaching hospital or not, and whether the unit is a general or specialized critical care unit. Each of these factors will be explored citing the differences and similarities. Figure 8.1 shows the role of various types of units in various hospitals.

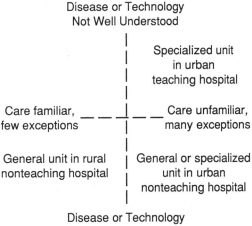

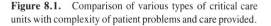

**Figure 8.1.** Comparison of various types of critical care units with complexity of patient problems and care provided.

## RURAL VERSUS URBAN SETTING

Intensive care units in rural settings are often four beds or less, adjacent to a nurses' station, at one end of the medical-surgical unit, or part of the postanesthesia recovery unit (PARU). These units provide close observation and "intensive" nursing care not available elsewhere in the hospital. Often nurses in rural settings have consultation available from critical care nurses at an urban referral hospital.

Remote cardiac monitoring (RCM) is an example of nurse-to-nurse consultation. RCM allows a rural hospital to provide coronary care without personnel experts in all aspects of coronary artery disease, cardiac rhythm interpretation, and current treatment regimens (3). There are 107 RCMs with a total of 213 beds in 15 states (Table 8.1).

**Table 8.1.** States with Remote Cardiac Monitoring Systems[a]

Arkansas
Colorado
Idaho
Illinois
Iowa
Kansas
Michigan
Minnesota
Mississippi
Nebraska
North Dakota
Oklahoma
Ohio
Texas
Wisconsin

[a]Adapted from Nottingham A, Camp V. Remote cardiac monitoring: nursing collaboration is the key. Dimensions of Critical Care Nursing, 1987; 6:176–180.

Many urban hospitals have more than one critical care unit. The most common unit designations are CCU and ICU. Urban critical care nurses often specialize in the care of specific patient populations. Clinical experts are often available in-house.

Knaus and associates (4) found that presence of a master's-prepared clinical nurse specialist to guide orientation and education in the ICU was one of two factors present at hospitals that had patient mortalities lower than that predicted by the Acute Physiologic and Chronic Health Evaluation score (APACHE II). The other factor that positively affected patient outcome in this study of 5030 patients at 13 hospitals was the level of interaction and communication between physicians and nurses. The patient outcome had little relationship to the administrative structure of the unit, amount of specialized treatment used, or the teaching status of the hospital.

The implications of this study for the nurse manager are that the quality of the relationships and communication between the physicians and nurses is very important. Additionally, the quality of orientation of nursing staff within the unit affects patient outcome. The nurse manager can foster physician-nurse relationships and support the unit-based critical care nurse educator or clinical nurse specialist's educational role. It may be fiscally impossible for rural hospitals to have master's-prepared specialists in-house for orientation of critical care nurses. When not available, nurse managers can obtain consultation locally from nurses in hospitals in nearby communities, schools of nursing, or clinical nurse specialists with practices providing consultation services.

## Demographics of Nurses

Many nurses working in rural settings work part-time. Of the nurses working in the CCU and ICU at the American Association of Clinical-Care Nurses (AACN) Demonstration Project (1) hospital, 68% work part-time. Few have advanced degrees or specialized training. This is due in part to the lack of educational opportunities. One clinical nurse specialist in the South reports being the only master's-prepared nurse for 100 miles (5).

Some rural and smaller urban hospitals have arrangements with university schools of nursing to offer degree programs (BSN, MSN) at the hospital. This arrangement helps the hospital by developing the expertise of current nursing staff and may help recruit younger nurses who would otherwise choose urban hospitals for the greater range of educational and advancement opportunities. Urban hospitals are more attractive to nurses in dual-career households because there are more opportunities for their spouses nearby.

Depending on the mix of nurses, the nurse manager will need to support a mix of educational advancement programs, including making the ICU available for student placement and providing child care facilities and sick child centers to recruit and retain nursing staff. If the hospital is located in a metropolitan area, the nurse manager should provide information about career opportunities to the relocation planning offices of large corporations whose employees from dual-career households are relocating to the area. Examples of corporations to approach are major industrial and manufacturing companies, retail store chains, large information and financial services companies, and universities. Some large realty firms also maintain relocation assistance offices.

## Patient Population

Patients in rural hospitals are usually local residents with routine health problems. Typically patients of all ages are admitted to the intensive care unit. They include those with chest pain, myocardial infarction, diabetic ketoacidosis, severe asthma or emphysema, gastrointestinal bleeding, drug overdose, and extensive abdominal surgery. Patients are not segregated by diagnosis, clinical service, or type of therapy. Because many are local residents, their families and others in their social support networks may visit and can participate in discharge planning. In contrast, patients in urban hospitals may be local residents or they may have traveled to the hospital to receive some specialized form of treatment not available at their local hospital. Their families may be away from home, be in need of affordable temporary housing, and lack their usual support networks. The nurse manager in the urban hospital should direct the nurse to a list or directory of housing options and community and social service agencies that provide assistance to patients and families from out of town.

In addition to the type of patient admitted to rural hospitals, patients are admitted to the ICU in urban hospitals for a variety of specialized nursing observation, therapeutic technology, and drug therapy. The nursing care requirements and the nurses' training in urban hospitals, therefore, is usually greater. For example, consider a patient who requires an extensive abdominal surgical procedure and suffers a massive myocardial infarction (MI) immediately postoperatively. The nurse must be able to balance care related to the MI with the fluid resuscitation requirements of extensive abdominal surgery.

### Specialization among ICU Nurses

Nurses in rural hospitals must be generalists, ready to cope with problems ranging from myocardial infarction and trauma to pregnancy-induced hypertension. Although skilled as generalists, nurses in rural settings may not encounter some problems often enough to develop the necessary specialized skills. When patient census is low, these critical care generalists often "float" to general care areas.

Nurses in urban hospitals specialize to a greater degree. They may be coronary care and intensive care nurses, medical ICU (MICU) and surgical ICU (SICU) nurses, or a combination of those above and/ or burn, trauma, pediatric, respiratory, neonatal, cardiothoracic, and neurosurgical ICU nurses. The degree of specialization depends on the hospital size, the degree of physician specialization, and the range of services offered by the hospital.

If "floating" is required, critical care nurses in urban hospitals are reassigned to another critical care unit. To minimize the "aggravation" experienced by nursing staff, the nurse manager may wish to implement a contingency staffing system using either a buddy unit or decentralized, self-sustained approach. If the buddy unit approach is used, a unit with similar patients should be chosen. Planning occasional educational and social events

with the buddy unit increases familiarity among the nurses and reduces the isolation frequently felt by the floated nurse. The decentralized system has the potential for providing the nurses with the most satisfaction. It eliminates floating. It does, however, limit the resources available to fill staffing needs and may result in higher personnel costs due to an increase in the use of temporary, outside agency nurses, which may be offset by retention of staff (see Chapter 6).

### Collaboration

Clinical practice in rural and urban nonteaching hospitals is often based on the medical model. This is due in part to the lack of nurses in advanced practice. In urban teaching hospitals a nursing/ collaboration model of practice is more common. Examples of collaboration include planning for expansion of the unit, developing admission and discharge criteria, orienting physicians in training, and developing clinical protocols. The "collaboration" model stresses that many patient problems are within both medical and nursing practice but recognizes separate spheres of activity as well (6). The distinction among cooperation, coordination, and collaboration is often unclear (7). Kilmann and Thomas (8) define collaboration as a combination of assertiveness and cooperation. Table 8.2 shows the result of combining varying degrees of assertiveness and cooperation. Assertiveness is behavior directed to achieve one's own goals. Cooperation is behavior directed to achieve another's goals. Thus, if collaboration = assertiveness + cooperation, collaboration results in a situation in which everyone wins. The nurse manager can facilitate collaboration among the physicians and nurses in the intensive care unit by clearly identifying the goals of each group and planning activities to achieve them. Devereux (9) proposed a model of collaboration that has five essential factors: communication, competence, accountability, trust, and administrative support. These factors might be represented by the establishment of joint practice committees, all-registered nurse (RN) staffing, primary nursing, encouragement of nurses to make individual clinical decisions, integrated patient records, and joint patient care review (10).

### TEACHING VERSUS NONTEACHING HOSPITALS

Teaching and nonteaching hospitals differ in many areas including fundamental priorities, degree of

**Table 8.2.** Relationship Resulting from the Interaction between Assertiveness and Cooperation[a]

|  | Assertive | Moderately Assertive | Unassertive |
|---|---|---|---|
| Cooperative | Collaboration | Compromise | Accommodation |
| Uncooperative | Competition |  | Avoidance |

[a]Adapted from Kilmann RH, Thomas KW. Developing a forced-choice measure of conflict-handling behavior: the "Mode" instrument. Educ Psychol Measurement 1977;37:309–325.

specialization, environmental actors and their arena of influence, and opinion leaders. The differences among hospitals fall on a continuum. A discussion of each follows.

### Fundamental Priorities

The priority for a nonteaching hospital is affordable patient care. The priorities at a teaching hospital include physician training (teaching) and patient care. Which of these is the first priority varies by institution. Usually the priorities in university medical centers are research, physician training, and patient care. The order of priorities in any given hospital may conflict with those of nurses who see patient care as the first priority. In all settings, the nurse, as the patient's advocate, must help the institution balance its priorities with the patient's needs.

### Environmental Actors

Environmental actors and their arena of influence vary by type of hospital. For example, a major employer and its choice of provider of health insurance coverage (indemnity, health maintenance organization, or preferred provider arrangement) have an impact on the hospital beyond any control the hospital can exert. This occurs in both teaching and nonteaching hospitals. Medical school faculty and their priorities, as well as those of the university at large, alter priorities in teaching hospitals but have little or no effect on nonteaching hospitals. The prudent manager identifies which environmental actors will affect his or her unit or hospital. The CCU manager may note a change in the recommendations of the American Heart Association and identifies how the recommendations will affect the CCU. For example, the recommendation may be that CCU nurses have classes in 12-lead electrocardiogram interpretation. At the same time the manager of the SICU notes these recommendations and determines they may not affect the SICU.

### Opinion Leaders

Opinion leaders are those persons whose support for a new program or change in a current one is necessary for success. Frequently opinion leaders do not hold administrative (line) positions. They may be academic faculty, clinicians, or influential others. Managers may not see the individuals as expert or powerful. If others perceive them as such, however, their opinion is essential. It is important to identify the opinion leaders among the physicians, the nursing staff, and support services. For example, the nurse manager, assistant nurse manager, clinical nurse specialist or educator, and medical director may decide that a particular practice must change and devise the optimal procedure. They will successfully implement the change if the opinion leaders concur. If, however, a senior nurse on the night shift, whose opinion less experienced nurses rely upon, does not see the need for the change, there will be significant resistance to implementing the new procedure. In nonteaching hospitals, physicians may be the majority of opinion leaders while in teaching hospitals, nurses and support staff play a larger role.

An opinion leader can be identified by answering "Whose opinion could severely hamper or stop implementation of the plan?" Once identified, involve these individuals in any planning for the critical care unit. Their input may be invaluable but their cooperation in implementing any program or change planned is essential.

### Physician Availability

Nurses often assume different roles when physicians are available and when they are not. At times, critical care nurses act as physician surrogates (11). The nurse in the nonteaching hospital assesses, diagnoses, prioritizes, coordinates, and intervenes when the physician is not present. When the physician arrives at the hospital, he or she expects the nurses to relinquish the roles they have assumed. This role strain can cause conflict between physicians and nurses. This can be a difficult problem for the nurse manager. The nurse manager should look for additional problems if role strain is the presenting complaint. Role strain often arises when the nurses perceive that their contributions are not valued by the physicians. For example, if a patient with a history of coronary artery disease and angina becomes acutely short of breath, the nurse may obtain an arterial blood gas, chest x-ray, and electrocardiogram and start low flow oxygen. During the daytime, the physician may object to the nurse using this initiative, while the same physician might berate a nurse for not instituting these measures if the incident occurred at 2:30 AM. The uncertainty about expectations leads to role strain. The nurse manager can reduce the risk of this type of role strain by working with the nursing staff and physicians to develop protocols or clinical privileges for the unit nurses.

In teaching hospitals, resident physicians are always present. The nurses have no difficulty in contacting a physician. Although this can help during emergencies, there are drawbacks. With physicians always present, they can physically be in the way at the nurses' station. Additionally, because they are present, it is easy for them to change "their orders." Transcribing, checking, and implementing the residents' orders can by very time consuming. To facilitate the ever present physician and minimize interference with the nurses, separate but adjacent charting and conference areas can be designated for the nurses and residents. To minimize interruptions with nursing care, some units set times for routine orders to be written and procedures performed. For example, the nurse manager could implement or facilitate the following:

All routine morning laboratory work, x-rays, and electrocardiograms should be ordered by midnight.

All transfer orders should be written by 8 AM.

All anticipated procedures (central line, arterial line, pulmonary artery catheter, and lumbar puncture) should be performed by 2 PM.

## GENERAL VERSUS SPECIALIZED UNIT

Many bright, assertive, technologically oriented, intervention-prone nurses choose critical care (12). They have a variety of critical care units to choose from. The general or medical-surgical ICU provides the nurse the opportunity to develop a wide range of assessment and psychomotor skills. Other nurses choose a specialized unit such as the coronary care unit (CCU), the medical intensive care unit (MICU), or the surgical intensive care unit (SICU). In large teaching hospitals the MICU and SICU may be further divided into the MICU and the respiratory intensive care unit (RICU), and

**Table 8.3.** Average Number of Direct Nursing Care Hours Provided per Patient Day by Type of Unit

| Unit | HPPD |
|------|------|
| CCU | 12–14 |
| MICU | 14–16 |
| SICU | 16–18 |
| CTICU | 18–24 |

the SICU may be divided into the general SICU, the neurosurgical intensive care unit (Neuro ICU), and the cardiothoracic surgery intensive care unit (CTICU or CSICU). In large hospitals there are pediatric intensive care units (PICU) and neonatal intensive care units (NICU). Each of these units has a different patient mix and requires a different expertise and level of care.

Table 8.3 lists the number of direct nursing care hours per patient day (HPPD) commonly provided in 1988.

The HPPD provided is adjusted depending on the severity of illness of the patients, the patients' care requirements, and the availability of support services. If support service personnel, such as respiratory therapists and unit clerical assistants, are not available, additional nursing hours are needed to provide these services. In December 1987, an expert panel for critical care nursing determined the range of nursing HPPD that will be required in 1988, 1990, 1995, and 2000 (13). The findings of this study are summarized in Table 8.4.

## CONCLUSION

Once the scope of services to be provided, environmental actors, and opinion leaders have been identified, resource needs can be identified. Regardless of the setting, physician-nurse communication and collaboration, expert nursing practice, nurses' accountability for their practice and patient outcomes, and caring are keys to creating a positive work environment that results in the best patient outcomes (4, 14).

**Table 8.4.** Range of Critical Care Nursing Hours Predicted by Expert Panel, December 13, 1987[a]

| Year | RN Hours per Patient Day |
|------|--------------------------|
| 1988 | 14.5–22.0 |
| 1990 | 18.0–24.0 |
| 1995 | 20.0–26.0 |
| 2000 | 22.0–26.0 |

[a]Adapted from American Association of Critical-Care Nurses summary analysis of critical care nurse supply and requirements. Newport Beach, California: American Association of Critical-Care Nurses, 1988.

REFERENCES

1. Mitchell P, Armstrong S, Forshee T, et al. American Association of Critical-Care Nurses Demonstration Project: Phase I report. Newport Beach, California: American Association of Critical-Care Nurses, 1988.
2. American Academy of Nursing Task Force on Nursing Practice in Hospitals. Magnet hospitals: attraction and retention of professional nurses. Kansas City, Missouri: American Nurses' Association, 1983.
3. Nottingham A, Camp V. Remote cardiac monitoring: nursing collaboration is the key. Dimensions Crit Care Nurs 1987;6:176–180.
4. Knaus WA, Draper EA, Wagner DP, et al. An evaluation of outcome from intensive care in major medical centers. Ann Intern Med 1986;194:410–418.
5. Hotter A. Personal communication, June 1984.
6. American Nurses Association. Nursing: a social policy statement. Kansas City, Missouri: American Nurses' Association, 1980.
7. Baggs JG, Schmitt MH. Collaboration between nurses and physicians. Image 1988;20:145–149.
8. Kilmann RH, Thomas KW. Developing a forced-choice measure of conflict-handling behavior: the "MODE" instrument. Educ Psychol Measurement 1977;37:309–325.
9. Devereux PM. Essential elements of nurse-physician collaboration. J Nurs Admin 1981;11:19–23.
10. National Joint Practice Commission. Guidelines for establishing joint or collaborative practice in hospitals. Chicago: Neely Printing Co, Inc.
11. Devereux PM. Nurse/physician collaboration: nursing practice considerations. J Nurs Admin 1981;11:37–39.
12. Torrens PR. Personal correspondence report to Edward A Shaw, May 12, 1981.
13. American Association of Critical-Care Nurses summary analysis of critical care nurse supply and requirements. Newport Beach, California: American Association of Critical-Care Nurses, 1988.
14. Hale JF. Caring: the key to recruitment and retention. Focus Crit Care 1984;11(5):44–47.

# Part III

# INTERVENING
### AND
# DIRECTING

# Chapter 9

# Communicating

ELIZABETH LEVSON
MARY ELLEN GUY

Communication is the lifeblood of any nursing unit. Barring everyone's presence at all times, it is the only way that nurses can make others aware of changes about to happen, events that have occurred, or information that needs to be known. Without communication, patient needs and responses, plans for nursing care, and physician requests cannot be known to others. Critical care nurses are especially dependent on communication as fast-breaking conditions change the levels of care required by critically ill patients.

Intervening and directing staff require an intimate knowledge of communication patterns within the nursing unit, as well as within and across divisions. Mastering communication channels is a skill as essential to the manager's effectiveness as the ability to staff units, motivate employees, and coordinate services. The nurse manager who has mastered organizational communication channels and utilizes them effectively is able to handle fast-breaking problems far better than the manager who fails to understand that communication is central to the smooth functioning of a critical care unit. Based upon recent research findings, this chapter explains the communication process, outlines the kinds of communication channels available to critical care nurse managers, explains which channels are appropriate for different types of messages, provides a list of barriers to effective communication, and closes with a list of rules to assist critical care nurse managers in communicating effectively.

## IMPORTANCE OF EFFECTIVE COMMUNICATION

The only way to learn and make staff aware of new information is through communication. Changes never end in the critical care area. Even at the most stable times, the number of patients on the unit is constantly changing; the patients' acuity levels and requirements of care change; staff rotations and shift changes bring different personnel every day and shift; and last minute problems with staff availability require sudden changes in staffing schedules. Beyond the predictability of these constant changes, other events produce even more change, such as arranging staffing during inclement weather; implementing hospital-mandated changes in personnel or patient care policies; preparing for an upcoming Joint Commission on Accreditation of Healthcare Organizations (JCAHO) review; or preparing to meet any of many other circumstances that are unpredictable and unstoppable. The only way to learn of these changes is through communication. The only way to notify staff and keep them abreast of what is happening is by communicating.

All kinds of things go wrong when a nurse manager fails to acknowledge the importance of communication, from minor misunderstandings to critical patient care issues. Communication provides a means for coordinating the activities of staff and giving clear instructions from one person to the next, and from one shift to the next. Inadequate attention to necessary information or assuming staff have knowledge they may not possess leads to risk and errors that usually could have been avoided.

The need to communicate effectively extends beyond patient care issues. It is integral to managing a unit because it serves to structure, guide, and reinforce the behavior of staff. The work of a manager is to coordinate and direct the work of others. In order to accomplish this, a manager must be able to communicate expectations to staff in a way that motivates them. Clear instructions and meaningful compliments encourage employees to be productive and take pride in their work. Both job satisfaction and job performance are improved by the presence of quality communication between supervisors and subordinates (1). Effective communication among employees satisfies a basic social need to relate to others and exchange both essential and nonessential information related to the work environment and requirements.

Although the importance of various communication skills varies across professions, there are five core communication skills that are very important regardless of whether one is a critical care nurse, a banker, an attorney, or an engineer. These are building relationships, listening, giving feedback, exchanging routine information, and soliciting feedback. These skills are necessary regardless of one's profession, position, or rank. Other communication skills vary according to the direction of the communication. Persuading and negotiating become important in communication with a superior. Advising, instructing, giving orders, and motivating become important in communication with subordinates (2). This means that particular communication skills are contingent on the direction of the communication. One's own rank, as well as the rank of those with whom one is speaking, affects the issues being discussed and the manner in which they are discussed.

## ELEMENTS OF THE COMMUNICATION PROCESS

Communication always involves four elements: a communicator, a message, a receiver, and the context in which the message is sent and received. The communicator is the one who sends the information. The message is the information passed through whatever channel is chosen. The channel and environmental conditions mediate the message. The receiver is the person or persons for whom the sender intended the message.

Communication is much more than a language process. It is a people process. As the originator of a communication, the sender must determine the best channel to use. In order to make this decision, the sender must assess the nature of the message, the speed necessary for making the transmission, the likely response of the receivers, and whether immediate feedback is necessary. Because the environment influences both sender and receiver, it plays an important role in the communication process. For example, in the context of a crisis, a message is treated quite differently than in the context of a casual lunchroom conversation (3). In a crisis, the essence of the message is received but details are lost in the frenzy of the moment. In a casual conversation, all sides of the issues are explored and pondered. Likewise, a pat

on the back and a compliment given in person from the nurse manager to the staff nurse is more rewarding than an impersonal memorandum addressed to all staff complimenting them on their work.

### Channels for Communication

The situation and the nature of the message dictate the appropriate communication channel. This means that form follows function (4). For example, some messages are communicated more clearly when a combination of channels is used. Communication in a hospital setting occurs either formally or informally. A formal message may be followed with informal communication to clarify the message, or an informal message may be followed by a formal message to document that the message was delivered.

The two categories, formal and informal, differ in terms of whether they are planned or unplanned and whether the message must be accountable and verifiable (5). Formal communications include written or oral messages that are sanctioned by the organization and travel along the chain of command. They include memoranda, policy and procedure statements, letters, logs, reports, minutes of meetings, and patient records. Face-to-face meetings and telephone conversations may be treated as either formal or informal communications. If the face-to-face meeting is recorded, what would otherwise be informal becomes formal. The same is true of telephone conversations.

There are several methods utilized by nurse managers for communicating with staff nurses. Policies and procedures kept in bound manuals on the unit are prime examples of written, formal communications. Newsletters, meetings, notices posted on bulletin boards, and attitude surveys provide additional formal channels for communicating. Newsletters are especially effective for developing a sense of identity with a unit. They are useful for announcing awards to staff, bragging about promotions, and introducing newly hired staff. They are also an effective means of notifying staff of changes in policies or procedures, changes going on elsewhere in the hospital, and updates on pay rates and benefits.

Formal communications are not limited to management-staff interactions. They are also helpful in communicating with patients' families. A newsletter written for patients' families lets them know of visiting policies; availability of the chaplain;

with whom to leave emergency phone numbers that may change daily; nursing policies, such as in primary nursing when a specific nurse is responsible for formulating a plan of care for a family member; and other pertinent information specific to that critical care unit. This form of communication can be an invaluable tool for lessening patient and family anxiety and enhancing visitor-staff rapport. As it is the nurse manager's responsibility to provide for communication in all areas of patient care responsibilities that occur on the critical care unit, a method for disseminating information to the patients' families certainly lies within those responsibilities. Additionally, improved staff-family communication may provide a method for lessening the ever-increasing legal actions prevalent in today's society, a goal desired by management at every level throughout the health care industry.

Although some issues are better handled through meetings, some are handled better through an exchange of memoranda and personal interviews. Meetings are appropriate when the information is nonroutine, while memoranda are the preferred channel for transmitting relatively simple, uncontroversial facts. For example, the nurse manager should call a meeting if the unit must eliminate two telephones and a management-staff decision is needed to determine which will go. However, a memorandum is a better use of a nurse manager's time for indicating that the switchboard numbers have changed. Call a meeting to discuss the proposal that shift hours be changed to an earlier or later starting time, but send a memorandum to verify that times have been changed once the issue has been decided.

When a nurse manager determines that problem solving meetings should be held, they should be treated as a formal communication process. Before conducting any meeting, such as monthly staff meetings, decide the overall strategy for the meeting. Decide what issues will be addressed. Plan the objectives of the meeting and state them clearly when the meeting is announced. Prepare an agenda and follow it during the meeting. This structures the discussion and ensures that the conversation will stay focused on the purpose of the meeting. Designate a recorder and keep minutes of the meeting. Select participants so that the group is as small as possible but is representative of those who will be affected by any decision made. For example, the charge nurse from each shift is the ideal rep-

resentative for decisions affecting only that particular shift.

Writing effective memoranda is easier said than done. They must be clear and to the point, include an adequate explanation, and yet not be too long. The ideas in the message should flow logically. They should be brief and preferably limited to one page so they can be easily posted on a bulletin board. Adjust the language so the intended readers will understand the message and still have all the information necessary. If the memorandum contains a directive, clearly specify what action must be taken, who is to do it, and what deadline applies.

Informal communications are oral, most often bypass the chain of command, and are called "the grapevine." Informal channels are used when peers engage in shop talk or supervisors and subordinates have off-the-record conversations. Transmission is by work of mouth through friendship networks (6). The grapevine supplements formal communication channels and provides access to information faster than formal channels. It activates when the formal system fails to respond quickly enough to a given situation. While investigating whether critical care nurses are more likely to use formal or informal channels for sending and receiving information, Levson and Guy found that critical care nurses are more likely to rely on formal channels for sending information but rely on the grapevine for receiving information. Despite its unverifiable nature, 55% of the nurses surveyed reported that they usually believe what they hear on the grapevine (5).

Communication may be spoken, written, or nonverbal messages transmitted with body language. Written communication is one-way because it does not allow the receiver to respond immediately to the message as face-to-face verbal communication does. The sender must wait for a response. The advantage of written communication is that it ensures better clarity. Because everyone who receives the communication receives exactly the same information, there is less variability in how the message is received. It is the most economical channel for groups, and it is permanently recorded. On the other hand, it allows no nonverbal messages, no immediate feedback, and it is time consuming to prepare a draft and have it delivered. The nurse manager could utilize written communication when notifying the staff of changes in policies or procedures, requesting specific sug-

**Table 9.1**  Formal versus Informal Channels

| Formal | Informal |
| --- | --- |
| Predictable | Flexible |
| Documented | Faster |
| Control over the message | Immediate feedback |
| Verifiable | More personal |

gestions for changes in policies, notifying other departments of changes in the policies of the critical care unit with regard to their dealings with the unit, requesting clarification of proposed policies from nursing or hospital administration, or requesting a meeting with management personnel in any area related to the critical care unit. Table 9.1 contrasts the advantages of formal channels with informal channels.

Spoken communication has two advantages over written communication: it allows for immediate feedback as to whether the message has been received as intended and it provides for nonverbal messages to be transmitted. This has the potential of being the clearest communication channel because confirmation, feedback, and clarification are immediate. It allows the listener to "listen between the lines." The disadvantages are that verbal, face-to-face communication may be less well planned than written communication, there is no record of the exchange of information, and it is the most time consuming of communication channels. Telephone conversations provide no permanent record unless they are tape recorded, and they are unwieldy for groups. On the other hand, they save time, provide an opportunity for confirmation and feedback, and some nonverbal messages can be communicated.

Verbal counseling of a staff member who has committed a relatively minor infraction may be appropriate for a first-time offense. Written counseling may be the more appropriate choice if the infraction is repeated several times or is more serious. In a more positive vein, verbal praise is the appropriate choice for a staff member who has made a special effort in some area. Written commendation is appropriate for a staff member who makes special efforts in any area over any period of greater than a few days.

Nonverbal communication are messages that do not involve the transmission of words. Some researchers estimate that almost two-thirds of human communication is nonverbal (7). Ceremonies and symbols are two ways of communicating messages

to employees. They have both verbal and nonverbal components. They serve to recognize exemplary employees as well as send a nonverbal message to others of what is considered exemplary performance. Other nonverbal messages are conveyed by a speaker's tone of voice, volume, gestures, facial expressions, and eye contact or the lack of it. Silence sends its own message. The time a sender takes to respond to a communication also sends a message to anyone waiting for a response.

Any nurse who has ever provided bedside care is familiar with the nonverbal communication that can occur with a patient who cannot speak and seems completely unresponsive, but responds to painful stimuli. The grimacing, body part withdrawal, and writhing in bed cease when simple comfort measures such as positioning, wiping the face with a damp cloth, and patting the patient gently are utilized. Similarly, managers are usually aware of the facial expressions and body positioning of employees when they engage in face-to-face communication. Arms folded across the chest and tight lips certainly convey a more negative message than arms held loosely at the sides with a smile on the face.

### Relationship between Spoken and Nonverbal Communication

Language is a system of words used to express ideas. However, the same words have different meanings for different people, and the manner of speaking the words intones different meanings. When a nurse manager says "Do it as soon as you can" the intent may be "Do it immediately." But the receiver may have assumed that the intent was "Do it when you get around to it." Speaking styles transmit a nonassertive, assertive, or aggressive tone to the communication. Neither nonassertive nor aggressive styles produce as clear a message as an assertive tone.

Nonassertive components of speaking send the message that the sender is not comfortable with the message and leaves the receiver with little confidence in the quality or sincerity of the message. Examples of nonassertive speaking behaviors are apologetic words, beating around the bush, and failure to say what the sender actually means. For example, "Well, would you do it as soon as you can?" transmits a weaker message than "Do it immediately."

Assertive components of speaking transmit a sense of confidence in the message. Examples of assertive speaking behaviors are straightforward statements of feelings that say what the speaker means. Saying "I need for you to do it as soon as you can, even if other things must wait for a while" is more assertive than saying "It would be nice if you would do it fairly soon."

Aggressive messages are different from assertive messages. An aggressive speaking style transmits a forceful message that is more often received negatively than positively. Aggressive speaking behaviors include accusatory language, "You" messages that blame or label, and a haughty or superior speaking posture: "I told you to do it!"

Nonverbal communication is perceived through the senses. While some gestures assist a message, some hinder it. When a supervisor says she wants to sit, talk with staff, and get to know them, but then proceeds to look frequently at the clock while others are talking, staff receive a message that the supervisor is eager for the session to be finished. This behavior stifles meaningful conversation and staff will not say very much because they are receiving a double message. The verbal message is that the supervisor is interested in them, but the nonverbal message is that the supervisor's words were not sincere. The contradictory message causes staff to withhold from full participation, telling far less about themselves than they would if the supervisor had appeared relaxed and interested.

Just as there are nonassertive, assertive, and aggressive styles that accompany spoken communication, these styles also accompany unspoken communication. Nonassertive behaviors that detract from a message consist of actions that indicate the speaker hopes someone will guess what the sender wants. These are manifested by a weak, hesitant, speaking voice; failure to make eye contact; a pleading tone to the voice; and being fidgety. Nonassertive behavior allows the receivers to choose for the sender and interpret the message however they please. This often results in the sender feeling angry and resentful because the receivers of the message do not respond as the speaker desired. Often nonassertive stands are taken because the speaker hopes to avoid unpleasant or risky situations and wants to steer clear of confrontation. Such behavior usually results in merely postponing a greater confrontation later. For example, nonassertive behaviors on the part of nursing staff include such actions as refusing to sign a list indicating order of choice for the major holidays, i.e., Christmas, Christmas Eve, and Thanksgiv-

ing, or refusing to indicate a preference between day/evening or day/night rotations. After managers have made the choice for them, managers are then confronted with an angry staff member who states that the manager "should have known" Christmas was a high priority or that child care difficulties make day/evening rotation impossible.

Assertive behaviors that strengthen a message include a generally assured manner that communicates caring and strength; speaking with a firm, warm, well-modulated voice; making eye contact but not staring; and using relaxed body motions. Assertive behaviors allow the speaker to stand up for legitimate rights without violating the rights of others; to communicate honestly and directly, expressing feelings, needs, and ideas; and they allow speakers to make their own choices. Speaking assertively allows one to own one's own feelings. The result is that this approach usually achieves the intended result. If it does not, at least the assertiveness reinforces positive feelings and improves self-confidence. The nurse who approaches the manager with a statement such as "I cannot work day/evening rotations due to child care difficulties but am willing to work more nights than days on a day/night rotation" communicates a sense of maturity to the manager.

Aggressive behaviors that detract from the message or alienate the receiver from the intent of the message and from the sender include a flippant, sarcastic style; an air of superiority; speaking with a tense, shrill voice; a cold "deadly quiet" presence; or expressionless eyes staring but not really "seeing" those being addressed. Aggressive behavior transmits a message that the sender wishes to dominate the sender. It creates a distance between the sender and receiver. For example, an aggressive response to a schedule conflict occurs when a nurse approaches the manager and states "I told you I won't work evenings because I can't get a babysitter, and if you don't like it, you can fire me. You're short-staffed already, and I can get a job anywhere." This sort of statement distances the receiver and engenders anger at the speaker.

## Communication with Different Levels

The nature of the message and the best channel to use differ according to the position and status of the sender and intended receiver. Communication flows in all directions. It flows up and down the hierarchy, horizontally among peers, and diagonally from a level in one unit to a different level in another unit or division. It penetrates any and all ranks in a hospital. Each level of the hierarchy has access to different kinds of information. Those at the top of hospital administration have a better picture of the total operation of the hospital. Those on a unit have a better idea of problems that affect daily patient care. Those in the middle have a better idea of where slowdowns in the system occur.

Unfortunately staff nurses often lack confidence in their ability to make decisions affecting daily patient care. It is important that the unit manager be able to communicate to staff that decisions affecting patient care at its most basic levels should and can be made by those providing direct care. Even changes in hospital policies directed toward all critical care areas are based on problems identified, evaluated, and solved by staff nurses. For example, a decision about collection of arterial blood gas samples falls under hospital policy, but determination of who will be allowed or required to draw those samples and the sites that will be utilized for collecting samples result from suggestions by staff nurses and physicians. A good manager should help staff appreciate the degree of influence they have on formulating such policies. In this way, an effective critical care nurse manager empowers the staff.

Communication needs vary according to the level within the hospital because the information within the message differs, the scope of the message differs, and the receivers and their frames of reference differ. Upper level management communication, which is interdivisional, involves communicating with the director of nursing, hospital administrator, divisional directors, chief of staff, budget director, and directors of ancillary services. The types of issues that require communication are of hospital-wide relevance. Examples are recruitment/retention, alternative staffing patterns, competitiveness of financial/staffing options, changes in policies, equipment needs, space requirements, construction needs, services needed from ancillary personnel, and federal/state legislation affecting delivery of care.

The most prevalent form of communication used in upper level, interdivisional decision making tends to be written communication, usually in the form of memoranda. For instance, assume that the nurse manager has been approached by staff regarding problems with accepting written orders for patient care from fourth-year medical students, even though these orders are written as verbal orders from the covering resident responsible for that medical student. As the problems are varied and constant over an extended period of time, the nurse manager decides to address the problem. Because staff's refusal to accept a written verbal order from the medical students involves a change in hospital policy, the medical director of the critical care unit, the nursing director of the division, the nursing director of the hospital, the medical director of the residency program, the medical director of the fourth-year medical students' program, and the hospital director are all involved in the decision. The problem must first be addressed in a memorandum to each of the parties and feedback obtained. Face-to-face meetings may be needed, or the entire problem may be handled by exchanges of written communication. An equitable settlement is obtained by the nurse manager when the agreement is reached among all of the involved parties that written orders will be accepted by the staff if the orders are cosigned by the resident physician before implementation of the orders by the staff nurse. The resolution of the problem is communicated to the staff by posting a memorandum from the medical director of the unit and by verbal communication from the nurse manager to the staff in a staff meeting.

Intradivisional communication involves communicating with divisional directors, other nurse managers in the division, medical director(s), staff physicians, and supervisors of ancillary personnel. The types of messages that are most prevalent involve staffing needs, support services needed, patient admission and transfer guidelines, equipment utilization/sharing, review of current policies, and budgetary requirements. For example, a nurse manager may find it necessary to contact the supervisor of a radiology technician when complaints are received from the staff nurses regarding the radiology technician's rudeness and rough treatment of patients. Or, the nurse manager may find it necessary to contact other nurse managers within the division when a particular piece of equipment would be beneficial to a small patient population seen on all of the patient care units but never in quantity to justify purchasing the equipment for a specific unit. Policies for storage, utilization, and priorities would have to be established among the nurse managers, as well as dividing the cost of the equipment among the units utilizing the equipment. Additionally, input from the nursing director of the division and the medical directors of the involved units would be needed.

Between units, the nurse manager must communicate with the physicians, ancillary personnel, and other unit managers. The types of messages that are most prevalent involve staffing needs, policy and/or procedural changes, patient admissions and transfers, equipment utilization and sharing, and utilization of ancillary personnel.

Within a unit, the nurse manager must communicate with staff, patients and their families, physicians, and ancillary personnel. Effective communication between a nurse manager and a staff nurse does not happen by accident. Unit goals and objectives are important for everyone to agree upon and understand. Communication skills are called upon daily. Bulletin boards must be kept up to date and placed in a position where they are easy to read. Mail boxes for staff provide an easy way to make sure than any daily communication to particular staff will be received. The walls in the staff restroom provide a place for brief notes of interest to the staff as well as quick information, i.e., "The new bedscales are here!" or "Name this cardiac rhythm."

Nurse managers also have a responsibility for encouraging intrastaff communications. Appropriate suggestions for the staff include communication books and individual pocket notebooks. Communication books exchange daily concerns among staff members and substitute for face-to-face communications that may have been forgotten during shift change. A pocket notebook prevents any staff member from forgetting to give someone a message. It also provides a way at the end of the shift for organizing one's notes and giving reports efficiently yet thoroughly.

Giving critical care nurses an opportunity to participate in making decisions increases commitment to the decision and is the most effective way to bring about change. Extensive communication between units can unfreeze resistance to change. When one unit rejects an innovation, the manager can arrange information exchanges with staff in equivalent units that have recently implemented similar policies. Even if a unit tunes out the manager who is bearing the message, staff are likely to listen to positive experiences of peers in other units. For example, technological advancements resulting in a change from handwritten documentation to computerized documentation may face less resistance

if staff have an opportunity to hear firsthand positive experiences from staff on the pilot unit. Almost everyone is willing to obey directives they have imposed on themselves, such as changing shift hours on a unit so there will be less difficulty finding a place to park, or agreement that everyone will wear a particular color scrub suit.

There is an optimal level of information that any one person can integrate and comprehend. With too little information, employees feel as if they are not being kept abreast of all that is happening. At the other extreme, too much information produces an overload. If employees are inundated with too much information, they cannot sort out what is important and what is not. Although research shows that job satisfaction increases with increasing amounts of information, it also shows that employees' job performance is rated lower by their superiors than is that of subordinates who are not overloaded with information (8). Error rates escalate when too much information is provided. In other words, past some optimal point, too much information leads to decreased decision making performance. When information overload occurs, staff have so much information that they are unsure what direction to take. Ambiguity and confusion occur as staff attempt to sort out what information is important and relevant to their work and what is not.

A nurse manager's communication with patients and their families serves at least four functions. It regulates behavior of the patient by explaining the need for them to comply with a treatment plan. It solicits their input into the plan so that the formulation of the plan will incorporate all aspects of patient needs, both physical and psychosocial. It comforts and soothes. It develops a relationship between the patient, the patient's family, and the nurse, and it transmits information (9). Although the most effective communication between a nurse and the patient and family is personal face to face, a printed brochure explaining procedures and policies can be very helpful. If that is not available, a unit newsletter can be used. It in no way replaces face-to-face communication but often serves to accentuate necessary information (10). Having a family member in an intensive care unit is stressful for both the patient and the family member, and having information in writing reinforces information that may be easily forgotten by a person undergoing stress.

Communication between nurses and physicians

is crucial to patient care. It is a part of the role of the nurse manager to facilitate the communication process between the physician and the staff nurse. As such, the nurse manager must emphasize to the staff nurse the importance of proper documentation and verbal communication. Simply writing in the patient's record will not suffice in many cases, the court has decided. "The nurse who documents critical observations in the patient's record but who does not communicate verbally to ensure the information is received will not be insulated against liability in the event that the patient suffers harm" (Ref. 11, p. 1597). Any information that the nurse receives that could result in a change of doctor's orders must be transmitted to the physician as clearly and quickly as possible. The nurse manager must also emphasize that the staff nurse has both a right not only to receive from the physician a decision regarding the information transmitted by the staff nurse but also a duty to document what that decision was, even if the decision was "I'll be right there."

Nurses often feel that they are left out of the decision making loop on critical care units. When life and death decisions must be made, physicians and nurses come into conflict over areas of decision making and role definition in highly stressful cases (12). Although studies show that no dichotomy exists between physicians' preferences and nurses' preferences when it comes to making life and death decisions, nurses often feel they have no voice in the decision making process. Critical care managers can help to enhance nurse-physician understanding by participating in such activities as serving on joint practice committees and jointly writing patient management policies and protocols.

Staff meetings are an opportunity for the manager to build, monitor, and maintain the communication network of the unit. Quarterly personal meetings with each staff member provide a means for individually coaching staff and encouraging them in their work (13), although this may not be feasible for managers of critical care units with a large number of staff members.

Effective management involves coaching employees to be as good as they can be. Employees have reasonable expectations of managers. They expect the opportunity to do their job; to be kept informed of matters affecting their work; to receive appropriate rewards for their contributions; to receive regular feedback about how well they are doing; and to receive whatever support, guidance, and training are necessary to do the job. To receive these, however, the manager must be able to communicate personal expectations of employees clearly and to give specific feedback on what they are doing right and what they are doing wrong. It is insufficient to rely on semiannual or annual performance reviews to iron out problems or compliment good work. Both compliments and corrections need to be given at the time the act occurs. Giving immediate feedback to staff lets them know what they are doing well and what needs to be improved. Such communication removes ambiguity and helps staff understand what is expected of them. This style of giving immediate feedback coaches staff and helps them improve their work habits before they make a mistake (14). Holding back from confrontation may be the easiest route to take when an employee has done a poor job in a task, but it is better to risk upsetting the subordinate and give feedback immediately after the behavior. It also allows the manager to determine whether the poor job is due to lack of understanding, lack of knowledge, lack of motivation, or lack of ability.

A way of highlighting good performance is through a "positive incident report." It can be instituted on the unit by the nurse manager so that all staff are encouraged to report positive acts they observe. A daily or weekly review of the positive incidents accompanied by positive feedback enhances the self-esteem of staff members at all levels and also fosters positive attitudes about the work environment in general.

## BARRIERS TO EFFECTIVE COMMUNICATION

There are a number of conditions that stand in the way of a message being clearly communicated. Although senders know the message they want to communicate, receivers interpret the message according to their own expectations, rather than the sender's. The list that follows explains barriers that block clear communication.

1. There may be perceived homophyly. People are more likely to speak with those whom they perceive to be similar to themselves. This is called *perceived homophyly*. When there are status or socioeconomic differences, they tend not to talk openly. This is true whether there is a nurse-patient communication, nurse-nurse communication, nurse-family communica-

tion, nurse-physician communication, or any level of employer-employee communication. Often administrators like to brag that they have an open door and any employee is welcome to drop in and talk with them whenever they choose. The reality of the situation is that this will rarely occur. Although it seems and sounds like a good idea, few employees will take advantage of open doors for two reasons. The first is that the person at the higher rank is perceived to be different from those at lower ranks. The second reason is that staff know not to bypass the chain of command. The nurse manager, often perceived by staff members as "not a real nurse anymore," may initially have to seek out staff members on an individual basis at frequent intervals if the manager's open door policy is to be realistically implemented. Additionally, the critical care nurse manager must recognize the position of the nurse manager as either a conduit or a barrier when the divisional manager has an open door policy for staff nurses as well as nurse managers.

2. There may be sanctions against circumventing the chain of command. Employees risk a great deal by appearing to take problems over their own supervisor's head. A better strategy for opening lines of communication is to take the initiative and sporadically visit all shifts. Nurses on the unit are flattered by visits and are more willing to express concerns when the manager has come to them. The critical care manager can further enhance communication opportunities by speaking to a few staff members on an individual, informal basis, such as saying, "I just came to look around and see for myself what a good job you've been doing. Is there anything on your mind you'd like to talk with me about? Anything you think I should be aware of?" Research shows that circulating among employees, talking with them, and observing conditions firsthand is much more revealing than sitting in one's office and receiving answers to direct questions in a planned interview (15, 16).

3. The message intended may or may not be the message received. There are three dimensions to communicating: the message intended by the sender, the message heard by the receiver, and the consequence of the message. The consequence may be desired action, undesired ac-

tion, or no action. A communication rarely means precisely the same thing to those who receive it as it does for the sender. People interpret messages in the context of their expectations about how others behave, what is expected of them, and how they are perceived by whomever is sending the message. It is fair to say that people "twist" communications to fit their own view of the world and of the people around them (5, 17, 18).

Total accuracy in communication requires that two persons have identical histories of shared experiences, much as identical twins who were raised together might have. This rarely occurs, of course. What does happen is what is called selective perception and selective reception. People perceive parts of the message and disregard other parts. The challenge to the communicator is to send the message in such a way that the message gets past the individual's internal filtering process. Studies indicate that managers shape their communications with employees in a manner consistent with what they expect their employees' reaction to be to the message (19). If a critical care manager expects staff to respond in a hostile manner to an announcement, the message is often delivered in an authoritarian style with little room for discussion. This is an example: "The nurse will notify the unit no less than 2 hours before the beginning of the shift if illness prevents working that shift. Failure to comply, except in an emergency, will result in a 3-day suspension without pay." However, if the expectation is that the message will be liked, then it is delivered in a relaxed tone: "We are pleased to announce that the Friday immediately following Thanksgiving Day will also be recognized as a holiday." The tone itself mediates the message, and in the case of a message that may be disliked, an aggressive tone compounds hostility from employees. Being aware that the tone of a message influences its reception helps the manager to soften unpleasant news or enhance good news: "We've had a problem with people calling in too near the beginning of the next shift to adequately give time to find someone to cover. I need to remind everyone that the hospital policy states that you must call in at least 2 hours before the beginning of the shift if you are unable to work, and that failure to comply except in an emergency will result in a 3-day suspension without pay. However, I'm certain we will all work together to be certain we don't leave our fellow nurses without enough help. I know everyone will do their best to cooperate so that no shift will be left having to scramble for help.'' This message, delivered in a positive, enthusiastic manner, will serve to help foster a cooperative and positive attitude of unity rather than an isolationist and hostile individual attitude.

4. Senders distort information to protect themselves. They will not send messages they judge irrelevant or harmful to themselves. On the other hand, they typically will send messages they believe are helpful to them. Thus a political dimension to communicating is present in any exchange of information. The nurse manager may receive good news from the staff while bad news is buried. The decision to transmit information is a personal decision, as is the text of the message. For this reason, good news flows freely up and down and across the hospital, while bad news remains trapped. Even when bad news is sent up the chain of command, the content of the information undergoes changes. Problems will be presented in their best possible light to diminish their impact, or they will be exaggerated to make a point, depending on how the sender hopes to benefit from the message.

By the time a message reaches the administrator it may have serious errors of omission or commission within it. As the message travels, it is mediated by receivers' and senders' expectations. Although employees want to be treated on a personal basis as individuals, the manager attempts to be impersonal and objective and to treat all employees uniformly. This gives rise to different interpretations and different inflections as the message travels from directors of nursing to critical care managers to bedside nurses. The result is that the unique meaning of the words as they were intended and used by the sender differs from how they are actually interpreted by the receiver.

5. Crises increase the probability that messages will be distorted. When the nurse is tense and overworked, almost any message can appear threatening. Rumors spread through the hospital grapevine, based on partial messages.

Having too little time complicates matters for busy nurse managers. A sense of urgency limits the time available to search for explanatory information when a quick decision is necessary. Relatively few people can be involved in making a quick decision, and personnel affected by the decision are insulted that they were not asked to participate in the decision making. The result is that there is an excessively narrow decision making process and there is no consensus that the solution reached is the best one.

### Example of a Crisis Decision

Consider the following situation: A patient is admitted to the hospital to await an organ transplant. The attending physician is known not only to be a competent physician but also a ruthless critic of the nursing staff. Additionally the physician is obsessive about each patient's medication protocol being followed to the minute, despite the policy of the hospital allowing a 30-minute leeway from the exact time. Because transplant patients are frequently on numerous potent medications, the staff understands the necessity for exact adherence to the protocols. The nurse managers of the' floors and the critical care units have repeatedly asked the physician to provide written guidelines that can be applied to all patients awaiting organ transplant. With a particular new admission, the resident covering the patient for the night has determined that the patient needs the closer monitoring of the intensive care unit as the patient's condition has become extremely unstable. The medication orders have been changed from the specific times noted by the attending physician on the admission orders to new times written by the resident. Previous orders are automatically canceled when the patient is transferred. New orders must be written by the physician ordering the transfer for every drug, meal, and activity.

In an attempt to be absolutely certain that the medication given is what the resident intended and at the time the resident intended, the critical care staff nurse telephones the resident and calls attention to the discrepancy between the original order and the transfer order with regard to medication administration times. The resident orders the medication to be given as the new orders state, and the nurse documents in the patient's chart that the resident was contacted for clarification and confirmation. The following day the critical care manager is contacted by an angry attending physician demanding to know why the medications were not given as originally ordered, including at the specific times ordered by the attending physician. The nurse manager assures the physician that the matter will be thoroughly examined, and additionally requests that the attending physician submit guidelines for medication administration of pretransplant medications to pretransplant patients so that a medication protocol for those patients can be established in that particular critical care area. In this transaction, without specifically stating it, the nurse manager managed to indicate to the physician that if the guidelines requested by the manager had been available to the resident and the staff, the problem could have been avoided. Conversely, had the real, not illusory, authority to change the medication schedule been delegated to the resident, there would have been no problem.

This case demonstrates that decisions often must be made under conditions of real or perceived crisis, that those decisions often may not involve all relevant parties, and that the decision reached, although perhaps understandable under the circumstances, may be erroneous. In this particular circumstance, the critical care manager had to deal with an attending physician who was angry at being eliminated from the decision making process as well as a staff nurse who was defensive about having carried out a legal order from a resident.

6. The presentation of the communication may be awkward. The presentation of a message serves as a help or a hindrance to communication. A long memorandum that is difficult to read will not be understood or remembered as well as a brief memorandum that gets directly to the point and clearly presents the information. Short paragraphs of three or four sentences are preferable to long paragraphs. Headings in a document make it easy for the reader to scan the page and find the information being sought. In oral communication, the speaker's style will be a major help or obstacle in ensuring that the message is received as intended.

7. There may be a perceived job threat. Barriers are inherent in a hierarchy. Employees are reluctant to speak up or disagree on issues because they may fear angering their supervisor and receiving a poor performance evaluation later, or even having their job threatened. They also may be uncomfortable challenging the nurse manager, or they may believe, whether or not it is true, that the manager is vindictive and will "get even" later. All of these barriers pose obstacles to communication and reflect a concern on the part of employees that messages given to a critical care manager or nursing administrator will not be received in an open, constructive atmosphere. Knowing how to disagree constructively with a supervisor or an employee is an important communication skill (20).

8. Mediated messages are altered with each new sender. Communication traveling down the chain of command can become as distorted as that traveling upward. Each link in the chain of communication is a place for modifying the message. Administrators send one message and assume it will be received by the unit nurse in the same form it was sent. But by the time it has been interpreted and paraphrased by intermediaries, it arrives on the unit with accumulated changes. Something as relatively straightforward as a new, written hospital policy will be subjected to oral interpretation of its meaning through the various levels of administration. When it reaches the staff nurse working on the unit, the interpretation given by the unit manager as to the meaning of the new policy may bear slight resemblance to the spirit of the original meaning. The unit manager merely reports the personal interpretation of the interpretation given by the divisional manager of the interpretation given by the interdivisional manager of the interpretation given by the nursing director of what the hospital director intended to say! It is important that the nurse manager allow adequate time for the staff to read new policies and then invite discussion to clarify any misconceptions as to the proper interpretation and implementation of the new policies. This may also require the manager to return to the appropriate administrator for further clarification, repeating the entire process as frequently as necessary to ensure full and appropriate interpretation and implementation of the policies.

9. Another barrier is erected when the communication is of one style while the receiver is expecting another. "Tell and sell," "tell and listen," and "problem solving" are three examples (5). "Tell and sell" communication are face-to-face communications in which the sender tells the nurse about an issue and proceeds to sell the nurse on an idea the sender has. It is an authoritarian approach that leaves little room for the receiver to respond. It is a one-way communication, such as: "Scrub suits, even white ones, will no longer be acceptable wear for work on this unit."

"Tell and listen" communications are those in which the sender tells the nurse information and then listens for the nurse's reaction. This form of communication requires active listening skills of the sender to hear and understand how the receiver responds. This method engenders less hostility and less tension than the "tell and sell" method. Consider this statement by the nurse manager: "Scrub suits that are being worn by many of the staff look sloppy. They're wrinkled and don't give the patients or their families a good impression." When a statement such as this is followed up by the sender listening to the receiver's reaction, then "tell and listen" communication is occurring.

"Problem solving" is an interactive method that requires presenting the problem and listening and responding constructively to the ideas put forth. "It looks like a lot of the staff want to wear scrub suits, but they come to work in wrinkled ones. The patients and the families don't get a very good impression of the professionalism of our unit based on the way the staff looks, even though I know everyone is very competent clinically. How can we improve our image while allowing some variety in uniforms?" This approach is one the nurse manager can use that is most likely to result in an improved appearance of staff.

10. Qualities of the receiver also influence the message. The receiver's values, perceptions, and perception of self as well as perception of the sender affect whether the message is evaluated positively or negatively. For example: "No one ever notices when I do a good job, but let me mess up and everyone comes down on me. I don't think administration really cares at all about us down here doing the real work, so why should I care what they have

to say?" This statement serves as an example of an employee whose supervisor has failed to communicate understanding of the demands and stresses employees must encounter every day. The perception by staff that the manager does not understand raises a communication barrier that blocks the manager's intended message from being received.

## HOW EFFECTIVE COMMUNICATION IMPROVES PRODUCTIVITY

Effective communication increases job satisfaction, which in turn enhances recruitment and retention of quality staff. This is because the quality of the communication determines the climate of the unit. The climate may be one of warmth and support or one of cold uncaring. The concept of climate is intertwined with communication, because it is largely communication that determines the climate. The amount of communication and degree of coordination on a unit affects how smoothly the unit operates and how much support there is for individual needs and concerns. In turn, the climate affects the turnover rate. In warmer, more supportive climates, staff are more likely to enjoy their work and want to remain. In colder climates there is less social fulfillment, and people are more likely to leave (21).

Climate is determined by a number of factors including the degree to which employees are given responsibility for their work, the degree to which the hospital gives appropriate rewards for work, the degree to which employees support one another in their work, the degree to which the hospital sets high standards for performance, and the degree to which conflicts are acknowledged and resolved (21). A positive, strong team spirit results from a supportive climate that rewards accomplishments.

Studies show that employees who report a high level of consideration from their supervisors perform significantly better than those who report their supervisors do not show them consideration. Employees who are shown consideration also report a greater degree of commitment to the organization (22, 23). This indicates that effective leadership is directly related to the ability to communicate a sense of caring to employees. Social support and closely related concepts of interpersonal warmth, trust, and openness are core dimensions of a constructive communication climate within a hospital. Using the "positive incidents report" mentioned earlier, along with a public recognition of the positive incident, communicates to employees that the manager is supportive of their work. This positive atmosphere promotes job satisfaction, a greater likelihood of better patient outcomes, and trust among staff. In turn, this promotes more sharing and more open communication and thus reduces the risk of unusual incidents and errors. Open communication also promotes a workforce that is more likely to be adaptable when changes are necessary because they have been kept abreast of events leading up to the necessary change. As communication increases between nurses, physicians, patients, and families, there is an additional payoff. The positive atmosphere reduces the potential for litigation because patients and families are kept informed about a patient's condition and treatment. All in all, a more positive attitude surrounds the unit. This translates into benefits for the hospital, as positive attitudes toward the workplace enhance recruitment efforts and lessen staff turnover.

Time spent communicating effectively is time well spent, similar to a sound investment that produces both short-term and long-term dividends. In order to communicate effectively, choose the best sender and best channel available to send information. The sender should transmit the message in a language and style that the receiver will understand. The communication process is an iterative one. After the message has been sent, the communicator becomes the receiver and listens for feedback. A list of six rules summarizes how to communicate effectively.

1. *Keep it simple.* A good rule of thumb is to use short sentences and paragraphs. Unnecessary words obscure the meaning. Use the shortest, simplest words to convey the meaning. "End" is just as effective as "terminate" and it is easier to read. Define terms whenever necessary to rule out alternative or contradictory interpretations. Be as concrete and specific as possible. Attractively package the message with clear readable type. A scribbled message is much less likely to be taken seriously than a neatly typed memorandum. Typographical errors, misspellings, and grammatical errors detract from the message.

    Remember that too much information is as bad as too little information. Tell people what they need to know and stop. The "golden rule" of communicating is to communicate to others as you would have others communicate to you.

Another golden rule is that the mind can absorb only what the seat can endure. Tell what needs to be told. If people want to know more, give them the opportunity to ask but do not inundate them with information that may obscure the essence of the message (24).

2. *Tell it like it is.* Beating around the bush only obscures the message. Clearly state the message. This goes hand in hand with the rule to keep it simple. Telling it like it is in language too complex for easy comprehension obscures the message.

3. *Validate before you communicate.* In other words, make sure the information you are about to give is accurate. Avoid having to rescind or qualify a memorandum you have just sent. If you send one message on Monday, then rethink your plans on Tuesday and Wednesday and send a new plan on Thursday, eventually staff learn to wait several days before implementing any directives you send. Although thorough validation will not guarantee that you will never have to retract information, consistent validation attempts will reassure the staff and minimize the number of retractions.

4. *Vary the methods utilized to send information.* Some messages are transmitted more effectively in face-to-face meetings while others are better when they appear in formal memoranda. Still others, especially those that are complex, are better when presented both orally and in writing. For example, the following case shows how a combination of channels work.

Communication through Multiple Channels

The posted notice states "The new pulmonary artery catheter insertion packs are here!" Each staff member receives a memorandum stating how to order the pack, where it will be kept on the unit, and what items are included in the pack. The critical care manager demonstrates the pack and utilization of its contents to the charge nurses for each shift and requests that the charge nurses demonstrate it to the staff at the beginning of the shift. The manager also identifies a location and times when a demonstration pack will be available for the staff to examine and become familiar with the contents. A method for feedback regarding problems, physician requests, additions, or alterations to the pack is identified and left in place for a specified period of time.

5. *Utilize humor where appropriate*. People tend to remember messages that have pleasant connotations and are more likely to disregard those that are unpleasant. A message wrapped with humor will help get it across and remembered. Consider whether a cartoon could be used to get the point across. Who could forget a green streetwalker named ''Sue DeMonas'' on an ''Unwanted'' poster, posted conspicuously on the staff restroom wall?

6. *Listen and clarify*. Active listening is a skill. Listen with a minimum of emotion to avoid biasing your interpretation of the message. Respond with positive regard, rather than dislike, inasmuch as the latter only causes the sender to become defensive. Be an unemotional and impartial audience. Use reflection and restatement to be certain you have clearly understood the message being sent. Be aware of allowing hostility and defensiveness to color both your reception and transmission of messages in potentially volatile situations.

Effective communication occurs when the message is clear and unambiguous. To achieve this, it must be expressed in terms that are easily understood. Both the words and the feelings which accompany them must be conveyed and received accurately. If a message is sent with warmth but is received in the context of hostility, it will result in a reaction far different from what was intended. The goal of communicating is to send a message that is received, understood, and acted upon just as the communicator intended. This is the challenge of communication for critical care nurse managers.

REFERENCES

1. Pincus JD. Communication: key contributor to effectiveness—the research. J Nurs Admin 1986;16(9):19–25.
2. DiSalvo VS, Larsen JK. A contingency approach to communication skill importance: the impact of occupation, direction, and position. J Bus Commun 1987;24(3):3–22.
3. Wurzell C. Putting communication skills into practice. Assoc Operating Room Nurses' J 1981;33:962–971.
4. Swanson E. Information channel disposition and use. Decision Sci 1987;18:131–145.
5. Schacter HL. Public agency communication: theory and practice. Chicago: Nelson Hall, 1983.
6. Levson E, Guy ME. Information channels for critical care nurses. Dimensions Crit Care Nurs 1987;6(1):40–46.
7. Randolph WA. Understanding and managing organizational behavior. Homewood, Illinois: Richard D Irwin, Inc, 1985.
8. O'Reilly III CA. Individuals and information overload in organizations: is more necessarily better? Acad Management J 1980;23:684–696.
9. Kasch CR, Lisnek PM. Role of strategic communication in nursing theory and research. Adv Nurs Sci 1984;7(1):56–71.
10. Jeffcoate JA. Improving communication in a special care baby unit. Early Hum Devel 1979;3,4:341–344.
11. Cushing M. Failure to communicate. Am J Nurs 1982;82:1597–1598.
12. Allen ML, Jackson D, Youngner S. Closing the communication gap between physicians and nurses in the intensive care unit setting. Heart & Lung, 1980;9:836–840.
13. Spicer, JG, Macioce VL. Retention: sound communications keep a critical care staff together. Nurs Management 1987;18(5):64A–64F.
14. Axmith M. Coaching and counseling: a vital role for managers. Bus Q 1982;47:44–53.
15. Andrews JR. On the horns of a personnel dilemma. Personnel J 1985;64:93–98.
16. Jones JW, McLeod R Jr. The structure of executive information systems: an exploratory analysis. Decision Sci 1986;17:220–249.
17. Chartier MR. Clarity of expression in interpersonal communication. J Nurs Admin 1981;11(7):42–46.
18. Klingner, DE. Public administration: a management approach. Boston: Houghton Mifflin Co, 1983.
19. McCallister L. Predicted employee compliance to downward communication styles. J Bus Commun 1983;20:67–79.
20. St John WD. Successful communications between supervisors and employees. Personnel J 1983;15:71–77.
21. Poole MS. In McPhee RD, Tompkins PK, eds. Organizational communication: traditional themes and new directions. Beverly Hills, California: Sage Publications, 1985:79–108.
22. Kirmeyer SL, Lin TR. Social support: its relationship to observed communication with peers and superiors. Acad Management J 1987;30:130–151.
23. Penley LE, Hawkins B. Studying interpersonal communication in organizations: a leadership application. Acad Management J 1985;28:309–326.
24. Eisenberg EM, Witten MG. Reconsidering openness in organizational communication. Acad Management Rev 1987;12:418–426.

# Chapter 10

# Retaining Qualified Staff

SUSAN L. CHAMBERLAIN
JANE RUZANSKI
SHIRLEY KOCZAN
ANNETTE M. PINGRY
CHERYL SIROIS

Retention of qualified nurses is a major concern at all levels of nursing leadership. Nationally, the average vacancy rate for hospital nursing positions is reported at 13–14% (1). This figure is even higher for critical care positions. At the same time vacancy rates are climbing, the demand for nurses is increasing and enrollment in schools of nursing is decreasing. Factors cited for the decline in enrollment include fewer young people of career age in the general population, a greater number of career choices available to women, and a devaluing of service-related professions in favor of more lucrative opportunities.

Even if nursing supply issues were not of concern, the loss of nurses through turnover has other serious consequences affecting both the budget and the delivery of high quality care. The recruitment and orientation of a critical care nurse is estimated to cost between $7000 and $8000 (2). This cost is based on recruitment expense plus a period of education and skill acquisition during which a nurse cannot contribute productively to the staffing of a unit. It does not reflect the additional costs for overtime or agency personnel when turnover has an impact on the numbers required for safe staffing.

Uncontrolled turnover can quickly affect the sense of cohesion and morale of a unit. Most nurses want to work with colleagues they know and trust, yet when frequent changes in personnel occur, familiarity and trust are undermined. Nurses can easily become dissatisfied, which limits energy available for patient care. Moreover, effective communication and collaboration have been identified as key variables influencing morbidity and mortality outcomes in critical care units (3). Interpersonal effort of this nature must have a firm foundation in group trust and cohesiveness.

The loss of qualified staff over time may result in a general decline in the level of competence on a unit making it difficult to maintain or improve standards of care. Failure to retain nurses who understand unit and organizational values will ultimately erode propagation of these values. When human values are not deeply entrenched in an organization, there are clear consequences for staff and the quality of patient care. To attract nurses initially, an institution must sustain a reputation for excellence and provide the kind of environment in which nurses choose to work.

Given the diminishing supply of nurses and the adverse effects of turnover, the successful nurse manager must assign highest priority to the retention of qualified staff. Effective retention strategies will be based on an understanding of the number and complexity of factors influencing nurse job satisfaction in the critical care setting. The ability to anticipate and plan for turnover will help to minimize the effects.

This chapter is intended to assist the nurse manager in identifying retention factors cited in the literature and corroborated by a survey of critical care nurses in a magnet hospital noted for its ability to attract and retain nurses. Next the chapter will explore the nurse manager's role in retaining qualified staff, including the impact of managerial style. Assessment and use of turnover statistics will also be discussed. Finally retention strategies of both a professional and institutional nature will be examined.

## RETENTION FACTORS: A REVIEW OF THE LITERATURE

Job satisfaction has been linked to turnover and found to be a key factor in retention of personnel. What satisfies or dissatisfies critical care nurses?

A review of the literature reveals a number of nursing studies that have identified factors relating to job satisfaction.

Larson et al. (4) correlated the level of job satisfaction with actual expectations. They found that high levels of job satisfaction were related to professional issues and that nurses were least satisfied with employment issues such as salary and staffing. They concluded that a "major focus should be placed on differential expectations at time of entry and the extent to which these are met or altered over the course of employment" (4). It is important to identify perceptions on entry to the job and provide sufficient information to avoid unrealistic expectations.

A study by Blenkarn et al. (5) examined the influence of primary nursing on job satisfaction. They found that job satisfaction increased on both of the two units studied. Increases were noted in the following areas: professional status, administration, nurse-physician relationships, and autonomy. The authors concluded that job satisfaction appeared to be positively influenced by primary nursing.

Simpson (6) conducted a study looking at sources of job satisfaction and dissatisfaction reported by nurses. Nurses at all levels overwhelmingly identified dissatisfaction with their work and work environment in the nursing service hierarchy. For the staff nurse group, the major dissatisfactions were social status, company policies and practices, advancement, creativity, compensation, working conditions, supervision, human relations, and recognition.

Mottaz (7) also found a lower level of work satisfaction when comparing nurses to other professional occupations. Correlates of the low level of work satisfaction were low levels of task autonomy, supervisory assistance, salary, and some lack of task involvement.

Hinshaw et al. (2) demonstrated that organizational job satisfaction for critical care nurses was strongly predicted by job stress, group cohesion, and control over practice in terms of personal resources. For both organizational and professional job satisfaction, the major stressor was found to be team respect. Professional growth and being recognized as professionals were also seen as producing high satisfaction and promoting retention.

In a study by Weisman (8), perceived autonomy was the strongest predictor of job satisfaction. Nurses were most concerned about control over their work

and the ability to make decisions on work conduct. Nurses were least satisfied with hours and scheduling, opportunity for advancement, and the prospect for future earnings.

Froebe et al. (9) based a study on Herzberg's "Motivation-Hygiene Theory" and Maslow's "Need Theory." They looked at the importance of motivators, hygiene factors, and the degree to which these were met in the nurse's workplace. Hygiene factors rated as very important were shift assignment, educational opportunities, supervisor and coworker relationships, and salary. Accomplishments, recognition, accountability, working in a clinical area, and nurse-patient ratio were the motivators rated as most important.

Alspach (10) reported results of a CRITICAL CARE NURSE readership survey on the shortage of critical care nurses. Reasons for staying in critical care were reported as (in ranked order): "(1) enjoy the challenge, (2) like 1:1 holistic care, (3) interested, learn a lot, (4) feel I can make a difference, (5) I like/love it, (6) like critical care patients, (7) like direct patient care, (8) prefer over floor nursing, (9) affords more autonomy, (10) need money to pay bills."

Reasons for leaving (also ranked in order) were as follows: "(1) burnout/stress, (2) understaffing, (3) work schedules, (4) salary too low for responsiblity, (5) receive no respect or recognition, (6) lack of administrative support, (7) physical and emotional fatigue, (8) poor nurse-physician relationships, (9) risk of contracting diseases, (10) political and bureaucratic hassles, (11) legal risks from working understaffed, (12) no opportunity for advancement" (10). Solutions proposed by readers to improve recruitment and retention of critical care nurses were in the following areas: salary, stress, staffing, stature, schedules, support, schooling, and status.

Ruffing et al. (11) identified several factors that could attract and retain nurses in hospitals: better salary, flexible hours, better staffing, educational opportunities and assistance, improved nurse-physician relationships, increased employee participation in decision making, and day care.

Career advancement programs have also been cited as an important recruitment/retention tool. Vestal (12) describes the multitrack career advancement program (PACE) at Hermann Hospital in Houston. Administration, clinical, education, and research tracks provide for upward and lateral mobility. PACE includes a residency program, performance appraisal system, and career consultant position.

An innovative recruitment/retention program is recounted by Wall (13). This program involves the role of the nurse recruiter in establishing an ongoing relationship with new employees. The recruiter conducts follow-up interviews, assists in the identification of problems, and provides feedback to administration.

Personal factors such as stress, burnout, and personal hardiness have been studied in relationship to nurse retention. These factors often lead to decreased job satisfaction and increased turnover. Hardiness is a personality characteristic of individuals who remain healthy after experiencing high degrees of stress. High levels of stress in critical care areas can also lead to emotional exhaustion and burnout.

Burnout in intensive care unit (ICU) nurses was looked at in a study by Bartz and Maloney (14). Their findings showed that the longer a nurse remains in nursing, the less she is likely to experience burnout. ICU nurses less prone to burnout are older, have less than a baccalaureate degree, and have civilian status.

McCraine et al. (15) studied the association between hardiness and burnout in both critical care nurses and non-critical care nurses. They found that nurses with less personal hardiness reported more burnout and those with more frequent work-related stress experienced more burnout. Hardiness appeared to reduce burnout but did not prevent burnout with high levels of job stress. The authors suggested it may be valuable to assess hardiness at the time of interview but cautioned that this strategy alone is not sufficient to prevent burnout. Organizational efforts to promote social support, improve staffing and scheduling, implement conflict management strategies, and improve organizational communication were recommended.

Values and characteristics of hospitals that have been successful in nurse retention are also important to review. Kramer and Schmalenberg (16) identify these values and characteristics in the magnet hospital study report. This follow-up study of the 16 magnet hospitals describes the characteristics of excellence present in each.

Institutions of excellence have a degree of fluidity and informality that allows for quick exchange of information and communication at all levels of the organization. Nursing leadership has the ability to solve problems quickly. A proactive stance and approachability of nursing leadership generate trust between staff and the leadership team.

Management in the magnet hospitals rewards the values of quality and service in their employees. Patients must feel that they are special; individualized, quality care is paramount. The extent and quality of support services enable the nurse to stay close to the patient and to deliver high quality care. Nurse managers care about the nursing staff with the same intensity that nurses care about the patients.

Autonomy and entrepreneurship are valued. Autonomy empowers nurses by enabling them to provide quality care. Nurses are encouraged to offer their ideas and opinions and to act within the full scope of their professional knowledge.

Respect for the individual is characteristic of the magnet hospitals. People are treated with dignity and provided with high performance expectations. Recognition and rewards for performance are key to productivity and high performance. Peer evaluation is valued and encouraged.

A major role of leadership is creating, instilling, and clarifying the value system of the institution, but success is dependent on the creation of a staff that shares the same values. Selection of new nurses who have a value system consistent with the institution is critical to perpetuation of the value system.

A decentralized nursing department with a minimum of administrative levels enforces autonomy of several small adaptive units. Nurse managers determine their own unit-based policies and standards within a larger institutional framework.

The magnet hospitals share simultaneous "loose-tight" properties. The climate is loose in terms of individual autonomy, flexible organizational structure, experimentation, copious feedback, and informality. It is tight in terms of a controlled set of rigidly shared values. Kramer and Schmalenberg (17) recommend that hospitals create conditions to prevent an "internal" nursing shortage (i.e., a shortage within their own institution) when the rest of the profession is faced with a severe "external" shortage.

An informal survey of critical care nurses at Beth Israel Hospital in Boston, Massachusetts, supports the literature (18). When asked what attracted them to the institution, nurses cited professional issues such as reputation, primary nursing, and professional work environment (see Table 10.1).

Nurses who have stayed in their units longer than 2 years were asked their reasons for staying.

**Table 10.1** Important Recruitment and Retention Factors of Critical Care Nurses Surveyed at Beth Israel Hospital, Boston, Massachusetts[a]

| Attraction to the Setting | Attraction to the Intensive Care Unit |
|---|---|
| Reputation | Primary nursing |
| Primary nursing | Surgical unit |
| Professional environment | Comprehensive orientation |
| Nurses like to work here | Increased opportunity for learning |
| Liked interviews | Challenge of an ICU |
| Attractive size hospital | Invasive monitoring |
| Nursing opportunities and benefits | Type of patients |
| Salary | Variety of patients |
| Close to home | Flexible weekend scheduling |
| Concept of earned time | 4-day work week |
| | Modern |
| | Clean |
| | Did not need previous ICU experience |

| Reasons for Staying | |
|---|---|
| *Practice Issues* | *Administrative* |
| Primary nursing | Nursing management style |
| Clinical ladder | Decentralized nursing department |
| Reputation of staff | Support of nursing administration |
| Respect for nurses | Care about employees |
| Professional growth | |
| Autonomy | |
| Participation in decision making | |
| *Education* | *Staffing* |
| Unit-based specialist | Type of patients |
| Continuing education (CE) opportunities | Better staffing than most |
| | Peer group |
| | Cohesive staff |
| *Scheduling* | *Pay and Benefits* |
| 4-day work week | Pay scale |
| Flexibility of schedule | Frequent pay raises |
| Shift overlap benefits | Earned time |
| Not floating | |
| Weekend schedule (every third weekend) | |
| *Environment* | |
| Clean, well-maintained | |
| Adequate supplies | |
| Free coffee | |
| Work environment satisfying | |

[a]From Shields A, Koczan S, Sirois C. Critical care retention survey. Unpublished survey, Beth Israel Hospital, Boston, Massachusetts, May 1988.

Practice issues cited were primary nursing, professional nurse recognition and advancement program, reputation of the nursing staff, autonomy, and participation in decision making. Overall they felt supported by nursing administration and liked the management style and decentralized nursing structure. From a developmental perspective, they found continuing education opportunities and presence of a unit-based specialist to be significant retention factors. Also mentioned were scheduling, pay and benefits, environment, and staffing. The nurses surveyed believed that their unit was better staffed than most and that having a cohesive staff was important.

## ROLE AND STYLE OF THE NURSE MANAGER IN RETAINING STAFF

Recent nursing literature is rich with data regarding cause of turnover in hospitals and suggested retention strategies. One theme that emerges consistently is the nurse's relationship with the manager. Campbell reports that 60% of the staff of a critical care unit saw leadership style as a major factor in job satisfaction and job-related stress (19). Prescott and Bowen (20) found that a major work-related reason for resignation "focused largely on head nurse characteristics and behavior." In a study by Duxbury et al. (21), burnout among ICU nurses was mediated by the leadership style of the head nurse. Vincent and Billings (22) studied ICU nursing personnel and reported that management of the unit was ranked as the major stressor by all respondents.

Managing nurses in critical care units poses a unique challenge. Critical care nurses usually have previous experience in another clinical area. They are older with more life experience and personal obligations. Critical care nurses are often confident in their clinical skills and need to be recognized for their achievements and knowledge. They want professional status and a work environment geared toward self-actualization. These needs must be met in the context of a setting that is fast paced, highly stressful, and confounded by ethical dilemmas and issues of serious illness and death.

Given the characteristics and context of critical care nurses, the successful ICU manager will adopt a collegial style, emphasizing consultation and support for staff. The nurse manager must provide a framework for the unit oriented in caring, professional practice, and commitment to group goals. Responsiveness to individual and collective concerns will further enhance effectiveness.

Fundamental to nurse retention is the nurse manager's role in creating a professionally enhancing work environment. Each nurse must understand group goals and the collective mission of the nursing staff. Establishing unit expectations and examining personal values and beliefs start with the initial employment interview. It is through this process that the nurse manager sets the tone of the professional environment or climate he or she wishes to promote.

Setting high, but achievable, expectations acknowledges individual worth and potential contribution to a unit. Clear goals and standards help to align new staff members around a common purpose from the very beginning. Each new nurse should understand the expectations regarding patient care, peer relationships, leadership, and communication. To avoid future disappointment, the nurse needs to know what to expect in terms of nurse/patient ratios, time scheduling, fringe benefits, and the culture of the unit.

Additionally, the nurse manager should clarify what the new employee can expect from the manager and the work environment. For example, in a primary nurse setting the new nurse can expect to give direct patient care and have authority and accountability for decisions. The nurse will also be guided to specific resources to help with this care. He or she can expect the nurse manager to assist in the nurse's personal growth and development through mutual goal setting, support, and evaluation.

Ultimately, it is incumbent upon the nurse manager and the interviewee to decide whether there is a "philosophical fit" between the needs of the nurse and the needs of the unit. To further strengthen group goals it is important to have staff members involved in interviewing candidates acceptable to the nurse manager. Staff feel empowered by the ability to influence group dynamics and to determine whether the individual meets their expectations and not just the nurse manager's needs.

In a professionally satisfying work environment, the critical care nurse must be supported in autonomous practice, defined as the full freedom to act within the scope of one's professional knowledge and skills. For the nurse manager this may mean giving up some traditional controls. Often the nurse manager is asked questions by physicians or others regarding the status or condition of a patient. She may know the answer but must direct the individual back to the primary nurse. This action emphasizes the primary nurse's role to others and reinforces accountability.

To support autonomous practice, the effective nurse manager must relinquish control over patient assignments. Given full professional accountability, experienced staff members will have more knowledge about patient care requirements than the manager. As managerial time is freed up from previous responsibilities, the manager will be more available for consultation, developmental needs, and overall coordination of the unit.

In addition to giving up control, the effective nurse manager must take a proactive stance in fostering collaboration and consultation among the staff and clinical resources. The nurse manager again may have the answer to a particular problem but is in a strategic position to foster and cement relationships by encouraging consultations. To illustrate, a new nurse in an ICU had a complex patient with many skin care problems. She sought the nurse manager for advice in managing the problem. Although the nurse manager could have easily supplied information, she suggested the nurse consult another nurse on the unit who had developed expertise in skin care. The nurse manager was influential in fostering relationships and emphasizing the value of nurse-to-nurse consultation. The unit "expert" in skin care experienced a sense of recognition for her achievements and helped the new nurse develop a plan of care for the patient.

In the kind of environment in which nurses choose to work, the nurse manager will encourage risk taking and honest admission of errors. Nurses need to know that individual judgment is more important than rules and that one must always ask the question "why or why not?" It is crucial for the manager to recognize the humanness of failed effort and to create a climate in which nurses can learn from mistakes.

The nurse manager's ability to model and to communicate caring has a powerful impact on nurses' perceptions of the unit environment. It is important that the staff, who are expected to give care, feel that they are cared for also. According to Miller (23), "Nurses in administrative roles have the power to assure that the caring philosophy, which forms the basis for nursing practice, is supported and enhanced."

To create a climate for caring, the nurse manager must advocate for individual and developmental needs of the staff. In a book entitled *Leadership Is an Art*, Max DuPree (24) comments on the leader's (or in this case, the nurse manager's) ability to focus on a "concept of persons." He believes this begins with an understanding of the diversity of people's gifts and talents and skills. Recognizing diversity acknowledges that one person cannot know or do everything. It is a way of connecting the unique strengths of individuals to the work and service of the organization. Moreover, it gives the manager the opportunity to provide meaning, fulfillment, and purpose in the workplace.

To this end, the developmental role of the nurse manager is pivotol. For example, in one critical care unit, a member of the staff had a strong interest in ethics and the many situational dilemmas she and her peers faced. Recognizing her particular interest, the nurse manager encouraged the nurse to contact the medical ethicist of the hospital, and together the nurse and the ethicist formulated monthly ethics rounds on the unit.

Another example is a critical care nurse who had an interest in organ donation and its implications for herself and her peers. She was encouraged to spend a day with the regional transplant coordinator and to share the information she gained with her peers. These two nurses are recognized by their peers and others as resources in their areas of interest, but equally important, recognition of individual diversity has professionally enriched the unit environment.

Personal issues ultimately affect performance and satisfaction in the workplace, so the successful manager must be highly sensitive to individual needs and requests. Time schedules are extremely important to nurses and every effort should be made to accommodate in this regard.

As the following examples demonstrate, a manager's openness to new possibilities clearly communicates commitment to nurse satisfaction and retention. In one instance, a critical care unit-based nurse specialist adopted a child. While on maternity leave, she decided she could not return to work full time. After consultation with the director of surgical nursing and the human resource department, the nurse specialist's manager offered the specialist an opportunity to job-share her position. Another unit-based specialist with similar needs applied for the job-share. The outcome satisfied both individuals and the nurse manager benefited by retaining experienced people in the unit specialist position.

In another ICU, after posting the schedule, the nurse manager assists staff in switching time with each other to meet personal needs, extend their time off, or work around unexpected events. One nurse in this unit received support to renegotiate her entire schedule around an unanticipated opportunity to travel.

A third example involves a nurse manager who was approached by a staff member with a proposal for a more flexible time schedule. The proposal identified 12-hour weekend shifts as a way of decreasing the number of weekends nurses in the unit would be required to work. Despite the nurse manager's concern about the potential for added difficulty when weekend sick calls occurred, she supported the nurse in presenting the proposal to the unit. When staff indicated their enthusiasm for the idea, the manager gave the nurse the opportunity to develop a 12-hour weekend schedule. Not only was the outcome satisfying for an entire group of nurses, but an individual learned the art of negotiating with her peers and collaboration with the nurse manager around fairness of the schedule and its congruency with unit goals.

The nurse manager's skill in team building and fostering group cohesion is one of the most important aspects of the role that can mean the difference in a stable staff versus constant turnover. To effectively promote group relationships, the nurse manager must have a sound understanding of group dynamics and show a strong commitment to staff participation in all unit decisions and issues that affect their practice. Group norms must be established that emphasize individual responsibility for peer feedback, problem solving, and good working relationships.

Successful team building is a product of the nurse manager's ability to shape communication within the unit. To achieve this end, adequate communication structures must be provided. Staff meetings should be frequent, particularly if the staff is large. The agenda should include dissemination of information, as well as recognition of individual and group accomplishments and staff input into unit issues and proposed changes. When decision making is effectively decentralized and staff participation highly valued, the nurse manager can be comfortable in a facilitative role, aligning staff around group goals rather than what the manager deems important.

In any group situation, cohesiveness cannot occur without clearly defined structures for resolving conflict. One very useful forum the nurse manager can provide is based on the notion of group support, or "psyche rounds." In this model, a clinical nurse specialist skilled in group facilitation and psychiatric nursing meets with the nursing staff of an ICU on a weekly basis. The psyche rounds can be used to help staff apply specific techniques and principles to address problems with patients, families, physicians, and peers. When supported by an open, caring nurse manager, the rounds can also be used to resolve issues with unit management.

For any forum designed to promote team building and communication, the nurse manager must show value for the forum through a consistent presence at meetings. The goals and procedural "rules" should be clear, and a climate of trust and nonjudgment established from the beginning. To keep meetings effective, the nurse manager needs to keep in touch with practice issues, interpersonal conflicts, and general morale on the unit. Most important is a willingness to bring these issues forward in a sensitive, honest manner.

Several other strategies are available to the nurse manager who is committed to a cohesive, productive group. A no-floating policy, maximizing numbers of full-time permanent staff and eliminating temporary or agency personnel where possible, are all-important steps in building trust and familiarity. The nursing staff's ability to depend on each other and to use each other's strengths in the best interest of patient care form the basis for collegial relationships and, thus, an effective team.

Stress among ICU nurses is a well-documented source of job dissatisfaction and often undermines group cohesion. Nurse-physician relationships and moral-ethical dilemmas rank high as stressors (24, 25). Nurse managers are vital links in providing a collaborative framework for nurse-physician communication. Not only can the nurse manager articulate the nurse's role in clinical decision making, but both nurse and physician can be assisted to understand the unique dimensions each brings to patient care.

Ethics rounds or team conferences provide an excellent forum in which to resolve ethical dilemmas and the stresses associated with these issues. A medical ethicist is an optimal resource to lead discussion. However, any interested staff member can be encouraged to develop expertise in this area and to facilitate ethical decision making based on moral principles rather than emotion or intuitive feeling.

The perceptive nurse manager will identify and listen to individuals who may be feeling stressed. With managerial assistance nurses can examine their situation for modifiable or controllable elements versus those requiring understanding and acceptance. The nurse manager can minimize stress by ensuring adequate staffing, providing needed time away from work, and recognizing when distance from a particular patient situation would be helpful. In one institution, despite the added cost, critical care nurses are supported in working four, 10-hour shifts. The additional day off is acknowledged as personal "recovery time" from the stresses of the critical care environment. The psychiatric nurse specialist is another resource the nurse manager can suggest to assist with ethical problems and other ICU-related stresses.

Answering the question "What style works best in retaining qualified staff?" defies a singular response. As DuPree (24) so simply states, "style is merely a consequence of what we believe and what is in our hearts.'' The successful nurse manager will apply caring practices in the workplace, recognizing that excellent leadership is firmly grounded in an understanding of human values.

Although no one style exactly fits, a nurse manager's actions and behaviors provide the strongest measure of the kind of environment the manager intends to create. In a climate that values nurses, the manager should be open and approachable to staff. He or she needs to be visible and involved in patient care. The manager needs to be action oriented, willing to take risks and admit error. The staff must have a sense of belonging and receive guidance without unnecessary controls. The manager should be sensitive to individuals' needs and recognize that personal and professional well-being go hand in hand. There must be frequent communication with staff focusing on the values of the unit and commitment to quality patient care, human relationships, and organizational goals. Most of all, for the nurse manager to be successful in retaining staff, effectiveness will come about through enabling nurses to achieve their full potential.

## ASSESSMENT OF TURNOVER DATA

Understanding turnover statistics is an important tool for the nurse manager in minimizing the effects of unwanted attrition. Turnover per se does not necessarily indicate a problem with management or working conditions. In fact, predictable, annual turnover can be essential to the maintenance of healthy, dynamic organizations. Nurses with new ideas and experiences in other systems challenge the status quo and promote organizational growth. Attrition also provides an opportunity to restructure and to eliminate ineffective roles. When turnover is anticipated and planned for, the nurse manager has greater control over the process and there is less associated anxiety both for the manager and the staff.

Turnover statistics can be derived from two types of data, quantitative and qualitative. Quantitative statistics give information about actual turnover rates, i.e., the number or percentage of individuals leaving a unit or institution in a given period of time. Statistics based on quantitative data can be obtained through methods that focus on the reasons nurses cite for leaving a position.

Calculation of turnover rates can be accomplished in several ways. The crude turnover rate is the most common methodology. This statistic,

reported as a percentage, is equal to the number of nurses who resign during a year divided by the average number employed during the year, multiplied by 100 (20). For example, if an intensive care unit has a budgeted complement of 40 nurses and 10 nurses resign during a year (assuming vacancies are filled in a timely manner), then the crude turnover rate would be 10 divided by 40 ($= .25$) $\times$ 100 $=$ 25%. If, however, vacancies were not immediately filled, the turnover rate would be somewhat inflated and less reflective of the actual situation.

Another method for calculating turnover rates looks at the number of nurses remaining in their same position at the beginning and end of a data collection period, usually 1 year. This figure is determined from retention rates and is not affected by prolonged vacancies. For that reason it provides a more accurate picture of turnover. The only disadvantage to this method is that it does not consider the employee who started and resigned between the beginning and ending dates of the data collection period. Therefore, it would not be useful in those areas of exceptionally high turnover where the average nurse's tenure is less than 1 year. To illustrate this method using the intensive care unit with a complement of 40 nurses, if 10 nurses resigned or transferred out of the unit during a year and 30 nurses remained in their same position, then the retention rate would be 75% (30 divided by 40 $\times$ 100) and the turnover rate would be 25%.

A third method incorporates two time frames and provides an average attrition rate based on turnover reported at the beginning and end of the year. For example, in the first time frame there are 100 nurses on staff and the number of resignations during the past year is 20. This means a 20% turnover rate at the beginning of the year. In the second time frame at the end of the year, there are 105 nurses on staff and 30 more have resigned. The year end turnover rate is 28.5% and the annualized average rate is 24.25%.

The third method is helpful when turnover is high, and it accounts for budgetary impacts such as additions to and deletions from approved complements. The disadvantages are that the method does not account for vacancies and it is calculated from two numbers that do not reflect comparable groups. In other words, institutional circumstances may be vastly different in each time frame.

Accessibility of turnover statistics based on qualitative information is critical to nurse manager effectiveness. Explaining why nurses leave a given position can be accomplished in a variety of ways. One involves an exit interview at the time of (or following) resignation. To ensure full disclosure, such an interview should be conducted by an open, supportive person who is not in a position of direct line authority to the nurse. The interviewer's ability to maintain values neutrality and to elicit both positive and negative responses is central to the process. A nurse recruiter, a representative of the human resources department, or a member of a recruitment/retention committee might be appropriate individuals to conduct the exit interview. Complete confidentiality must be guaranteed, or the nurse's permission obtained, if the interview content will be shared with others. Despite assurances of confidentiality, the one disadvantage of the interview approach is a nurse's reluctance to fully disclose her reasons for leaving. If a nurse is made to feel comfortable in honestly discussing her experiences, this approach is superior to all others in the richness of data obtained.

As exit interviews are completed over time, a content analysis of the data can be done to isolate variables related to job satisfaction and reasons identified for resignation. Simple mathematics can be applied to show the frequencies for each variable. Data should be generated that is both unit and institution specific. In decentralized nursing services, divisional and departmental data may also be helpful.

An alternative approach to the exit interview is the completion of confidential questionnaires by nurses after they resign. One type of question is a rank ordering of favorable and unfavorable aspects of a job or work environment. This type of questionnaire is easy to administer and analyze but limits spontaneity. An open-ended type of question would query a nurse's reasons for resignation or specific incidents precipitating their decision (26). Responses to open-ended questionnaires can then be analyzed for content in the same manner as exit interviews. Although open-ended methods allow for richer data than forced choice methods, neither provides the opportunity to probe, clarify, or observe nonverbal responses.

## Use of Turnover Data

Average annual turnover rates currently range from 11 to 30% nationally (1). Because of this wide variability, the nurse manager should compare his or her own figures with regional or local data. State hospital associations or local chapters of the American Association of Critical-Care Nurses (AACN) may be good sources of information or data collection.

Turnover statistics can assist the nurse manager in predicting an annual, average rate of turnover for a given unit. Peak periods of turnover can be identified and recruitment initiated in advance of expected vacancies. In areas where critical care positions are difficult to fill, advance hiring may be less costly than the use of overtime pay and agency personnel when vacancies are prolonged. When change in unit leadership is anticipated, hiring of new staff nurses should commence immediately as high turnover is often associated with unit instability.

Turnover rates can also be used to determine when there may be a problem in the immediate work environment. For example, if a unit has experienced an annual turnover rate of 20% and attrition suddenly increases to 30% or more, then the nurse manager will want to carefully examine factors within his or her own unit and leadership style. In this scenario, access to unit turnover data is an essential element for change.

For the nurse executive, turnover statistics provide vital information in a number of ways. Comparison of turnover rates among local hospitals offers a crude measure of the success of the recruitment and retention programs of an institution. From an economic perspective, annual turnover figures are useful in justifying the cost of such programs. To illustrate, suppose hospital A has a budgeted complement of 100 RN full-time equivalents (FTEs) and it reduces turnover by 10% in one year. If the cost of replacing one nurse is $8000, then the annual savings to the hospital is $80,000 (100 RN FTEs × .10 = 10 nurses not requiring replacement × $8000). This savings should be reported as an offset to the cost of any program aimed at retention (27).

Critical analysis or turnover factors should provide a major vehicle for targeting retention strategies and implementing organizational change. Nurse managers and nurse executives must know what nursing staff want in terms of benefits, recognition, and a positive work environment. Unit statistics and total nursing service data must be considered both in isolation and collectively. If, for instance, a problem with managerial style was identified frequently on a particular unit, then intervention would be focused on a single nurse manager. If, however, leadership issues were reported across several units, a management development program might be indicated for the aggregate.

Discussion of the use of turnover data should not conclude without mention of turnover within an organization itself. Internal transfers from one unit to another do not necessarily signal a problem and are often an indication of career advancement and mobility in a healthy institution. Greenhalgh's (28) career matrix pictured in Table 10.2 provides a useful composite of turnover for individual units and for the nursing division. Comparison of retention rates by unit and movement within the organization can be determined. On the vertical axis, individual units are listed by name. On the horizontal axis, units are identified by number. The sequence for units is the same on each axis; thus, unit A corresponds with number 1 and unit B corresponds with number 2, etc. The diagonal of the matrix signifies retention percentages for each unit. Above and below the diagonal there are percentage figures to show where nurses have transferred during the year. The four columns on the right are, respectively, transfers to nonnursing departments (OT), total terminations (TT), total percentage of turnover (TU), and total number of employees (TE).

The career matrix is an extremely valuable tool for nurse managers and nurse executives, particularly as data are gathered and reported from year to year. Answers to questions can be sought, such as why some units have higher retention rates than others, what makes certain units desirable for internal transfer, and how many nurses can be predicted to move within the institution versus leave the institution each year. Annual trends can be shown as well.

## PROFESSIONAL STRATEGIES FOR NURSE RETENTION

Professional retention strategies are designed to support the nurse in achieving expression of the full professional role. One strategy is the method of nursing care delivery itself. It is well documented that nurses are no longer satisfied with the mere performance of tasks, nor will they remain in systems that promote fragmented, uncoordinated care. Alternatively, nurses seek opportunities to maximize their knowledge and skills and to realize the outcome of their efforts through a constant care relationship with patients and families.

Primary nursing is widely recognized as a practice system that provides a coordinated approach to care and supports the nurse's search for autonomy, active participation in clinical decision making, and recognition and respect by medical colleagues and others (29). In the critical care setting, the nurse has 24-hour accountability for the patient (and the patient's family's) care from the time the patient is admitted to the unit through transfer to another primary nurse's care in a less acute environment.

Accountability for assessment and care planning, as well as consistent assignment to the patient, enables the primary nurse to understand the unique needs of each patient and family. In the primary nurse's absence, associate nurses deliver care based on the information and plans supplied by the primary nurse. This continuity of care allows the development of one-on-one relationships and forms the basis of trust between the primary nurse and patient. Satisfaction results from improved quality of care, being recognized and valued by the patient and family, and the ability to

**Table 10.2.** Greenhalgh's Career Transition Matrix[a]

| Unit | 1 | 2 | 3 | 4 | 5 | 6 | 7 | 8 | OT | TT | TU | TE |
|------|----|----|----|----|----|----|----|----|----|------|------|------|
| A (1) | 69 | | | 3 | 3 | | | 6 | | 21 | 33 | 39 |
| B (2) | 2 | 65 | 13 | | | | | | | 20 | 35 | 46 |
| C (3) | | 5 | 73 | | | | | | | 23 | 28 | 22 |
| D (4) | | | | 90 | | | 10 | | | | 10 | 10 |
| E (5) | | | | | 88 | | | | | 12 | 12 | 12 |
| F (6) | | | 2 | | 4 | 72 | | 12 | | 9 | 27 | 43 |
| G (7) | | | | | | | 93 | | | 7 | 7 | 15 |
| H (8) | | | | | | | | 88 | 4 | 8 | 12 | 48 |
| | | | | | | | | | .5 | 12.5 | 20.5 | 26.5 |

[a]From Greenhalgh L. A longitudinal study of nurses' organizational career decisions: development and application of the Dartmouth nursing inventory (faculty working papers). Hanover, The Amos Tuck School of Business Administration, Dartmouth College, 1982. Figures in each cell are percentages except total employees, TE. OT, transfers to nonnursing departments; TT, total percentage of terminations from the institution; TU, total percentage of turnover; TE, total number of employees.

link care outcomes with an individual nurse. A sense of recognition and respect arises from the primary nurse's role as a central resource for her patients' care and progress.

The retention strategy success of primary nursing is contingent upon the totality of the practice environment in which it occurs. The method of nursing care delivery is only one element contributing to the expression of a nurse's full professional role. Decentralized decision making and an organizational structure that supports five dimensions of practice—caregiving, teaching, consulting, leadership, and research—have been identified as significant contextual factors for nurse satisfaction (30). Nurses want and need opportunities to develop professionally within each of the practice dimensions. And, when the environment supports and expects professional growth, nurses will respond and achieve accordingly.

Central to caregiving is the acquisition of basic competencies fundamental to effective performance in the role. Initial experience for a nurse is critical to the development of confidence and professional self-esteem. Therefore, a successful and satisfying orientation contributes to overall nurse retention.

In the ICU setting, a competency-based orientation program guided by an experienced preceptor is a cost-effective way to meet the needs of both new and seasoned nurses. The competency-based program requires each unit to develop its own objectives founded on a list of technical, critical thinking, and interpersonal skills frequently used in the unit or necessary to master because of their "high risk" nature (31). The orientee works with the preceptor until all of the objectives on the orientation check list have been met. The program helps to focus clinical experiences and emphasizes validation of learning, rather than what has been taught.

Experienced nurses (new to the institution) can progress through competency-based orientation quickly, while nurses new to the ICU environment will require more time. As key competencies and skills are highlighted, both preceptor and orientee can feel confident in the new nurse's ability to function independently when orientation is complete. Advanced knowledge and skills can then be delineated and added to the foundation (see Chapter 15).

The preceptor role is fundamental to the development of the teaching and leadership dimensions of professional practice. Preceptors are selected by nurse managers for the preceptor's skills in each of these areas, as well as the ability to model the primary nurse's role. Preceptors assume full responsibility for a new nurse's orientation and learning experiences. This responsibility is an obvious source of professional status, recognition, and achievement for the preceptor.

The nurse manager's skill in pairing the new nurse with a compatible preceptor strongly influences the success of the orientation. Consideration must be given to the unique needs and personality characteristics of each. The preceptor and new nurse spend a flexible amount of time together, usually 4 to 6 weeks, assigned to the preceptor's normal work schedule. The preceptor selects daily patient experiences that foster development of the orientee's competencies. Throughout the orientation, the preceptor provides feedback to the new nurse and allows for increasing independence as competencies are demonstrated. The continuity and consistency of this one-on-one relationship are nurturing to the new nurse and communicate a sense of caring and that he or she is valued in his or her environment.

Preceptor-guided orientation contributes to nurse retention in yet another more global way. The one-on-one relationship allows the new nurse to learn the unit culture while observing the preceptor's actions and behaviors in the workplace. The values of professional accountability, clinical excellence, resource utilization, risk-taking behavior, and continued learning and growth are passed on. Transmission of these values supports the maintenance of a professionally satisfying work environment.

Attention must also be given to the specific educational needs of critical care nurses. They are committed to advanced clinical knowledge, often a reason they chose an ICU setting. The critical care nurse manager must ensure not only that orientation needs are met, i.e., basic skills to deliver safe care, but must provide for ongoing education and learning as components of practice that ultimately affect and improve patient care.

Continued development of practice is largely dependent on the availability of nurse-to-nurse consultation and a variety of educational opportunities. One resource, the unit-based specialist role, has been instrumental in meeting these goals. In this model, each unit has a master's-prepared clinical nurse specialist with expertise in the speciality area of the unit. The nurse manager and the unit-based specialist are responsible for assessing and planning for the educational needs of the staff. An educational needs assessment survey is distributed annually so the nursing staff can prioritize what they perceive as learning needs. Unit program planning is based on the information gained in the survey.

Particularly valuable is the unit-based specialist's availability for one-to-one consultation and assistance with problem solving and education at the patient's bedside. It is here that real learning can be applied, enhancing a nurse's sense of accomplishment.

In addition to individual consultation and more formal classroom presentations, the unit-based specialist plays an important role in developing the professional nurse's clinical teaching skills. With coaching from the unit-based specialist, staff nurses can learn to participate in the planning and presentation of unit in-services and advanced educational offerings, both unit-based and hospital wide. As examples, a surgical intensive care unit presents a yearly all-day seminar on shock; a postanesthetic care unit has developed an annual 2-day course on anesthetic agents. These two units combine with other critical care units to organize six advanced cardiac life support classes each year. The classes are planned and many of the lectures given by staff nurses in conjunction with the unit-based specialists from the respective units. Models of this nature maximize rewards and achievements while expanding resources available to the institution.

Centralizing the clinical nurse specialist's role (through accountability to the nursing director or vice president for nursing services) may be more expedient in small hospitals and when the nurse specialist's expertise transcends multiple patient populations. As with the unit-based specialist, nurse satisfaction is best accomplished when the specialist role emphasizes consultation and development, rather than direct intervention where skills are lacking. Encouraging nurses to identify and seek out appropriate resources for patient care increases control over practice.

Career advancement programs are another professional strategy for nurse retention. Among others, one successful model is the Clinical Advancement and Recognition Program at Beth Israel Hospital in Boston. Through this program, professional nurses are provided opportunity for career development recognition for advancement in their area of practice. Four levels of clinical practice are currently described. Advancement through the levels requires excellence in clinical practice, development of expertise in a defined practice area, and a willingness to assume increased responsibility within the nursing department. Advancement largely relates to the nurse's ability to integrate clinical competency with other professional activities—teaching, consultation, leadership, and research. Recognition for advancement comes from peer acknowledgment, a 4% salary increase, a title change, and many other intrinsic rewards.

In addition to the teaching and precepting activities already discussed, the following are some examples of clinical achievements that have led to individual recognition and advancement through the Beth Israel Advancement and Recognition Program. In one ICU, nurses are given the opportunity to participate in clinical nursing rounds. The rounds are designed to present a complex patient situation to a group of peers and clinical experts. The nurse responsible for presenting the patient invites appropriate nurse specialists and other clinical resources who can offer expertise. The nurse manager and unit-based specialist attend rounds to give feedback to the nurse on her presentation skills and to participate in discussion of patient care management. Peer input is actively solicited. Clinical rounds are an excellent forum in which to promote learning, expert consultation, individual achievement, and improved patient outcomes.

In another unit, nurses interested in development of management/leadership skills are designated as clinical and administrative resources on the off-shifts and in the absence of the nurse manager. Chosen for their objectivity, communication skills, and resource utilization, these individuals are given the opportunity to participate in problem solving and decision making for the unit. Individuals receive peer and managerial feedback regarding their performance in this role and gain a sense of achievement as their evolving leadership capacity is recognized.

Clinically expert practice can be acquired as exemplified by a critical care nurse who identified her interest in developing more knowledge about skin care. The nurse was given a professional day to do a literature review on the topic. The nurse manager then arranged for the nurse to spend time with a clinical nurse specialist whose area of expertise included skin care problems. In addition, the nurse selected primary patients requiring skin care interventions. As the nurse's knowledge increased, she presented educational progams and served as a skin care resource to her peers.

Recognition for research activities has occurred through a nurse's participation in nursing research studies or through more basic research that begins with the evaluation of clinical practice. In yet another example, interested nurses can seek appointment as the quality assurance coordinator of a unit. These individuals convene other members of the staff to conduct chart audits and patient/family interviews and to evaluate predetermined aspects of practice. The coordinator compiles the audit results, gives feedback to the unit during staff meetings, and plans for educational activities based on needs identified through the audit. The quality assurance role emphasizes unit autonomy, development of skill in peer review, and systematic evaluation of practice.

## INSTITUTIONAL RETENTION STRATEGIES

Institutional strategies for nurse retention can be examined using Herzberg's classic "motivation-hygiene theory" as a framework (see Chapter 12). Herzberg identifies two types of conditions important to job satisfaction in the workplace. One set of conditions, referred to as motivational factors, relates to the human need to experience psychological growth. Sources of job satisfaction in this category include achievement, recognition, the work itself, responsibility, and advancement.

Another set of conditions Herzberg calls hygiene factors because of their preventative role in avoiding human psychological pain or distress. Although the hygiene factors are not inherently motivating, their absence or inadequacy can induce job dissatisfaction. Traditionally, these factors include pay and benefit structures, company policy, and other characteristics of the work environment (32). Elsewhere in the chapter, retention strategies based on an understanding of motivational factors have already been discussed. Attention must now be given to those strategies requiring full institutional commitment and participation. Nurse retention strategies of this nature fall largely in the "hygiene" domain.

### Salary

The issue of nurses' salaries has been given extensive consideration in both the media and the professional literature. Low starting salaries have been identified as a reason for the lack of attractiveness of nursing as a career choice. For nurses already in the profession, the highly compressed ranges make continued salary advancement an unreality. The national average for starting salaries is $22,000 and the average maximum is $30,000 (3).

Some experts argue that rigid adherence to economic principles cannot be applied to recruitment and retention problems of nursing. They identify salary issues as secondary in importance to nurses' concern for the motivational factors like gaining professional status, sharing authority for decision making, and acquiring opportunities for advancement and recognition (11, 34). Although this may be true, salary cannot be viewed simply as a hygiene factor. For nurses on staff in an organization, substantial yearly pay increases are a meaningful symbol of institutional recognition.

Kramer and Schmalenberg (16) reported that in the Magnet hospitals, pay scales are competitive but not exceptionally high. A growing trend seems to be the commitment of budget dollars toward increasing salary maximums for experienced nurses. In a shrinking market there is no logical choice but to emphasize retention through economic reward. Starting salaries must be stabilized at acceptable levels and continued focus given to improving step increases and raising maximums consistent with the notion of a professional career.

Some hospitals are moving into full salary models as a way of promoting nursing as a professional discipline and similarly influencing nurses' attitudes toward themselves. At Beth Israel Hospital in Boston, nurses are assigned a salary (or "compensation category") based on the percentage of time worked in off-shift and weekend hours. Specific formula tables assist the nurse manager in assigning salary categories. Not only has the program moved the institution into a professional salary model for nurses, but it has been useful in recruiting and retaining nurses for unpopular schedules.

Salary differentials for critical care have been identified by ICU nurses as a desired institutional retention strategy (10). Although there may be no option where critical care vacancies are inordinately high, such differentials can devalue nursing practice in other specialties and set up artificial status differences. If salary scales are established to recognize experienced nurses and critical care positions carry an experience requirement, then critical care nurses will be paid at higher rates absent a differential. Salary increments tied to clinical advancement programs provide an excellent alternative to differentials based on practice areas. Because of the seniority and competence of many critical care nurses, they are often ideal candidates for advancement.

## Benefits

A benefit package of an institution may play more of a role in attracting nurses to a particular hospital than in retaining them (26). As with salary, however, for nurses already on staff, any improvements in the benefit package can be a significant indicator of institutional recognition. Benefits cited as important to nurses include: flexible scheduling, child care, tuition reimbursements, and support for educational activities (11, 20). Critical care nurses have identified and added to the list the need for more time off and better vacation benefits (10).

Flexible scheduling should include management support for individual circumstances and requested days off. More commonly, it refers to a variety of creative scheduling patterns designed to decrease shift rotations and to minimize weekends and holidays worked while maximizing time off. Twelve-hour shifts are gaining in popularity as they reduce the number of nurses needed in a 24-hour period. Using a 12-hour weekend model, the number of weekends worked can be decreased from the traditional every other weekend to one of three. The 12-hour shift is also useful in reducing the number of nurses needed on holidays. In some areas, a schedule of three 12-hour days (often paid as a 40-hour week) has been offered as a recruitment/retention strategy. Caution should be used in implementing this model due to its impact on continuity of patient care, the difficulty in building cohesive group relationships, and nurse fatigue.

For an institution that values the competence and development of its nurses, educational benefits are extremely important. Tuition reimbursement should be standard in any benefit package and many hospitals are increasing allowable amounts. On-site workshop offerings and paid time for participation in educational and project activities are important vehicles for recognizing the nonclinical components of the professional nurses' role. In the magnet hospitals, most offered at least 1 to 3 education days per nurse per year (16). As entry into practice requirements become established, those hospitals wishing to retain qualified staff will need

to provide on-site degree programs through cooperative arrangements with local or regional colleges of nursing.

Child care can no longer be ignored as a priority concern of women in a female-dominated profession. On-site, hospital-sponsored day care is still largely unavailable although many institutions are moving in this direction. A few trend-setting organizations are offering 24-hour, on-site child care. Arrangements of this nature must be the wave of the future as nurses become an increasingly scarce commodity.

An attractive alternative to on-site care is the availability of day care subsidies as part of the flexible benefit program of an institution. Flexible benefits allow nurses to choose from a menu of benefit options offered to them. Other benefit choices might include a variety of health insurance options, dental care, long- and short-term disability, and life insurance. National and local consulting firms can assist hospitals in developing these packages.

To meet nurses' needs for time away from today's stressful hospital environment, many institutions are recognizing the demand for "earned-time" programs. These programs combine allowable paid sick days, vacation days, and holidays into a single earned-time bank. Individuals accrue a certain number of hours each week to be used as paid time off, regardless of the circumstances. In addition to vacations, nurses have used their time bank for paid maternity leave, to care for sick children and aging parents, and to pursue advanced degrees.

Institutional strategies for nurse retention include some important characteristics of the work environment. Availability of adequate support personnel is essential in eliminating nonnursing responsibilities from the professional nurse's role. Studies indicate that nurses spend significant time in nonclinical activities and that nurse satisfaction decreases when nurses are required to perform tasks that take time away from patient care and do not allow full expression of professional knowledge and skills (10, 35). Nurse managers should be accountable for monitoring any activity taking nurses away from the patient's bedside and for working with others in the institution to develop systems that maximize the amount of nursing time spent in the delivery of high quality care.

Finally, the institution must value nurse participation in decision making at all levels of the organization. A decentralized organizational structure should effectively create autonomous, independent nursing units having significant control over the immediate practice environment within a framework of institutional goals and values. Staff nurses must be given a strong voice in policy and procedural changes and any other decisions affecting their practice. To achieve this goal, nurses must be included in the membership of all hospital and nursing service committees and be recognized as essential resources in institutional problem solving for all matters of patient care.

Ultimately, success in retaining qualified nurses will not arise from the implementation of a few "proven" retention strategies in isolation. Rather, there must be a long-term institutional commitment to a total package of strategies and factors representing the kind of professionally satisfying environment in which nurses choose to work. Operationalizing this "package" at the unit level is the singular challenge of the nurse manager.

## REFERENCES

1. American Hospital Association. Report of the hospital nursing personnel survey, 1987. Chicago: American Hospital Association.
2. Hinshaw A, Smeltzer C, Atwood J. Innovative retention strategies for nursing staff. J Nurs Admin 1987; 17(6):8–16
3. Knaus W, Draper E, Wagner D, et al. An evaluation of outcome from intensive care in major medical centers. Ann Intern Med 1986;104:410–418.
4. Larson E, Lee P, Brown M, et al. Job satisfaction. J Nurs Admin 1984;14(1):31–38.
5. Blenkarn H, D'amico M, Virtue E. Primary nursing and job satisfaction. Nurs Management 1988;19(4):41–42.
6. Simpson K. Job satisfaction or dissatisfaction reported by registered nurses. Nurs Adm Q 1985;9(3):64–73.
7. Mottaz C. Work satisfaction among hospital nurses. Hosp Health Serv Admin 1988;33:57–74.
8. Weisman C. Recruit from within: hospital nurse retention in the 1980's. J Nurs Admin 1982;12(5):24–30.
9. Froebe D, Deets C, Knox S. What motivates nurses to join and remain with an organization? Nurs Leadership 1983;6(1):22–33.
10. Alspach J. The shortage of critical care nurses: readership survey results. Crit Care Nurse 1988;8(3):14–21.
11. Ruffing K, Smith H, Rogers R. Factors that encourage nurses to remain in nursing. Nurs Forum 1984;21(2):78–85.
12. Vestal K. Nursing careerism. Nurs Clin North Am 1983;18(3):473–479.
13. Wall L. Plan development for a nurse recruitment-retention program. J Nurs Admin 1988;18(2):20–26.
14. Bartz C, Maloney J. Burnout among intensive care nurses. Res Nurs Health 1986;9(2):147–153.
15. McCraine E, Lambert V, Lambert C. Work stress, hardiness, and burnout among hospital staff nurses. Nurs Res 1987;36(6):374–377.
16. Kramer M, Schmalenberg C. Magnet hospitals: part I. J Nurs Admin 1988;18(1):13–24.
17. Kramer M, Schmalenberg C. Magnet hospitals: part II. J Nurs Admin 1988;18(2):11–19.
18. Shields A, Koczan S, Sirois C. Critical care retention survey. Unpublished survey, Beth Israel Hospital, Boston, Massachusetts, May 1988.
19. Campbell R. Does management style affect burnout? Nurs Management 1986;17(3):36–40.
20. Prescott P, Bowen S. Controlling nursing turnover. Nurs Management 1987;18(6):60–66.
21. Duxbury M, Armstrong G, Drew D, et al. Head nurse leadership style with staff nurse burnout and job satisfaction in neonatal intensive care units. Nurs Res 1984;33(2)97–101.
22. Vincent P, Billings C. Unit management as a factor in stress among intensive care nursing personnel. Focus Crit Care 1988;15(5):45–49.
23. Miller K. The human care perspective in nursing administration. J Nurs Admin 1987;17(2):10.
24. DuPree M. Leadership is an art. East Lansing, Michigan, Michigan State University Press, 1987:9.
25. McCloskey J, McCain B. Satisfaction, commitment and professionalism of newly employed nurses. Image J Nurs Sch 1987;19(1):20.
26. Prestholdt P, Lane I, Matthews R. Predicting staff nurse turnover. Nurs Outlook 1988;36(3):145–147.
27. Marquis B. Attrition: effectiveness of retention activities. J Nurs Admin 1988;18(3):26.
28. Greenhalgh L. A longitudinal study of nurses' organizational career decisions: development and application of the Dartmouth nursing inventory (faculty working papers). Hanover, The Amos Tuck School of Business Administration, Dartmouth College, 1982.
29. Clifford J. Will the professional practice model survive? J Prof Nurs 1988;4(2):77.
30. Clifford J. Consultative role of Beth Israel nursing division. Unpublished paper submitted to Linda Aiken for a grant proposal (Robert Woods Johnson Foundation), 1988.
31. Del Bueno D, Weeks L, Brown-Stewart P. Clinical assessment centers: a cost-effective alternative for competency development. Nurs Econ 1987;5(1):21–26.
32. Herzberg F. Work and the nature of man. In: Simpson K, ed. Job satisfaction or dissatisfaction. Nurs Adm Q 1985;9(3):65.
33. Curran C. Viewpoint. The nurse executive. Newsletter of the American Organization of Nurse Executives, 1987;12:10.
34. Moss J. May 31, 1988. [Quoted by Milt Frendenheim, ed. Nursing shortage is costing billions.] The New York Times, D2.
35. Aiken L. Unpublished grant proposal to test an innovative model of restructured hospital nursing designed to attract and retain an adequate complement of professional nurses to assure high quality patient care. Robert Wood Johnson Foundation, 1988:82.

# Chapter 11

# Mentoring

MARY BLICHFELDT O'BRIEN

Next to stand was Mentor, comrade in arms of the prince Odysseus, an old man now. Odysseus left him authority over his house. . . .

Homer
*The Odyssey* (1)

Before departing on his 10-year odyssey, Odysseus also asked his friend, the wise old Mentor, to watch after and advise his son Telemachus. Mentor offered the young boy guidance, support, and love until his father returned. (1) Today, a mentor is defined as a "trusted counselor or guide," (2) a "guru, teacher, advisor, sponsor." (3) What place does the concept of mentoring have in the professional development of today's nurses?

Newspapers, magazines, and professional journals today are filled with evidence of the growing nursing shortage. Enrollment in nursing programs has reached an all-time low. For those of us who remain active in nursing, effective, long-term solutions to the shortage are needed more than ever. Some important concepts are related to nurse recruitment and retention. For example, for over a decade we have heard from Marlene Kramer (4) about "reality shock" and the role that it plays in nurse burnout and attrition. We have also learned from Benner (5) about the five stages of development within nursing "from novice to expert" and the importance of recognizing and rewarding expert nursing practice. We have yet to fully appreciate the role that mentoring can play within the professional development of nurses. This chapter will explore these concepts and the role that mentoring can play in preventing reality shock and burnout, and in developing professional nurses from novice to expert.

Mentoring is defined as a "patron-protégé system whereby those more experienced and further along in their careers (mentors) serve as role models, teachers, promoters, supporters, and door openers for the newer, less experienced people [protégés] in the profession. They could also be called 'creators of competence' " (6). In their classic and often quoted article, Collins and Scott (7) suggest that "everyone who makes it has a mentor." They describe the mentor relationships of three successive Chief Executive Officers who played an important role in shaping the Jewel Companies. They concluded that a one-on-one mentor relationship was necessary for the development of leaders and that every manager must be a sponsor.

In a survey of top executives mentioned in the "Who's News" section of the *Wall Street Journal*, nearly two-thirds of the respondents had a mentor. The number of mentoring relationships was growing, and those who had a mentor earned more money at a younger age and were happier in their career progress (8).

In a 1980 study, Larson (9) sought to determine whether nursing leaders in hospitals had mentor relationships and if these relationships affected their job satisfaction and subsequent mentor relationships. The study revealed that having mentor relationships resulted in greater job satisfaction for both parties in the relationship (9).

In studying nurse educators and nursing service administrators, Hess found that mentors were valued at the beginning level positions and during specific transition periods in their careers (10). Nursing as a profession encompasses the roles of practitioner, teacher, researcher, and administrator, roles that require different but complementary areas of expertise. For this reason Hess believes, as others do, that multiple mentors may be necessary. Mentoring can advance the practice of nursing by "cultivating dynamic leaders who will then influence health care policy and its delivery system, will promote the control of nursing practice through intraprofessional collegiality and networking, and will foster a clearer professional identity among nurses'' (10). Hess believes that if the concept of mentoring could develop in nursing as it has in other professions, the results would be increased numbers of competent, successful, and satisfied professional practitioners.

Gunderson and Kenner (11) examined the socialization of newborn intensive care (NIC) nurses through the use of mentoring and described five distinct phases through which NIC nurses pass in their clinical growth and development. She observed that for NIC nurses the environment itself is stressful, as is the transition into a new role. Therefore, ''mentoring provides the support necessary to foster a positive transition and ultimately gives the nurse an incentive to stay in such a supportive atmosphere'' (11). The result is a productive staff member who desires to stay within the institution, thus improving retention. If the mentoring process is successful, nurses make the transition into independent and capable practitioners. ''Generally when role congruency accompanies feelings of self-worth and self-esteem, job satisfaction results'' (11). Gunderson concluded that the professional development of NIC nurses could be enhanced through the mentor-mentee relationship.

Based on the previous citations, there is support for the notion that mentoring can have a positive impact on the professional lives and career development of those involved in the mentoring process. How can the concept be further applied within critical care nursing?

### Reality Shock

In her work with new graduate nurses, Marlene Kramer (4) discussed reality shock as an unsettling, anxiety-provoking realization that all in the real world is not as it is perceived in the academic world. The new nurse's perception of what should be is often devastated by what is. The new graduate, during the transitional phase, may experience anxiety, disillusionment, and fear bordering on terror when it becomes clear that the real world of nursing is different from the world seen as a student. ''Mentoring relationships could ease this transitional period for new nurses, strengthening both individuals and the nursing profession'' (12). During this period, new graduates might be assisted in making the transition from the world of academia to the world of every day practice by a mentor—''a wise, experienced, caring and supportive person who takes this new nurse 'under wing' and guides both the personal and profes-

sional growth of the individual'' (12). Mentoring is an active process. Unlike being a role model, whereby a person can unknowingly be admired and emulated from afar, a mentee must seek out a mentor and a mentor must agree to ''serve.'' Once this committment is made, both people can grow, share, give, and take. Beyond the adjustment from the new graduate to beginner nurse, mentoring has implications for the life-long development of all nurses.

### From Novice to Expert

In her descriptive research, Benner (5) identified five levels of competence in clinical nursing practice: novice, advanced beginner, competent, proficient, and expert. Her book *From Novice to Expert* is based on dialogue with both beginning nurses and experienced nurses recognized for their expertise. Over and over again, expert nurses described their perceptual abilities using phrases such as ''gut feeling,'' a ''sense of uneasiness,'' or a ''feeling that things are not quite right.'' Although these descriptions make educators, clinicians, and physicians uncomfortable, the expert nurses had come to realize that if they allowed themselves to listen to these perceptions, the confirming evidence that they needed and that eventually leads to a more definite evaluation would be forthcoming. Benner asserts that perceptual awareness is central to good nursing judgment, and that this awareness begins with vague hunches and global assessments that initially bypass critical analysis. In emphasizing the role that expert hunches play in nursing practice, Benner states ''there is much to learn and appreciate as practicing nurses uncover common meanings acquired as a result of helping, coaching, and intervening in the significantly human events that comprise the art and science of nursing'' (5).

Benner describes the movement of clinical nurses from novice to expert as being based on a model of skill acquisition uncovered in studies of chess players and airline pilots (13). This model suggests that in acquiring and developing a skill, a student moves through the five levels of proficiency previously mentioned and that these levels reflect changes in three aspects of skilled performance. One is a movement from reliance on abstract principles to the use of past concrete experience as paradigms. The second is a change in the learner's perception of the demand situation, in which the situation is seen less as a compilation of equally relevant bits and more and more as a complete whole in which only certain parts are relevant. The third is a passage from detached observer to involved performer (5). Skilled practice includes skilled nursing interventions and clinical judgment skills. Benner clearly states that she is *not* referring to psychomotor skills demonstrable in a skills laboratory outside the normal practice arena but rather refers to the applied skills of nursing in actual clinical situations.

How is it that nurses move from novice to the expert, "skilled" practitioner? Clearly experience is important, but not only in terms of the passage of time. More importantly, it is "the refinement of preconceived notions and theory through encounters with many actual practical situations that add nuances or shades of differences to theory (5). Formal models, decision analysis, and process models cannot adequately describe the holistic, rapid decision making exhibited by experts. It is precisely because the practice of expert nurses is not easily explained, standardized, interpreted, or taught that we need mentors in nursing. Teaching the science of nursing is difficult enough. Teaching the art of nursing and developing a nurse skilled in both is our challenge. A French artist once said that what really matters about art cannot be explained. So it is with much of what constitutes the expert nurses' practice.

Kramer, Benner, and others cited previously support the notion that mentoring has application to clinical nursing. Others have observed the positive impact that mentoring can have in nursing *education* (10, 14–16), *management* (9, 10, 16–26, 45), and *research* (27, 28). The time has come for the concept of mentoring in nursing. It deserves a closer look.

## WHAT MENTORING IS AND IS NOT

### Functions of a Mentor

A mentor is a teacher, counselor, advisor, and sponsor. "Mentee" refers to the protégé(e) or the person being mentored. Mentoring, the process of serving as a mentor, is defined in terms of the relationships and functions it serves. Levinson (3) has identified five functions of a mentor:

1. teacher: one who develops and enhances the mentee's intellectual and technical skills;
2. sponsor: one who uses his influence to ease the mentee's entry into and advancement in the work organization;

**Table 11.1** Nine Functions of a Mentor[a]

1. Provide upward career mobility.
2. Boost self-esteem.
3. Share dream.
4. Give vision.
5. Provide advice, counsel, support.
6. Introduce corporate structure, politics, players.
7. Teach by example.
8. Impart valuable information.
9. Give feedback on progress.

[a]Modified from Collins, NW. Professional women and their mentors: a practical guide to mentoring for the woman who wants to get ahead. Englewood Cliffs, New Jersey: Prentice Hall, Inc., 1983:22–29.

3. host and guide: one who welcomes the mentee into the professional community, acquainting him with its values, customs, resources, and cast of characters;
4. exemplar: one who models a way of life and professional achievement;
5. counselor: one who provides moral support, advice, constructive criticism, and affirmation, especially in times of stress.

Levinson also identifies a sixth and most important function of the mentor—to support and facilitate the realization of "The Dream" (3). He describes The Dream in its primordial form as a vague sense of self-in-adult world. It has the quality of a vision. It is an imagined possibility that generates excitement and vitality. "At the start it is usually poorly articulated and only tenuously connected to reality, although it may contain concrete images such as winning the Nobel Prize (3).

Further description of the functions of a mentor can be found in *Professional Women and Their Mentors* (29). In this book, Collins describes the mentor functions extrapolated from her survey of over 400 professional women. These are listed in Table 11.1. Some similarities and overlaps with Levinson are obvious. Collins describes a mentor as someone who provides upward mobility to the mentee's career and boosts the mentee's self-esteem by believing in him or her. A mentor shares the mentee's dreams, gives vision, and teaches how to think big. A mentor provides advice, counsel, and support. A mentor introduces the mentee to the corporate structure, its politics and players. This includes telling the mentee whom to trust, when to fight for an idea and when not to, which contacts to develop, and how to use them. "Mentors develop leaders that will be the next 'generation' to take over the corporation'' (29). A mentor can serve as a role model, but a role model is not a mentor due to the lack of personal involvement of a role model. A mentor imparts valuable ''inside'' information that is not readily available. A mentor gives feedback on the mentee's progress and lets the mentee know how others see him or her. This helps the mentee to modify his or her style in everything from wardrobe to voice pitch and public speaking skills (29).

## What a Mentor Is Not

Collins (29) also describes what a mentor is *not*. A mentor is not a role model. A role model is someone who can be observed and admired from a distance and the desired behavior of the role model emulated by the observer. The role model need not be aware of the admirer's observation and imitation. A new staff nurse may consider a senior staff nurse a role model and may pattern his or her behavior on that of the experienced staff nurse. If there is no commitment by both to work together to develop the new nurse, then the senior staff nurse is not serving as a mentor, although he or she is—knowingly, or not—serving as a role model. A mentor, on the other hand, is selected and must agree to serve verbally or more often implicitly.

A mentor is not ''automatically a pal'' (29). If the relationship grows, the mentee may eventually be included in the mentor's personal life and receive social invitations to mix with family and friends. This should not be expected or taken for granted by the mentee, however, as it may never happen. If the nursing manager has established a mentoring relationship with the vice president for nursing, their relationship may or may not extend beyond the hospital walls or working hours.

A mentor is not ''on call'' to listen to imagined grievances or real frustrations (29). For example, a nurse manager who has established a mentoring relationship with the director of staff development should avoid ''dropping in'' without an appointment to discuss the latest problem on the unit. A mentor can be counted on to discuss major problems and tactics but should not be imposed on to listen to and counsel the mentee in all minor ones.

A mentor is not ''exclusively yours'' (29). Inasmuch as mentors are usually selected because they are successful and competent, they are frequently busy and may be mentoring more than one person at a time. When choosing mentees, a mentor takes note of people with superior performance

in their assigned work and takes an interest in potential mentees who ''distinguish themselves as intelligent, competent, diligent, good humored and tactful'' (29). Consequently a mentor may have more than one mentee at a time. For this reason, the nurse manager should assume that his or her mentor is busy. Appointments should be made to discuss issues, and the mentor's time should be respected and not abused. This includes judicious use of ''hallway conferences'' should the nurse manager run into her mentor at a time when a problem or issue needs to be discussed.

Bolton (30) analyzes what a mentor relationship is and is not and reminds us that it is not an apprenticeship. Although both the mentor relationship and the apprenticeship may serve to develop the novice occupationally, the mentor relationship is much less formal and more personal. A senior critical care staff nurse may be assigned to serve as a preceptor for a new staff nurse. Although the preceptor role is clearly defined, this relationship is more of an endorsed apprenticeship than it is a mentoring relationship. In a mentor relationship, perhaps equally as important as the learning that takes place in the individual are the impressions that are created on others. The unspoken message from the mentor is that 'this person is O.K. because I have taken him or her under my wing. They are worthy of my attention and are therefore worthy of yours'' (30). By giving such a blessing to the mentee, acceptance and advancement within the organization usually follow. The nurse manager who has established a mentoring relationship with the vice president for patient care services or the chief operating officer may be singled out by his or her mentor at professional or social gatherings and may be personally introduced by the mentor. This personal introduction and interest does communicate acceptance of the nurse manager by the mentor.

## Contributions of Mentors and Mentees

A mentor provides, by example, a model for successful behavior (31). The organizational climate may be difficult for a new worker to understand and respond to, particularly with regard to communication and behavior. A mentor can make observations and offer advice, especially regarding individual techniques and competencies that a mentee needs to develop. At the bedside, this may mean assisting the new staff nurse to become an active participant in morning rounds, moving from observer to interested, informed caregiver and then to patient advocate. As a manager, this may mean assisting a new nurse manager to successfully present a proposal for an alternative time schedule at a department-wide meeting. The mentor would be certain to advise the nurse manager as to the homework to do and data to collect before the meeting, the best method for presenting the proposal, how best to facilitate open discussion, who supporters and opponents are likely to be, and what strategies are most likely to succeed in that arena.

A mentoring relationship is not one sided. Just as the mentor has certain functions and can be expected to provide counsel, advice, information, feedback, guidance, and support, so the mentee can be expected to provide certain things to the mentor (31). The mentee, through open respect and admiration, can make the mentor look and feel good. The mentee's public approval can increase the visibility of the mentor. Because the mentoring relationship is a two-way relationship, the information flows back and forth. The mentee may bring as much valuable "bottom-up" information from the organization as the mentor may bring "top-down." Consider the nurse manager who has established a mentoring relationship with the vice president for human resources. In working together, they both might be extremely interested in the successful implementation of a clinical career ladder in their institution, both for recruitment and retention purposes. The vice president for human resources will bring important organizational, financial, and regulatory information to their discussions on the implementation of the ladder. The nurse manager will bring equally important information from the grass roots of the organization related to staff nurse perceptions, priorities, questions, and concerns about the clinical ladder.

As a protégé of the mentor, a mentee may help to perpetuate the ideas and values of the mentor. For example, a new staff nurse who is interviewed by the nurse manager is hired because of his or her belief in and commitment to holistic care or primary nursing (or whatever the mentor values highly). This can help to perpetuate those values and ideas, thus extending the mentor's sphere of influence. The mentee can also provide some relief to the mentor. By accepting delegated duties and responsibilities, the mentee not only obtains useful training and experience but also may relieve the mentor of those duties that were successfully delegated.

The mentoring relationship offers mutual rewards, and each member of the pair stands to gain from the experience. There is a bonding that occurs in a mentoring relationship. This bonding—the process of holding together for common strength and good—does not mean that one controls or holds a bond *over* the other. Rather, "mutual admiration and respect are the basis for the pact" (31). Consider for example the critical care nurse manager who has taken an interest in quality assurance (QA) and who has established a mentoring relationship with the director of nursing QA. The manager has developed a new critical care QA monitor with the potential for hospital-wide application. The director of QA can assist the nurse manager with his or her plan for implementation of the monitor in critical care. Should the nurse manager use a written memo to outline plans for establishing this monitor on the unit or use a personal appointment and conversation with the hospital QA coordinator? Should the memo be copied to the medical director of the unit? Should the monitor be discussed with the medical director first? A mentor who knows the system and the personalities involved can guide the nurse manager. Both the director of nursing QA and and the critical care nurse manager recognize that if the nurse manager is successful in introducing the QA monitor in critical care, the "next step" toward hospital-wide-implementation will find them functioning as a team to develop that implementation plan.

## MENTORS FOR THE NURSE MANAGER

"Cheshire-Puss," she began . . . "would you tell me, please, which way I ought to go from here?" "That depends a good deal on where you want to get to," said the Cat. "I don't much care where" said Alice. "Then it doesn't matter which way you go" said the Cat.
Lewis Carroll
*Alice in Wonderland Through the Looking Glass* (32)

As is clear in the above quotation, if you do not know where you are going, any road will take you there. But for the nurse manager who has a career path in mind, a mentor (or mentors) can help you get where you want to go. One of the major barriers to advancement by women and minority group members is the fact that they rarely have mentors (33). This makes it difficult for them to learn many managerial skills and to become a part of the informal communication network. "Much of management is still an art . . . and must be learned through the medium of apprentice-master relationships'' (33).

The development of mentor relationships can be an important tool for nursing leaders to use in advancing their careers. Larson states that with a mentor's guidance and counsel, an individual can develop his or her resources and skills so that personal goals are met (9). Collins' nine functions of a mentor all have application to the nurse manager and will be addressed individually (see Table 11.1).

1. A mentor can provide upward mobility to your career. By speaking highly of you, giving you access to information and exposure to people you would not normally have, a mentor can help you to get ahead. Assume that you are currently the nurse manager of the surgical intensive care unit (SICU) but have developed an interest in outpatient surgery. You have shared this with your mentor who is the nursing director of outpatient services. One way that your mentor might provide upward mobility to your career would be to invite you to attend a brainstorming sesson regarding development of a new outpatient surgery department. Although you would, by all appearances, be a legitimate part of the session due to your expertise in post surgical patient care, your mentor knows of your developing interest in outpatient surgery and has provided you an opportunity to be in on the ''ground floor'' of the new department.

2. By believing in you, the mentor boosts your self-esteem. As a nurse manager in critical care, one of your primary areas of interest is pain management. You may have some thoughts about the implementation of patient-controlled analgesia (PCA) for your hospital. You have established a mentoring relationship with the director of marketing in the past. Your mentor has supported your ideas and abilities on prior projects, and you expect that this assistance and advice will help you to be successful in the exploration, development, and implementation of PCA. Your mentor may be able to see far-reaching positive outcomes for the hospital if PCA becomes available. For example, he or she might describe for you the marketing that could be done to promote PCA ideas to patients in the community who would choose to have surgery in your hospital because of the PCA program. By believing in your expertise and

ability to develop the concept, as well as assisting you, your mentor can build the self-confidence and self-esteem you need to take risks, be creative, and dare to succeed. This belief and mentor support can give a feeling of security.

3. A mentor shares your dreams. If a mentor believes that your dream is worthwhile, it can make a difference. Levinson says the most crucial function of the true mentor is to foster the young adult's development by believing in him or her, sharing The Dream, giving it his or her blessing, helping to define the new self, and creating a space in which the young person can work on a reasonably satisfactory life structure that contains The Dream (3). Perhaps your dream is to develop a critical care course in collaboration with the area university. Historically, both the university and the hospital have neither expected nor encouraged students to rotate through critical care, let alone to take a semester-long course devoted to critical care. You believe that exposure to critical care nursing in the undergraduate program is vital to the development of an interest in critical care nursing as a career choice. Your mentor, the director of continuing education at the university, can share your dream, encourage you, and help you to develop and define this dream. Although the course may be several years in the making due to the history of nonsupport by both the hospital and the university, your relationship with your mentor will also span several years and help you to keep the dream alive.

4. A mentor gives vision, teaching you to ''think big'' and expand your horizons. By setting high standards and encouraging curiosity and open mindedness, a mentor can set the stage for this kind of perspective throughout your career. A nurse manager may be faced with the prospect of closing ICU beds due to declining census or accepting a new patient population (post-angioplasty) on his or her unit. If managing with vision and ''thinking big,'' the nurse manager will seize the opportunity to provide the new service, seeing this as a new opportunity to serve and excel.

5. A mentor provides advice, counsel, and support. Whether in times of crisis or times of great opportunity and advancement, a mentor can provide advice and then support your decision. It is important to note here that although you

are not bound to follow a mentor's advice, it is wise to do so or to explain why you chose not to in order to preserve the relationship. For example, your mentor is the director of emergency nursing services. He or she has assisted you in the development of a student nurse aide position in the emergency department and critical care. Due to the current nursing shortage, your mentor suggests that paramedics also be hired to fill the position of student nurse aide. Because you have developed, implemented, and promoted the student nurse aide concept as a hospital-sponsored clinical pathway in nursing, you are reluctant to use paramedics in this position. Your staff has been very vocal about *not* using paramedics due to the potential for role conflict. You choose not to follow your mentor's advice on this issue but share your reasons openly and honestly.

6.  A mentor introduces you to the corporate structure, its politics and players. In nursing even more than many other professions, there is a language that exists, and each organization has its own quirks and idiosyncrasies of communication. For example, you may find through the help of a mentor that the politicking and consensus building in your department occur before the monthly meeting of the nursing executive council. This meeting is more a rubber stamping and pass/fail point for most of the proposals and decisions that are being made behind the scenes before the meeting. Your mentor can share this information with you, teach you who the heroes and villains are within the department, whom to trust for actual support at the executive committee table, and who typically fails to come through supportively on controversial issues. Your mentor can also use his or her knowledge and influence to facilitate your appointment to the powerful and/or prestigious committees within your institution, thus increasing your exposure and your opportunity to excel and be noticed.

7.  A mentor teaches by example. It was noted earlier that a role model is not a mentor and a mentor is more than a role model. However, a mentor can be a role model—by personal conduct in meetings, and ideas, choice of persons for network building, and even presentation and social behavior. Suppose your mentor is a faculty member in the graduate nursing program at the local university. He or she has submitted a proposal for a study of spouses of myocardial infarction (MI) patients. Specifically, the goal is to determine the spouses' knowledge of signs and symptoms of an MI. Data collection is to occur in the coronary care unit (CCU) where you are nurse manager. You are invited to accompany your mentor to the human subjects research committee, and your attendance has been approved by the committee chairperson. You accompany him or her for presentation of the study for approval. Your mentor is dressed in a business suit. You are introduced as his or her guest at the committee meeting, and your mentor states that your support and that of your staff will be crucial for the success of this study. During the presentation of the study, your mentor's advance preparation, clear purpose and hypotheses, strong nursing focus, openness to questioning, collaborative approach with physicians in the CCU (before and during the meeting) and astute replies to questions are a living example for you of the "right way to do things."

8.  A mentor imparts valuable information. This "inside" information that a mentor has access to and shares with you can include background information related to an idea that you want to try that previously failed, and why (e.g., the undergraduate critical care course mentioned earlier). It can also mean giving you feedback about the anticipated reaction of a supervisor to a proposal being developed. If you are careful not to violate your mentor's trust, this "inside information" can help protect you from getting burned as you develop as a manager.

9.  Finally, a mentor gives feedback on progress. This feedback may be offered freely or solicited by the mentee. It can include everything from the appropriateness of your dress and the speed of your speech to how you are interacting with your peers or how assertive to be with the human subjects research committee. Your mentor, if he or she is not your boss, has little to lose in giving you candid appraisals of your management style. Because all managers were new managers at some point in their career, an objective critique can help you develop a management style that is best for you.

In weighing the pros and cons of finding a mentor, Collins' (29) previous nine mentor functions and their benefits can help you realize what you stand to gain from a mentoring relationship.

## Who Can Mentor the Nurse Manager?

There are dangers in having your boss as mentor, primarily because of the employer/employee relationship that exists and that brings hiring, firing, and promotion into it. Some authors advise that you never select your boss, because you need a mentor with whom you can discuss your own boss and your objective relationship with him or her, especially if there are personality conflicts (29). This relationship makes it difficult to nurture a mentor/protégé(e) relationship that is separate and unaffected by the boss/subordinate relationship. Although men almost never select their boss as mentor, women select their boss as mentor about 50% of the time (29). Within the world of working women, and particularly within nursing, it may be difficult to find a suitable mentor other than your boss or someone on the organizational chart in line with you and your boss. Who, then, is a suitable mentor?

Typically a mentor is someone higher on the organizational chart or corporate ladder than you, who is an authority in his or her field and influential in the organization. The mentor you select should be interested in your growth and development and willing to commit time and energy to the relationship (29). You have made the decision to seek a mentor because you realize you need coaching, development, and grooming. You must be willing to look for someone who can provide it and you should not be timid about aiming high. You may not be able to get the vice president for patient care services, chief executive officer, or chief financial officer to be your mentor, but you can try. A mentor should have access within the organization.

## How to Select a Mentor

After determining who potential mentors are, the nurse manager is faced with the question of how to select a mentor. It is helpful to first understand what elements are vital in a mentoring relationship. After interviewing 150 people (50 nurses and 20 physicians), Darling (17) determined that three elements were vital: attraction, action, and affect. Attraction includes the desire to establish a relationship with a potential mentor. A natural aftermath of this initial attraction is the need for mutual admiration and respect as a basis for the pact of mentoring (31). Action means the mentor is willing to invest time and energy in a mentoring relationship. Affect refers to the positive,

respectful feelings that must be present for a mentoring relationship to be satisfying (17).

Pilette (34) describes mentoring as "an encounter of the leadership kind" and believes that the most basic human need is to believe in oneself. Mentoring relationships can promote and support the growth of both the personal and professional self. Pilette describes four basic stages: invitational, questioning, informational, and transitional. These are highlighted in Table 11.2. In the invitational stage or the early stage of mentor/mentee encounters, the mentee is encouraged to try out thinking and test dreams within the bounds of a nurturing relationship. Questioning is characterized by anxiety and self-doubt on the part of the mentee, with the mentor assisting by clarifying concerns and identifying realistic goals. During the informational stage, the new nurse "learns the ropes" in the chosen area of clinical, education, or management nursing. This necessitates learning the formal and informal power structures. Finally, the mentoring relationship enters the transitional stage in which the mentee realizes resources that are his or hers alone and begins to assume some ownership for them (34). Because the mentoring relationship is nurturing, the mentee has become self-reliant, self-responsible, and a colleague. Pilette believes the most natural end to a mentoring relationship is friendship.

In analyzing potential mentors, and determining how to go about establishing a mentoring relationship, realize that there are select people who can help you, depending on your area of need. You have to identify the things you need assistance with and who can specifically help you with them. Once you have identified both the need for a mentor and a qualified and acceptable slate of candidates, how do you select a mentor and get the relationship growing? "You should choose someone for whom you feel admiration, affection, respect, trust, and even love in the broadest sense. These feelings should outweigh any negative emotions such as a feeling of lesser importance, envy, or being threatened. These feelings can be especially present in competitive women when someone outranks them" (29).

When you have identified a potential mentor, you do not actually say, "Will you be my mentor?" This would "show a lack of sophistication or organizational understanding" (29). Mentor relationships take time to develop and they develop gradually. As you are working, seeking advice and

**Table 11.2.**  Four Stages in the Evolution of a Mentoring Relationship[a]

| Stage | Characteristics of Mentor | Characteristics of Mentee |
|---|---|---|
| Invitational | Invites mentee to try out new thinking<br>Helps decrease mentee's reistance to change<br>Energizes/renews mentee<br>Shares secrets of success<br>Is a visionary leader—enkindles a pioneering spirit in mentee<br>Exhibits charisma | Demonstrates willingness to learn<br>Tests dreams with mentor |
| Questioning | Directs goal clarification<br>Helps mentee define and prioritize goals<br>Helps mentee project herself into future<br>Helps mentee develop a realistic plan for goal achievement<br>Affirms mentee's renewed self trust | Experiences dissonance, anxiety, and fear related to goals and expectations<br>Copes with self-doubt, which leads to deeper self-discrimination and goal analysis<br>Analyzes the internal war between hope and fear and negotiates a plan to resolve it |
| Informational | Provides information to assist mentee in establishing effective communication network<br>Bolsters mentee's survival skills<br>Serves as mentee's advocate<br>Serves as mentee's guide to the power structure | Learns the game plan of the institution<br>Tests reality<br>Gains insight<br>Learns the formal/informal power structure |
| Transitional | Transfers more responsibillity to the mentee<br>Fosters more independence in mentee | Develops increased self-assurance<br>Becomes more self-reliant<br>Defines professional and personal capabilities more clearly |

[a]Modified from Pilette P. Mentoring: an encounter of the leadership kind. Nurs Leadership, 1980;3(2):22.

guidance, and growing in your new role as manager, you can be evaluating potential mentors as you build a relationship with them. Exactly when one of those relationships evolves into a mentor/protégé(e) relationship may be hard to pinpoint, but it happens gradually and by mutual assent. This does not mean you should become passive and disinterested about finding a mentor—just be persistent and open minded as you work with your mentor candidates on a day-to-day basis.

Once you have identified your primary mentor candidate, how can you develop a mentoring relationship? One way is to share ideas. As you become more familiar with potential mentors and are exposed to them in different settings, you will have the opportunity to exchange information and get to know one another. By sharing ideas, you can test the waters of compatibility to see whether this potential mentor is someone you would *like* to work with.

Another way to select a mentor is to *ask for help*. Your potential mentor is someone who you have determined to be a source of information, support, advice, counsel, and power. By asking for help, you tap into that source and begin to

establish a relationship. For example, imagine that you have identified the vice president for human resources as your potential mentor. As you are writing performance appraisals for the first time, you might make an appointment to carefully review the tool of your institution with the vice president for human resources. You might also discuss with this potential mentor the mechanism for determining salary increases based on the performance appraisal. From these early meetings, you will have shared ideas and asked for help. After completion of several appraisals, you might go beyond the asking for help phase and ask for specific feedback. You could make an appointment with the vice president, your potential mentor, to review your completed appraisals. Did you use objective, descriptive terminology and sufficient anecdotes? Is your scoring more or less rigid than other managers by comparison? Can he or she suggest methods for improving your completion of the appraisals? Asking for specific feedback from the vice president exposes this potential mentor to your work, allowing you to be seen as talented, competent, and ambitious. It is at this point that your active interest in him or her may become mutual.

As a mentoring relationship develops, the mentee and mentor share ideas and communicate in an ongoing, give and take way, both gaining from the relationship. You will each gain added perspective from your discussions. As a nurse manager, you can share the operational, reality-based perspective you bring to all discussions of staff motivation and performance. As vice president for human resources, your mentor can share an organizational ''bigger picture'' and provide the counsel, advice, support, and door opening described previously. Both of you gain from this ongoing sharing. Your first thoughts about the performance appraisal form of your institution may have been that it was lengthy and not sufficiently related to the job description. Having established a mentoring relationship with the vice president for human resources, you will have a resource person with knowledge and interest in the performance appraisal process to assist you in revising the evaluation process within the department of nursing. Not only that, but you will have facilitated crossing the first barrier toward department-wide implementation of a revised performance appraisal form.

### When Should the Nurse Manager Have a Mentor?

Some would say you *always* need a mentor unless you are content with the status quo or the organizational chart is firmly in place (29). If you have aspirations of ''going somewhere'' or work in a typical health care organization of today, you need a mentor, particularly if your peers and your boss have one. In his survey of top executives, Roche (8) determined that most executives view the first 15 years of their career as the learning and growing period. This is the time when they seek mentors. Studies have shown that successful men at the top echelon of their organization believe mentors determine who gets ahead (7, 8). Having a mentor is crucial if you want to ''make it.'' Although men seek mentors aggressively, women are not as sophisticated, and over 50% who had found mentors fell into it (29).

There comes a point in time when all relationships must end, and so it is with the mentoring relationship. This may or may not coincide with a job change. Mentors can be outgrown intellectually. You may come to feel that you have learned almost all you can from a mentor. At this time the mentoring relationship needs to be terminated and

a more distant relationship—with the two almost as colleagues—put in its place. Men know a mentor relationship is more or less temporary and transitional. They tend to seek a mentor, gain all they can, and let go sooner than women. Men's mentor relationships tend to last about 3 years, whereas greater than 34% of women state their relationships lasted 5 years or more (29).

A good mentor has your interests at heart, is proud of you, and feels somewhat responsible when you are promoted. The mature mentor will help you assess when your mentoring relationship should end and when you are at a point in your career that you no longer want or need a mentor's advice. Collins (29) believes that when you cut the mentor relationship, the support and loyalty can continue (29). This may not always be the case, however, and some mentoring relationships may end on less than positive terms. It is interesting to note that for men, the reason for terminating a mentor relationship is conflict or a geographic move. For women, conflict is rarely mentioned (29).

### NURSE MANAGER AS MENTOR

Although the nurse manager is seeking to grow in the role and has identified a mentor for him- or herself, this individual may indeed be in the position to mentor others. Why should the nurse manager invest the time in such a relationship? At first glance, the answer seems obvious. If we are to build a new generation of nurse leaders, then we must all be willing to assume the mentor role at some time to bring that new generation along. In the role of nurse manager, a particular set of skills needs to be developed. Some of these skills and related areas of management concern are listed in Table 11.3. By sharing knowledge and skills in our own field, we can all teach others, whether they be managers, practitioners, educators, or researchers. When asked if he thought being a mentor was part of his managerial responsibility, CEO of the Jewel Companies Donald Perkins replied, ''Every manager must be a sponsor'' (7). In nursing, professional nurturance through mentor-protégé(e) relationships can advance practice by cultivating dynamic leaders.

Nurse managers serve as role models for all of their staff. To move beyond that uninvolved, detached observer role to an interactive mentor relationship means identifying potential protégé(e)s and being receptive to those who ask for information, help, and feedback. ''Since nursing as a

**Table 11.3.** Selected Management Functions

Strategic planning
Budgeting
Patient Classification
Patient care delivery systems
Staffing
Alternative work schedules
Competency-based position descriptions
Employee interviewing
Recruitment and retention
Motivation and job satisfaction
Participative management
Self-governance
Progressive discipline
Conflict resolution
Continuing education
Professional development

profession can encompass the roles of practitioner, teacher, and researcher, which require different yet complementary areas of expertise, multiple mentors may be in order'' (10). To this list one must add the nurse *manager*. We need nurse managers as mentors if we are to build a next generation of nurse managers and begin to fill the hundreds of vacant positions for nursing management positions that currently exist across the country, and that were open before the current nursing shortage existed.

Beyond this professional obligation to develop a next generation of nurse managers, why else should a nurse manager agree to mentor? One reason is because it is good for the manager as well. Larson (9) studied job satisfaction of nursing leaders with mentor relationships and found that those who reported being mentors to others had higher job satisfaction scores than those who were not mentors to others. The mentor relationship can assist nurse leaders in career advancement, job satisfaction, and management staff development.

The nurse manager can serve as mentor to new nurses, particularly in the management arena. Depending on the setting and organizational structure, the manager's role may or may not involve direct patient care. The trend seems to be moving the nurse manager away from the bedside and into an organizational and resource management arena. However, as the first ''boss'' to a new clinician, the nurse manager is in a position to serve as a mentor in the management arena and to set the scene for that nurse's organizational experience. The nurse manager represents the first professional relationship a new nurse has within the profession.

In such an influential position, the nurse manager can set the stage for a positive, supportive relationship. On the other hand, the nurse manager can also set unclear or unrealistic expectations and demonstrate inflexibility. The questions ''Do nurses eat their young?'' has been raised (35). When it comes to dealing with our young nurses, some would say we commit a kind of genocide. Rather than accepting new graduates as beginners, knowledgeable and anxious to achieve but with untested judgment and organizational skills, some managers expect performance equaling that of experienced employees. Nurse managers who do not support new nurses' beginner status can contribute heavily to the professional frustration, burnout, and dropout of these new nurses (35).

The nurse manager can have a lifelong impact on a new nurse by fostering a positive, supportive, goal-directed relationship. Beyond this initial relationship, the nurse manager can be a mentor to new nurses in the management arena. Because most nurses must manage others at some level, (including new graduates who must manage nurse aides, orderlies, licensed practical nurses (LPNs), paraprofessional assistants, and eventually other nurses), the nurse manager is in a position to serve as a mentor for this area of the new nurses' development.

The seeds of a mentoring relationship can be planted at the initial employment interview and cultivated during the orientation period. The new nurse is most concerned with delivery of safe, competent bedside care. In order to do that, however, there is a need to rely on the assistance of others who work with and under the new nurse, and he or she will need to manage these human resources. Although management techniques may not seem of paramount importance to a new nurse, they quickly will become so, particularly when the nurse leaves the security of the day shift and finds him- or herself quickly in charge on the off shifts. The nurse manager may be conscientious about assuring that an adequate clinical orientation is conducted, yet the management of human and material resources must be incorporated into that orientation. Time may be spent with the head nurse, charge nurse, unit secretary, or others ''picking up pieces'' of these management functions. The management orientation can, more preferably, be organized in a systematic way. It can include progressive exposure to and assimilation of these management functions, recognizing that these nurses represent the future managers, educators, researchers, and clinicians. Whether or not a new nurse *chooses* the management track may well depend on the exposure to and expertise developed in the management arena early in their careers.

How should the nurse manager go about fulfilling the mentor role? Some basic assumptions about management first need to be established. Assume that your expectations alone can influence the behavior of others. "Successful managers recognize that people achieve more when they know exactly what is expected of them" (36). This means establishing explicit goals and clear expectations, offering feedback, reinforcement, and meaningful rewards, assigning individual responsibility, and establishing an atmosphere of trust. Remember to use the orientation period to make your expectations clear and to provide answers to often asked questions. You know that new nurses have questions regarding everything from hospital and unit policies and procedures (written and unwritten) and personnel management to scheduling and visiting hours. New nurses will get their questions answered somewhere—hopefully from you. As the nurse manager, you will be in a position to not only provide answers but also to reinforce your expectations.

Above and beyond these basic management functions, how should the nurse manager incorporate the concept of mentoring into her management role? Important functions that assist a manager to become a more mentoring manager include stimulating enthusiasm, maintaining high expectations, giving credit for performance, being approachable (especially to new ideas), providing information, encouraging risk taking, assigning challenging tasks, and reinforcing achievement (23). Establish a climate of excellence in your unit or department, and set yourself up as a source of inspiration and support to your staff. Make it clear to them that they are worth the investment of your time and energy, and that you will protect and defend them publicly within the organization while correcting or questioning them in the privacy of their own area or unit. Having said and done all that, begin your search for the staff member(s) you would like to mentor.

As a mentor, you will help the staff members to plan their career path, share the benefit of your experience, and help them to get where they want to go. That means selecting staff who are motivated and who seem receptive to your advice. Be-

gin to offer your mentees some *specific aid*. As they come to you with questions or requests for action, assist them to take action themselves. For example, a potential mentee approaches you and identifies a problem with delayed transfers of patients out of your surgical ICU, with subsequent back up of postoperative admissions to your unit. This results in a high number of patients going to the recovery room rather than being admitted directly to the SICU, as is desired by the nurses and surgeons. The staff nurse expresses an interest in trying to investigate and correct this situation. You can offer to sit down with him or her and review the situation and develop an action plan to investigate the causes of the backlog, along with any potential solutions. You can also inform your staff at the next staff meeting that this nurse is undertaking a study of the delayed transfer situation with your assistance and support. You can provide regular contact and assistance to the nurse as he or she addresses the problem. Ongoing feedback to the staff also reinforces the interest you have taken in this staff member and his or her exploration of the problem.

This may lead you into the next step of developing a mentoring relationship that is *offering protection* (29). In working on the delayed transfer problem, the staff nurse may discover that the bottleneck is occurring on the step-down surgery unit to which your SICU patients are transferred. Evidently, nurses on this unit are keeping beds logged into the computer as occupied or dirty, even after they are emptied and cleaned. The reason is apparently to assure adequate time for lunch breaks for all staff by delaying SICU transfer until after lunch, and frequently until late afternoon. In making this discovery, your staff member may be subject to criticism and disfavor from the step-down staff, perhaps even from SICU staff who have friends on the step-down unit. It is here that your support, protection, and endorsement become crucial. If you do not provide it, your staff member may never "stick his or her neck out" for you, the unit, or the patients again. It is important to sit down with this nurse and plan strategies for discussing, validating, and resolving the situation.

As a mentor you can help your potential mentees with *long range assistance* to their career by setting them up for success. As you identify readiness for a staff nurse to assume charge nurse responsibilities, you can assure that he or she receives information, orientation, and supervised experience in the charge nurse role before "turning the nurse loose" on his or her own. You may also see to it that this staff nurse is appointed to the charge nurse committee of the department or is provided relief to attend the charge nurse support sessions. As this staff nurse progresses in the role of charge nurse, you can discuss his or her needs for further management development on a regular basis and provide feedback on performance in the role.

The nurse manager as mentor performs many functions. Just what do nurses want in a mentor? Darling (17) addressed this question and identified 14 characteristics as significant to guiding the growth of nurses. These 14 functions appear in Table 11.4. This table can assist you in analyzing your previous experience with a mentor and your potential for serving as a successful mentor. High mentoring potential is indicated on the Measuring Mentoring Potential (MMP) tool by achieving a rating of 4 or 5 in the following roles: investor, supporter, and at least one of the inspirer roles (model, envisioner, energizer). High ratings in several of the other nine mentoring action roles (especially 4 or 5) identify a well-rounded, valuable mentor.

There are two important points to keep in mind as you seek to incorporate mentoring into your management role. First, recognize that people can be what Darling refers to as mentor resistant or mentor dependent. "At one extreme are those people who strongly resist the notion that anyone can teach them anything and at the other end are those who strongly resist the notion that they can learn anything on their own" (24). Second, the nurse manager must differentiate between temporary and permanent inequality between mentor and mentee. At all times, strive to develop a mentoring relationship that does not foster permanent inequity between mentor and mentee. This would result in dominance, subordination, and oppression.

## STAFF NURSES AS MENTORS

> I hear and I forget
> I see and I remember
> I do and I understand
>
>                              Confucius (37)

If you had your choice of completely staffing your unit with 20 experienced critical care nurses who had an average of 12 years of experience or with 40 new graduate nurses, which would you choose? If you are looking beyond the immediate "open full-time equivalent (FTE) positions," you will most likely choose the 20 experienced nurses.

Why? What is it that these nurses bring to the bedside that twice as many new graduates do not? If you could bottle it and sell it, you know you would be rich. "It" is what Patricia Benner (5) refers to as expertise. Expertise develops when nurses test and refine their hypotheses and expectations in actual practice. Expertise results "when preconceived notions and expectations are challenged, refined, or disconfirmed by the actual situtation" (5). Experience is therefore a requisite for expertise. Expertise in complex human decision making, such as nursing requires, makes the interpretation of clinical situations possible. "The knowledge embedded in this clinical expertise is central to the advancement of nursing practice and the development of nursing science" (5).

Is there value in seeking to retain nurses long enough to witness their move from the novice to the advanced beginner, competent, proficient, and finally the expert stage of practice? Can patient outcomes and economics be improved when care is delivered by expert nurses? There is evidence to support the role that expert nurses can play in improving patient and financial outcomes for health care. As these are discussed, the underlying premise to remember is that mentoring is one method of retaining nurses and moving them from the novice to the expert stage of practice. As the following discussion reveals, this is an extremely desirable goal.

The position of advanced nurse clinician has developed in recent years in response to a changing health care environment. To improve quality of care, administrators seek expert nurses to develop programs ensuring quality care. Because of increased numbers of master's-prepared nurses, as well as attempts to reward excellent staff nurses, advanced clinical positions have developed (e.g., clinical nurse specialists, and clinical ladder levels of practitioners). Although there is a great need for multiple research studies to demonstrate the impact of these roles, evaluation of the impact of advanced nurse clinicians can occur initially on theoretical grounds and using empirical evidence (38). For example, advanced clinicians may assess situations that would be missed by others with less sophisticated skills. This assessment information can be used by nurses and physicians to (a) improve therapeutic maneuvers, potentially reducing length of stay and (b) determine appropriateness of therapy required to achieve optimal outcomes, which may reduce unnecessary tests/therapies (38).

**Table 11.4**    The Darling MMP: Measuring Mentoring Potential[a]

The following characteristics have been identified by nurses as significant in their guidance and growth. Use this questionnaire to assess your mentoring potential or to assess the mentoring potential of other nursing leaders.

|  | Low | | | High | | |
|---|---|---|---|---|---|---|
| 1. Model | 1 | 2 | 3 | 4 | 5 | "I'm impressed with her ability to . . . "; "really respected her . . . "; "admired her . . . " |
| 2. Envisioner | 1 | 2 | 3 | 4 | 5 | "Gave me a picture of what nursing can be"; "enthusiastic about opportunities in . . . "; "sparked my interest in . . . "; "showed you possibilities" |
| 3. Energizer | 1 | 2 | 3 | 4 | 5 | "Enthusiastic and exciting"; "very dynamic"; "made it fascinating" |
| 4. Investor | 1 | 2 | 3 | 4 | 5 | "Spotted me and worked with me more than other nurses"; "invested a lot in me"; "saw my capabilities and pushed me"; "trusted me and put me in charge of a unit"; "saw something in me" |
| 5. Supporter | 1 | 2 | 3 | 4 | 5 | "Willing to listen and help"; "warm and caring"; "extremely encouraging"; "available to me if I got discouraged and wondered if I was doing the right thing" |
| 6. Standard-prodder | 1 | 2 | 3 | 4 | 5 | "Very clear what she wanted from me"; "pushed me to achieve high standards"; "kept prodding me if I allowed myself to slack off" |
| 7. Teacher-coach | 1 | 2 | 3 | 4 | 5 | "Taught me how to set priorities"; "to develop interpersonal skills"; "guided me on patient problems"; "said 'let's see how you could have done it better' " |
| 8. Feedback-giver | 1 | 2 | 3 | 4 | 5 | "Gave me a lot of positive and negative feedback"; "let me know if I wasn't doing right and helped me examine it" |
| 9. Eye-opener | 1 | 2 | 3 | 4 | 5 | "Opened my eyes; got me interested in research"; "helped me understand the politics of the hospital";" . . . why you had to look at the total impact something has on the hospital" |
| 10. Door-opener | 1 | 2 | 3 | 4 | 5 | "Made inservices available"; "included me in discussions"; "said I want you to represent me on this committee; this is the information, this is our view"; "would delegate to you" |
| 11. Idea-bouncer | 1 | 2 | 3 | 4 | 5 | "Bouncing things off her brings things into focus"; "eloquently speaks for professional issues; I like to discuss them with her"; "we would discuss issues, problems, and goals" |
| 12. Problem-solver | 1 | 2 | 3 | 4 | 5 | "Let us try new things and helped us figure it out; always had a pencil and calculator"; "we looked at my strengths and created a way to use them to benefit nursing" |
| 13. Career counselor | 1 | 2 | 3 | 4 | 5 | "Got me started on a 5-year career plan"; "I went to her when I was trying to sort out where I wanted to go in my career"; "I could trust her" |
| 14. Challenger | 1 | 2 | 3 | 4 | 5 | "Made me really look at my decisions and grow up a little bit"; "she'd challenge me and I'd be forced to prove my point; I found out if I believed what I recommended" |

[a]From Darling LAW. What do nurses want in a mentor? J Nurs Admin 1984;14(10)42–44.

In the area of critical care, if the advanced nurse clinician's assessment of patients receiving mechanical ventilation results in fewer complications and/or a 1-day decrease in length of stay, substantial cost savings would result. Evidence suggests that a clinical nurse specialist in cardiovascular nursing or wound care management can suggest changes in practice that can decrease length of stay, number of clinical interventions, and complications. This can result in significant savings (38).

Preliminary data from at least two studies suggest that experienced critical care nurses make a difference in patient outcomes, quality, and cost effectiveness of care (39, 42). In a study of 5030 ICU patients at 13 tertiary care hospitals, actual and predicted (Apache II) death rates were compared after stratifying patients on several variables (39). Outcomes of care varied significantly among hospitals. The ICUs with the better patient outcomes did not appear to be better because of the amount of specialized treatment used, teaching status, or administrative structure. Rather, it was the interaction and communication between physicians and nurses that appeared to be one of the major determinants of the difference, as were well-defined clinical protocols, comprehensive nursing education, and independent responsibilities for the ICU nurses (39).

In its Demonstration Project, the American Association of Critical-Care Nurses (AACN) set out to study the cost effectiveness of critical care nursing (42). Several factors were shown to have a positive impact on both patient care and cost. These included physician-nurse collaboration, use of critical care standards, an all-registered nurse (RN) staff, nurses with specialized knowledge of critical care (CCRNs) and participative management. Results of the Demonstration Project can be summarized as follows:

1. There was an unusually high quality of care.
2. Mortality was 50% below the prediction.
3. Job satisfaction of nurses was high, and turnover was 40% below the national average.
4. All of this was accomplished at low cost.

How important was the contribution of nursing expertise in these two studies? Could the same high quality of care, mortality rates significantly less than predicted rates, low nurse turnover, and low cost be assured if the nursing staff had been less experienced and less expert? It is doubtful.

Pyles and Stern (40) have developed a theory of Nursing Gestalt to explain the cognitive process used by experienced critical care nurses in making assessments and judgments. They defined Nursing Gestalt as a "matrix operation whereby nurses link together basic knowledge, past experiences, identifying cues presented by patients, and sensory clues including what nurses call 'gut feelings.' Using this matrix, nurses . . . arrive at diagnoses on which they base their care" (40). In their analysis of interviews with critical care nurses, the authors discovered that *new* critical care nurses learn to make assessments, diagnoses, and sound judgments about care from a more experienced nurse who supports and teaches them the Nursing Gestalt during a mentoring relationship. They call this mentoring relationship the Gray Gorilla Syndrome, a descriptive term that refers to the characteristics of the Silverback primate who serves as a leader-teacher-protector-role model for his group (41).

In terms of patient outcomes, new critical care nurses need experienced critical care nurses to "teach them the ropes" and to help them develop from the novice stage. In terms of financial impact, it is also clearly worthwhile to keep these critical care nurses at the bedside to develop along Benner's continuum. It is estimated that replacing an RN in a hospital now costs $20,000 and that nursing turnover now costs over $3 billion nationally (43). If nurses can have a positive impact on economic and patient care outcomes, and if replacing nurses is a multibillion dollar health care expenditure, then clearly a goal for all health care professionals would be to promote the retention of nurses at the bedside in order for them to develop the skill and expertise that come with experience. Developing expertise in critical care nursing can be facilitated by mentoring.

The mentoring process can be promoted in a number of ways. The first is through the establishment of a clinical career ladder that recognizes and rewards nurses not for the years of service but rather for their developing expertise and contribution to patient care. Staff nurses can be mentor and mentee at the same time. As they move along the continuum from novice to expert, at each level along the way they may be able to benefit from the rewards cited previously for mentor and mentee. The Darling MMP Inventory (Table 11.4) can assist staff nurses to evaluate not only potential mentors but also their potential as mentors.

The second way to promote mentoring is through the establishment of formal orientation programs with subsequent preceptorships in which willing (and able) experienced and expert nurses volunteer to serve as preceptors to new critical care nurses for an assigned period of time. This preceptorship promotes the development of the new nurse by providing a formal resource person. The preceptor could develop into a mentor for the new nurse, should both agree to such an ongoing relationship after the preceptorship time period is completed. While serving as a preceptor, the experienced nurse helps the new nurse learn to analyze data, consider variables, consult other people, make decisions, understand the risks involved in clinical decision making, and come to accept the inevitable moments of uncertainty. The foundation for a mentoring relationship can be laid in a preceptor program.

The concept of an internship program for senior nursing students has been successfully implemented (44). The authors described the process for implementing a nurse intern program, whereby senior nursing students were provided a supervised work experience with an experienced RN during their last term in a baccalaureate nursing degree (BSN) program. The internship was structured to provide a gradual increase in responsibility, promote integration of theory with clinical experience, and develop leadership abilities. The program was perceived as a way to prepare the senior students to assume the responsibility of staff nurse. Program participants believed the program successfully facilitated the role transition from student to RN practitioner.

Both internships for student nurses and preceptor programs for newly hired RNs can serve to promote mentoring. Such a relationship, once formed, may grow into a mentoring relationship if both parties agree to it.

## SUCCESS TIPS FOR MENTORS

In embarking on a mentor relationship, the nurse manager can keep several points in mind. Do not wait to be asked to be a mentor. Rather, actively seek the nurses you wish to mentor. Recognize that there are mentor resistors (those people who think that no one can teach them anything) and nurses who are mentor dependent. Identify talented, enthusiastic, ambitious nurses early and establish a positive relationship from the beginning. Look for mutual attraction. Give specific feedback and aid. Inspire, invest in, support, protect, and defend your mentee(s). Fulfill the 14 roles of a mentor identified in Table 11.4. Feed the relationship with ongoing communication, support, challenges, and feedback.

Keep your mentee's best interests at heart. Remember that you are not a parent or a peer, but a combination. Recognize that your mentee(s) may have more than one mentor at a time, and that the mentoring relationship is temporary. Know when to end the mentoring relationship. While you are busy mentoring tomorrow's nursing leaders, do not forget to have your own mentor!

## CONCLUSION

There is support for the notion that mentoring can have a positive impact on the professional lives and career development of critical care nurses involved in the mentoring process. This chapter has explored the role that mentoring can play in preventing reality shock and burnout, and in developing professional nurses from novice to expert. The need for experienced nurses in all areas of professional nursing has never been greater. As nurses seek to act both as mentor and mentee, they will support The Dream for nurses. If, as Eleanor Roosevelt stated, "the future belongs to those who believe in the beauty of their dreams" (46), then mentoring has a role to play in the future of nursing.

*The author gratefully acknowledges Barbara Fitz, Deborah Shields, R.N., and C. Michael O'Brien, M.D., for their editorial assistance in the preparation of this manuscript.*

REFERENCES

1. Homer, The odyssey, translated by Robert Fitzgerald. Garden City, New York: International Collectors Library, 1961.
2. Webster's ninth new collegiate dictionary. Springfield: Merriam Webster, Inc, 1983:742.
3. Levinson DJ. The seasons of a man's life. New York: Alfred A Knopf, 1978:97.
4. Kramer M. Reality shock: why nurses leave nursing. St Louis: CV Mosby, 1974.
5. Benner P. From novice to expert: excellence and power in clinical nursing practice. Menlo Park: Addison-Wesley, 1984.
6. Vance CN. Women leaders: modern day heroines or social deviants? Image 1979;11:40.
7. Collins EGC, Scott P. Everyone who makes it has a mentor. Harvard Bus Rev 1978;56(4):89–101.
8. Roche GR. Much ado about mentors. Harvard Bus Rev 1979;57(1):14–28.
9. Larson BA. Job satisfaction of nursing leaders with mentor relationships. Nurs Admin Q 1986;11:53.
10. Hess B. Mentoring aids professional growth. Washington Nurse 1986;16:21.
11. Gunderson LP, Kenner CA. Socialization of newborn intensive care unit nurses through the use of mentorship. Clin Nurse Specialist 1987;1:20–24.
12. Shields DA. Mentoring relationships. Unpublished Master's Thesis, Wright State University, Dayton, Ohio, 1986:3.
13. Dreyfus SE, Dreyfus HL. A five stage model of the mental activities involved in directed skill acquisition. Unpublished report supported by the Air Force Office of Scientific Research (AFSC), USAF (Contract F49620-79-C-0063), University of California at Berkeley, 1980.
14. Megel ME. New faculty in nursing education. J Nurs Educ 1985;24:304–306.
15. Pardue S. The who-what-why of mentor teacher/graduate student relationships. J Nurs Educ 1983;22(1):32–37.
16. May K, Meleis A, Winstead-Fry P. Mentorship for scholarliness: opportunities and dilemmas. Nurs Outlook 1982;30(1):22–27.
17. Darling LAW. What do nurses want in a mentor? J Nurs Admin 1984;14(10):42–44.
18. Darling LAW. Mentor matching. J Nurs Admin 1985;15(1):45–46.
19. Darling LAW. Can a non bonder be an effective mentor? J Nurs Admin 1985;15(2):30–31.

20. Darling LAW. Mentor types and life cycles. Nurse Educator 1985; 10(2):17–18.
21. Darling LAW. Mentors and mentoring. J Nurs Admin 1985;15(3):42–43.
22. Darling LAW. What to do about toxic mentors. J Nurs Admin 1985;15(5):43–44.
23. Darling LAW. Becoming a mentoring manager. J Nurs Admin 1985;15(6):43–44.
24. Darling LAW. The case for mentor moderation. J Nurs Admin 1985;15(7–8):42–43.
25. Darling LAW. Cultivating minor mentors. J Nurs Admin 1985;15(9):41–42.
26. Darling LAW. Endings in mentor relationships. J Nurs Admin 1985;15(11):40–41.
27. Kim MJ, Felton G. Research mentoring. J Prof Nurs 1986;2(3):142.
28. Werley H, Newcomb J. The research mentor: missing element in nursing. In: Chaska NL, ed. The nursing profession: a time to speak. New York: McGraw Hill, 1983:202–215.
29. Collins, NW. Professional women and their mentors: a practical guide to mentoring for the woman who wants to get ahead. Englewood Cliffs, Prentice Hall, Inc., 1983.
30. Bolton EB. A conceptual analysis of the mentor relationship in the career development of women. Adult Education 1980;30(4):195–207.
31. Fenn M. In the spotlight: women executives in a changing environment. Englewood Cliffs, Prentice Hall, Inc, 1980.
32. Carroll L. Alice in Wonderland & Through the Looking Glass. Cleveland, The World Publishing Co, 1946:79–80.
33. Levinson H. How adult growth stages affect management development. Training HRD 1977;May:42.
34. Pilette P. Mentoring: an encounter of the leadership kind. Nurs Leadership 1980;3(2):22.
35. Meissner JE. Nurses are we eating our young? Nursing 86 1986;16:52–53.
36. Lancaster J. Creating a climate of excellence. J Nurs Admin 1985;15(1):18.
37. Patillo MM. Students in the ICU. Am J Nurs 1988;88(5):713.
38. Ahrens T, Padwojski A. Economic impact of advanced clinicians. Nurs Management; Crit Care Management Ed 1988;19(6):64C–F.
39. Knaus W, Draper E, Wagner D, et al. An evaluation of outcomes from intensive care in major medical centers. Ann Intern Med 1986;104:410–418.
40. Pyles SH, Stern PN. Discovery of Nursing Gestalt in critical care nursing: the importance of the Gray Gorilla syndrome. Image: J Nurs Scholarship 1983;15(2):51–57.
41. Fosse D. More years with mountain gorilla. National Geographic 1971;140:574–585.
42. White S, Ed. AACN demonstration project results released at 1988 NTI. AACN News 1988;July:2.
43. Department of Health and Human Services Interim Report, Secretary's Commission on Nursing, US Government, July, 1988, vii.
44. Talarczyk G, Milbrandt D. A collaborative effort to facilitate role transition from student to registered nurse practitioner. Nurs Management 1988;19(2):30–32.
45. Dotan M, Krulik T, Bergman R, et al. Role models in nursing. Nurs Times 1986;82:55–57.
46. Great quotes from great women! Great Quotations, Inc, 1986, Lombard, IL, W44.

# Chapter 12

# Motivating

SUSAN G. OSGUTHORPE

Today's health care system is complex and changing rapidly as social and economic forces challenge the manager to maintain quality patient care in a financially constrained environment (1). Can we achieve a system that provides adequate health care coverage, enhances quality of care, and encourages technological innovation while remaining fiscally prudent and accountable (1)? As the business of healthcare changes the provision of nursing services must change. Facilitating change to assure the delivery of effective and efficient nursing services for people is the primary goal of nurse managers, and this requires utilization of sound management theory and practice (2).

Managing change is defined by Mackenzie (3) as "stimulating creativity and innovation in achieving goals." This definition is significantly related to motivation of professional nursing staff as the nurse manager assumes the role of change agent "to persuade and inspire people to take desired action" (3). The purpose of this chapter is (a) to examine theories of motivation and change in terms of significance for the nurse manager in achieving change within the health care organizational structure and (b) to enhance the change process through effective motivation of professional nursing staff.

## CHANGE THEORY

If one defines change as a verb it means "to cause to become different, alter, transform, or convert" whereas defining change as a noun infers "the act or process of substitution, alteration, or variation" (4). Rowland and Rowland (2) describe structural change, technological change, and people-oriented change in the healthcare system. Structural change affects the organization process, i.e., organizational charts, budget process, or policies and procedures; technological change affects the physical environment, work practices, or systems; and people-oriented change affects the performance and conduct of employees (2).

Structural, technological, and people-oriented change can be effected through the change process described by Lewin (5) as unfreezing, changing or moving, and refreezing. Forces in the system act on the homeostatic forces of equilibrium to allow unfreezing of the status quo and create "environmental and individual readiness" for change to occur. Changing allows the exploration of alternatives to the status quo that will effect a new equilibrium. Implementation and integration of the selected alternative as the new norm refreezes the system (5, 6). Lewin (7) used force field analysis to examine the change process. A balance of driving (promoting change) and restraining (inhibiting change) forces exists to achieve equilibrium that can be broken to facilitate change (6, 7).

## THE NURSE MANAGER AS A CHANGE AGENT

Spradley (8) described planned change as "a purposeful, designed effort to bring about improvement within a system, with the assistance of a change agent." As a change agent, the nurse manager actively applies change theory and strategies to implement effective change. The nurse manager can employ empirical-rational, power-coercive, or normative-reeducative strategies to achieve the structural, technological, or people-oriented change toward a preferred future or target (9, 10). The empirical-rational strategy assumes people are rational and will adopt a change if it is rationally justified and the proposed change will effect a perceived gain. The manager determines what needs to be changed and focuses energies in providing the necessary knowledge for the individual(s) to make a rational choice (9). Key points for the nurse manager to remember are that the change must be useful, and the advantages must be perceived as greater than the disadvantages by the nursing staff (11).

In the following example of the empirical-rational strategy, the change is beyond the control of the nurse manager. Although the staff may not be convinced of the value of the change or fully understand the reasoning behind the change, the staff may be convinced that the change must be made and resistance can be decreased (12).

A critical care nurse may not value a new requirement of completing a nursing history and care plan within 8 hours of a patient's admission, however, regulatory bodies require the documentation and nursing management supports this requirement through specific hiring, evaluation, and reward practices. The critical care nurse may justify a continued lack of compliance with the new requirement as not practical in the critical care unit because of physical life-threatening priorities. The nurse manager agrees that many patients will require other nursing interventions immediately upon admission, however, she points out that few patients remain in crisis throughout their critical care stay and that many patients are admitted for monitoring rather than immediate intervention. As the discussion with staff progresses, a colleague states that a written plan of care in complex patients allows other health care professionals to follow the current patient priorities. The nurse manager indicates that many nursing observations relative to the patient and family may not be written anywhere else in the patient record but directly affect the ability to transfer or discharge the patient from the hospital. If no family members or friends are available to assist a patient with limited ability to complete normal activities of daily living or a confused mental status is a barrier to patient education and compliance with the medical plan of care, the nursing goals and interventions change. Involving other health care providers in effective discharge planning may still allow timely discharge rather than a longer hospitalization.

In this example, the nursing history and care plan would document these patient problems. If the nurse identifies that the history and care plan facilitate nursing care and positively affect patient outcomes, the nurse is more likely to support this "requirement."

The power-coercive strategy assumes people with less power will comply with the leadership, direction, and plans of individuals with greater power (9). This strategy is less effective in managing health care professionals as the manager not only iden-

tifies the proposed change, but utilizes specific direction, pressure, manipulation, coercion, or force to effect the change (9). Key points for the nurse manager to remember when utilizing the power-coercive strategy are to clearly communicate the reason or need for the directive change, especially when time has been a real constraint to employing other strategies, and remain empathetic to the needs of the nursing staff to share their views if the change significantly affects them (11). The most effective change occurs gradually, therefore the nurse manager must expect greater resistance to change that is rapid or power-coercive in nature (11). The hospital may determine that a new payroll plan requires that employees be paid on a given day of the week and announce the change with a proposed effective date. The staff are not consulted about the change, but the manager can inform the staff of the proposed change as early as possible to minimize staff dissatisfaction with the change.

Of the three change strategies, the most effective is the normative-reeducative strategy that is participative in nature and supports both growth and autonomy in the health care professional (9). The individual(s) affected by the change participate in identifying the problem, choosing alternatives, and implementing the change (9). This strategy assumes that people are guided in their actions, roles, and relationships by social norms, personal meanings, habits, and values. The change occurs as people are reeducated to change personal meanings, alter norm perceptions, and value the proposed alternative. The change requires a decrease in the commitment to an established norm or value and the adoption of the alternative as the new norm (9, 10).

In a large metropolitan hospital the critical care unit has experienced a sustained peak census requiring significant overtime from the staff. The hospital has utilized critical care agency nurses to supplement the staff overtime to maintain adequate staffing. As the situation extends into months, the nurse manager observes increasing sick time utilization, decreasing morale, and poor communication as some of the overt signs of stress in the staff.

The nurse manager requests volunteers from each shift to participate in a staffing and retention task force. The task force members will need to participate in 2-hour weekly meetings starting immediately to formulate strategies to resolve the situation. At the first meeting, the staff identify the most important problems as inadequate scheduled staff to meet continued high census needs, inadequate staff to meet significant acuity or census changes during a shift, altered standard of care related to use of agency nurses unfamiliar with the hospital, unit, and patient care standards, and decreased morale related to long hours, excessive overtime, and inadequate pay compared to the agency nurses. During the next several meetings, the staff draft a proposal utilizing 12-hour shifts and an extensive on-call schedule with a double-time rate of pay for on-call worked by full-time nurses and time and a half for on-call worked by nurses hired at half time or greater but less than full time. The staff felt that this was adequate for nurses working most of the overtime, and it would decrease the number of staff leaving the hospital to work in critical care agencies.

The proposal was presented in staff meetings. Most staff supported the plan, however, some staff indicated they were unable to work 12-hour shifts. The nurse manager explained that a mix of 12- and 8-hour shifts was possible. Nurses with specific scheduling problems were to meet with the nurse manager over the next several days. The staff brought up other staffing issues that were noted as long-term goals for the task force. The nurse manager completed supporting documents to accompany the proposal for the hospital administration to review. The nurse manager submitted staffing information indicating the number of nurses needed, scheduled by shift over a 2-month period, as well as the number of agency nurses hired and at what cost to the hospital. The proposal included sample schedules for the 12- and 8-hour shift mix and the on-call.

The nurse manager was able to document a significant estimated savings to the hospital based on decreased use of agency nurses and increased retention despite the proposed rates of pay for on-call worked. The hospital administrator approved the proposal for immediate trial and evaluation over the next 90 days. The administrator indicated that hospital-wide scheduling changes would be based on the outcome of the trial and congratulated the staff on a timely proposal.

This strategy was successful because it utilized the change principles identified by Kosen and summarized in Table 12.1 (11).

## RESISTANCE TO CHANGE

Resistance to change should be expected as a natural human response to a threat to the organizational or individual equilibrium. McConnell (12) identified

**Table 12.1.** Principles of Change[a]

1. The change must be useful.
2. The change must be communicated.
3. The manager must be empathetic.
4. Employees should participate when possible.
5. The benefits must be stressed.
6. Timing must be considered.
7. Change must be gradual.
8. Resistance to change must be anticipated.

[a]Modified from Kosen S. The human side of organizations. New York: Harper & Row, 1978.

the five changes in work organizations that generate resistance:

1. organizational changes in which the reporting relationships of managers and departments are altered;
2. management changes in which one is left reporting to a new superior;
3. changes in work methods and procedures and in the policies of the organization;
4. job restructuring in which task responsibilities are added or taken away; and
5. the introduction of new technology and equipment.

McConnell related the resistance in these organizational changes to concern about the unknown (see Table 12.2). In each of the examples, involved individuals affected by the change in the change process would mitigate the unknown. The proposed changes would all require assessment and planning before implementation and evaluation. The degree of participation by staff in some changes may be limited by the nature of the change or time, however, in these situations, the nurse manager should maintain excellent communication with the staff during the planning process. Staff should be able to provide direct or indirect feedback during the change process for the most effective change to occur.

Not only is the type of change likely to influence resistance, but the conditions related to the change can increase resistance when (13):

1. The nature of the change and its effects are not clearly communicated and understood by those affected.
2. Staff are not prepared for change.
3. Staff have not been consulted regarding the need for change or included in discussions of alternatives.
4. Information is distorted, particularly if staff have been threatened in past work situations.
5. The change is made on personal grounds rather

**Table 12.2.** Resistance in Organizations[a]

| Change | Example | Operating Unknown |
|---|---|---|
| Organizational change | Reorganization of critical care units in the organization by product line | Unfamiliarity with product line, change in reporting relationships, different from status quo, loss of current critical care department identity, change may not work as well, those charged with the change may fail, or unclear need to change |
| Management change | Selection of a new clinical director (CD) for critical care | Staff may not recommend same individual as management, staff liked previous CD, new CD may have different management style and practices, individual's informal power base may change, some things will be different and may not be as effective |
| Change in work methods, policies, and procedures | Introduction of primary nursing (PN) in critical care unit | Unfamiliarity with PN, current method works, perceived disadvantages, lack of perceived advantages |
| Job restructuring | Hospital proposes nursing assume the responsibility for respiratory therapy evenings, nights, and weekends to decrease costs | Increased responsibility for complex intervention, more work, less time, less available resources, possible decrease in standard of care, and increased liability |
| Introduction of new technology or equipment | Hospital announces it will start a new cardiac transplant program in 6 months | Lack of knowledge relative to cardiac transplantation, need to learn new skills, need to deal with ethical dilemmas, how the new program will be planned and implemented, how current units and staff will be affected. |

[a]Modified from McConnell CR. Managing the health care professional. Rockville, Maryland: Aspen Systems Corporation, 1984.

than impersonal group or institutional requirements.

6. The change ignores established group norms or customs.
7. Excessive work pressure or stress is involved in the change.
8. Planning fails to consider in detail how the change will occur.
9. Insufficient anticipation of problems, solutions, and alternatives occurs.
10. There is fear of failure or the change is ineptly managed.
11. It is not obvious why the change is needed or what was wrong with the old way of doing things.

Returning to the example of the power-coercive strategy involving the hospital proposal and implementation of a new payroll plan, many of these conditions existed. Staff were not consulted, the nature or reason for the change was not communicated, staff may be inadequately prepared, rumors would probably circulate and increase concerns, personal financial stress may be anticipated by some staff, the traditional pay day will change, insufficient anticipation of problems for

individuals may have occurred, the change may be poorly managed for those on vacation or sick leave, and finally, a majority of staff may not perceive a need to change the current system. The nurse manager may be able to resolve some of the resistance to the change through good communication in staff meetings, with individuals and using written notices, however, staff and organization stress will be increased. If the payroll plan goes into effect with relatively few problems, the organization will move on. However, if major problems are encountered that were not anticipated, significant organizational energy will be required to manage the stress. Staff will be more likely to distrust future organizational changes if this occurs.

## OVERCOMING RESISTANCE TO CHANGE

Bennis et al. (14) described methods managers could use to manage change. These include:

1. using resistance as a diagnostic symptom to get at its cause;
2. using feedback, the release of feelings, and ventilation to identify resistance and get it out in the open;
3. allowing the group to make some decisions

within defined limits on the implementation of the change and problem solving;

4. building a trusting work climate;
5. communicating, discussing, and encouraging feedback to help individuals identify the need for change within their own framework of reference and needs;
6. using group norms and customs in planning and implementing change; and
7. using a feedback loop to help those affected by the change to develop
   a. their understanding of the need for change,
   b. explicit awareness of how they feel about the change, and
   c. understanding of what can be done about their feelings.

If the nurse manager anticipates resistance related to change, it is possible to develop an implementation plan resulting in change with only nominal resistance. Although the most effective approach in managing change with a professional nursing staff involves the staff in assessing the need for change and in determining the form and substance of the change, organizational or regulatory mandates and time may preclude utilizing this approach (12).

Workman and Kenney's (6) Planned Change Model incorporates Lewin's (5) change theory and nursing process (see Tables 12.3 and 12.4). Nurse managers can use the Planned Change Model to achieve successful change toward a preferred future. Viewing the change process as a challenging opportunity rather than a burden assists in the promotion of a positive and progressive organizational climate and promotes the concept of empowerment at all levels.

## ORGANIZATIONAL CLIMATE AND LEADERSHIP STYLE

The organization itself and the leadership style of the nurse manager also influence the change process. Change toward a preferred future is not random, it is brought about by forces in the organization (2). Beyers (15) states that change involves unfreezing attitudes to gain acceptance of the need to change and attributes movement in the change process to the establishment of relationships conducive to change. Organizational climate can promote relationships conducive to change and foster change in the organization (15). Organizations that encourage staff to make suggestions and discuss alternatives with first line, middle, and top level management in scheduled group meetings or forums, in writing through an employee suggestion program, or individually through their immediate supervisor clearly value staff input. Directly rewarding utilized suggestions monetarily or through verbal and written recognition encourages staff participation in such an exchange of ideas. Many organizations have experienced significant financial savings by listening to ideas from staff working most directly with their respective work specialty.

The nurse manager then strives to create a nursing climate within the context of the organizational climate to foster growth and development (15). Bennis et al. (14) assert that the willingness of employees to change behavior is based on the climate established by the nurse manager and top organizational management.

Organizational approaches to change include the unilateral approach, the shared power approach, or the delegated power approach (16). The unilateral approach employs authoritative decision

**Table 12.3.** Planned Change Model[a]

| Nursing process | Planned change process: internal and/or external stimulus | Problem solving method |
| --- | --- | --- |
| Assessment | Recognize the need for change: unfreezing | Problem identification<br>Problem definition |
| Planning | Plan for change: moving<br>• assess organizational climate for change<br>• identify various alternatives<br>• analyze pros and cons of alternatives by assessing the driving and restraining forces<br>• select the best alternative | Alternative solutions<br><br>Recommended action |
| Implementation evaluation | Implement change: moving<br>Evaluate effectiveness of change and either:<br>• accept and stabilize change: refreeze<br>• reject change and revise plans | Implementation evaluation |

[a]From Workman RJ, Kenney MBA. The change experience. In: Pinkerton SE, Schroeder P, eds. Commitment to excellence. Rockville, Maryland: Aspen, 1988.

**Table 12.4.**    Applying the Planned Change Model[a]

| Nursing Process | Example |
| --- | --- |
| Assessment | During sustained high census period the manager observes increasing sick time utilization, decreasing morale, and poor communication. |
| | During first staffing and retention task force meeting the staffing problem is specifically defined as: |
| | • inadequate scheduled staff to meet continued high census needs |
| | • inadequate staff to meet significant acuity or census changes during a shift |
| | • altered standard of care related to use of agency nurses |
| | • decreased morale related to long hours, excessive overtime, and inadequate pay compared to agency nurses |
| Planning | The task force determines that there are two options or alternatives. These include drafting a proposal that resolves the problem in a timely and cost effective manner or waiting for another 30 days to see if the high census period ends. As the staff, unit manager, and hospital are unable to continue much longer without significant financial liability, legal liability, and loss of staff occurring, the task force decides to draft a proposal. |
| | The proposal includes implementation of 12-hour shifts, implementation of an on-call schedule with significant remuneration depending on number of hours regularly scheduled. |
| Implementation | Proposal is presented at staff meetings for discussion and suggestions. The proposal is amended to include both 8- and 12-hour shifts. |
| | The nurse manager meets with individuals to address specific individual needs. |
| | The nurse manager provides staffing information from the past 2 months, sample schedules, and an estimate of the financial impact or savings anticipated with implementation of the proposal. |
| | The hospital administrator reviews the program and recommends a 90-day trial. |
| Evaluation | The proposal is evaluated at the end of 90 days based on ability to provide adequate staffing, meet on-call needs, and increase staff satisfaction and retention with reasonable financial expenditures. |

making at the top of the organization to announce decisions by decree; the shared power approach uses group decision making and problem solving; and the delegated power approach uses case discussion and sensitivity sessions to move the group toward self-initiated change. The selection of a change strategy may then be organizationally directed in approach as well as individually directed by leadership style and group maturity, or determined situationally (14, 16, 17).

Examples of the unilateral, shared power, and delegated power approach used by organizations are presented in Table 12.5.

A continuum of leadership and subordinate decision making authority was initially described by Tannenbaum and Schmidt (17) (see Fig. 12.1). They identify forces in the manager, subordinate, situation, and environment as the determinates affecting leadership style. Examples of the decision making continuum in the nursing environment by Sheridan et al. (18) are given in Table 12.6.

## MOTIVATING STAFF TO CHANGE

Forces in the manager, subordinate, situation, and environment affect the motivation of an in-

dividual or group as well as leadership style (17–20). Motivation is a relationship between people and their environment that is characterized by needs or expectations, behavior, goals, and some form of feedback (19, 20). Individuals have needs, desires, and expectations that create a state of disequilibrium (21). The desire to reduce the internal state of disequilibrium and the anticipation or belief that specific actions will accomplish this cause individuals to behave in a certain manner to achieve their goal (20, 21). As the individual takes action, internal or external environmental feedback causes the individual to continue or modify his or her behavior to satisfy the need or desire and reestablish equilibrium (20, 21).

Building on this concept of motivation, the nurse manager is charged with managing organizational change or "stimulating creativity and innovation in achieving (organizational) goals" using their ability "to persuade and inspire people to take desired action (3). Managers can improve this ability by applying theories of motivation.

The three major motivational theory groups are Need, Cognitive, and Reinforcement Theories (20). Examination of the concepts within each of these

**Table 12.5.**  Organizational Approaches to Change

| Problem | Approach | Example |
|---|---|---|
| The hospital has experienced an increase in complaints from patients and their families. | Unilateral | The hospital administrator hires a patient relations firm to implement their product over the next 90 days after a brief review of products on the market. |
| | Shared power | The hospital administrator designates a manager as chairperson to convene a task force of different hospital employees. The task force is to review the problem and make recommendations to him or her within 90 days. |
| | Delegated | The hospital informs middle and first line managers of the problem and requests departmental and unit-based recommendations within 90 days. Department, unit-based, and hospital strategies are to be combined in a hospital plan to resolve the problem. |

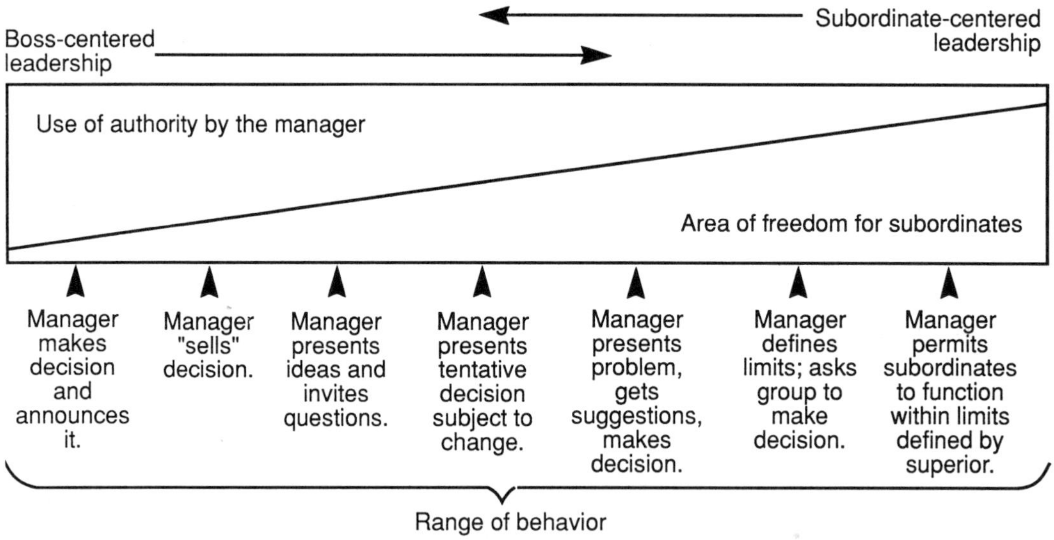

Boss-centered leadership ——————————————→     ←—————————————— Subordinate-centered leadership

Use of authority by the manager

Area of freedom for subordinates

| Manager makes decision and announces it. | Manager "sells" decision. | Manager presents ideas and invites questions. | Manager presents tentative decision subject to change. | Manager presents problem, gets suggestions, makes decision. | Manager defines limits; asks group to make decision. | Manager permits subordinates to function within limits defined by superior. |

Range of behavior

**Figure 12.1.**  A continuum of leadership behavior. Reprinted with permission from Tannenbaum R, Schmidt WH. How to choose a leadership pattern. Harvard Bus Rev 1958; March-April: 96.

three major motivational theory groups will assist the nurse manager in the application of these motivational theories.

### Need Theories of Motivation

The need theories of motivation are primarily individual theories of motivation emphasizing characteristics within the individual that contribute to work behavior (20). Well-known need theories include Maslow's Need Hierarchy, Alderfer's Modified Need Hierarchy, Murray's Manifest Needs Theory, and Herzberg's Motivation-Hygiene Theory. In Maslow's Need Hierarchy, the individual is motivated by a desire to satisfy physiological, safety, belongingness, esteem, and self-actualization needs that are universal across populations and hierarchically arranged. Once a need is satisfied it is no longer a motivating force (unless it is activated again), and the individual is motivated to satisfy a higher level need (20, 22, 23).

A staff nurse is working for a critical care agency while returning to school for a Master's degree in nursing. The agency allows very flexible hours arranged on a weekly basis and the highest rate of pay available in the area relative to hours worked. The nurse is meeting basic physiological needs in terms of time and available energy expended relative to the financial

**Table 12.6.** Decision Making Styles and Examples of Their Appropriate Use[a]

| Possible Styles to Use in Each Situation | When to Use | Examples |
|---|---|---|
| Manager makes decision and announces it. | Emergency<br>Down-the-line communication that is clear | You are the manager, and you walk into a patient room when a cardiac arrest is in process. You see that CPR is being done by one nurse. You tell another nurse to assist. As two other nurses enter the room, you tell one to call the operator to announce the code and have the other nurse bring the "crash cart." |
| Manager "sells" decision. | Tense climate<br>To keep moral up<br>If you anticipate difficulty with decision | Due to financial cuts mandated in an economic recession, tuition reimbursement benefits were decreased. You explain that this reduction was preferable to cutting nursing positions. |
| Manager presents ideas and invites questions. | When group cannot change but may need clarification | You receive five vacation requests for Christmas holiday, but safe staffing on your unit allows only three people to be out. You announce your decision, explain rationale, and invite questions. |
| Manager presents tentative decision subject to change. | Relatively set but there may be some information you have not considered | A recent resignation of a night shift RN needs to be covered. Until a new RN is hired and oriented, you need to schedule staff to fill this slot. You tentatively schedule three nurses to rotate for coverage. This plan is presented to them for their approval or changes subject to your final approval. |
| Manager presents problem, gets suggestions, makes decision. | Adequate time<br>There may be more than one solution<br>You want group to "buy into" participation management<br>People expect it because it is a group norm | Linen usage has escalated on your unit with subsequent large (negative) budget variances. You present this problem to a small group of interested staff members for suggestions to decrease linen use. |
| Manager defines limits, asks group to make decision. | Often used in committees given a specific charge<br>Report format<br>Decision has strong implications on group and manager trusts group to make a good decision | For change of shift report, give guidelines, length of time, who must attend, some statement about type of information to be exchanged. Let group decide on format. |
| Manager permits subordinates to function within limits defined by superior. | Informal/social | A $300 check is given to a nursing unit in gratitude for care by a family. Manager reiterates family wishes that the money be used to benefit all unit nurses in some way. |

[a]Adapted from Tannenbaum R, Schmidt WH. How To Choose a Leadership Pattern. Harvard Bus Rev 1958;36:96. By Sheridan DR, Bronstein JE, Walker DD. The new nurse manager. Rockville, Maryland: Aspen Systems Corporation, 1984.

remuneration that allows the nurse to meet financial obligations while returning to school. The nurse is experiencing some frustration related to belongingness, esteem, and self-actualization that she did not experience while working in her last critical care staff nurse position. The hospital develops a hospital-based critical care agency to recruit and retain nurses. The nurse decides to return to work for the hospital and regains a sense of group identity or belongingness working in her former unit, experiences increased self-esteem as peers seek her as a mentor, and begins to focus on self-actualization of her long-term goal to be a clinical nurse specialist for the critical care unit. The nurse manager is aware of a possible position opening and approaches the nurse to apply for the position.

Alderfer collapses Maslow's five hierarchical levels into existence, relatedness, and growth needs (ERG Theory) and also uses a satisfaction-progression process from lower to higher order needs (20, 24). Alderfer postulated a frustration-regression process in his theory as well as suggesting that more than one need may be operative or activated simultaneously (20, 24).

The nurse is selected by the staff and management as the new clinical nurse specialist. Six months into the new position the nurse manager asks to meet with the clinical nurse specialist for an interim evaluation. During the evaluation, the clinical nurse specialist describes her increasing frustration with changing several unit practices and prevalent staff attitudes of nonsupport. She states that it is taking 10-hour days and much of her time off just to get the ''basics done.'' The nurse manager asks the clinical nurse specialist to return in a week with a prioritized list of projects, tasks, and assignments she is working to complete. The nurse manager assists the clinical nurse specialist to retain primary accountability for some projects and tasks, delegate others to small groups of staff interested in the projects, and place others under long-term goals to be accomplished in the next year. While working with the staff nurse groups, the clinical nurse specialist reports a renewal of staff support for her role, an increase in the number of simultaneous projects rapidly coming to conclusion, and a sense of regaining control of her work place life and hours. The clinical nurse specialist experienced a regression to existence needs because of excessive time worked, a frustration and regression in relatedness needs as the staff support decreased, and, finally, a frustration of her growth needs in the new clinical nurse specialist role related to overextension and taking on too many projects at once. The nurse manager was able to assist the nurse in managing these frustrations to reestablish positive need satisfaction and progression.

Murray described achievement, affiliation, aggression, autonomy, endurance, exhibition, harm avoidance, nurturance, impulsivity, order, power, succorance, and understanding needs that may be inferred from observed behavior in an individual (20, 25). Each need has a qualitative or directive component that represents the object toward which the motive is directed and a quantitative or energetic component that signifies the strength or intensity of the motivation (20). Several needs can be operative simultaneously and may be conflicting (20).

Finally, Herzberg categorized factors related to the job as factors inherent in the work that may be true motivators and factors in the environment that influence employee satisfaction when they are not present (12, 26). He described sources of motivation as the opportunity to learn or acquire new knowledge; to achieve or perform work that is interesting and challenging; to do meaningful work; to assume responsibility; and to become involved in determining how the work is done (12, 26). The environmental factors can be grouped into five categories including communication, growth potential, personnel policies, salary administration, and working conditions (12). Environmental communication factors include appreciation of one's efforts or praise when it is due, knowledge of the activities and intentions of the organization, inclusion in the employer's goals and plans, knowledge of where one stands with the organization at any given time, confidentiality in personal dealings with management, and tactful discipline with reasonable privacy. Environmental growth factors include the opportunity for advancement and encouragement in growth and advancement. Environmental personnel policies include reasonable accommodation of personal needs, reasonable feeling of job security, organizational loyalty to employees, respect for an individual's origins, and fair and consistent treatment of employees. Salary factors are a fair salary and benefits relative to others in the organization, community, and occupation. Environmental working factors are the physical working conditions relative to what is expected or desired (12).

**Implications of need theories for nurse managers** include understanding important differences in the application of Herzberg's Theory in the workplace between motivators of professional nursing staff versus nonprofessional health care providers. McConnell (12) states that the professional is more likely to:

1. aspire to growth within both the organization and occupation;
2. aspire to earn more money;
3. be driven by a stronger need for accomplishment;
4. be more dedicated to the aims of one's occupation;
5. harbor a stronger liking for the work itself; and
6. have a strong need for occupational security that can be more completely met by a profession than by a job.

The professional is more likely to place greater emphasis on higher order needs than the non-professional employee (12). These motivating needs include:

1. placing more emphasis on learning and achieving;
2. preferring work that is interesting, stimulating, and challenging;
3. desiring a sense of accomplishment related to doing the meaningful work; and
4. seeking opportunities to assume responsibility and determine how work is done.

It is important for nurse managers to review the staff nurse job description and role expectations in light of the intrinsic motivators for the professional nurse. This would enhance motivation when environmental factors are simultaneously addressed by the organization, department, and unit to ensure quality of work place life.

### Cognitive Theories of Motivation

Three related cognitive theories of motivation are the Expectancy/Valence Theory, Goal-Setting Theory, and Equity Theory (20). Vroom states in the Expectancy Theory that motivation is a combined function of (*a*) the individual's perception that effort will lead to performance and (*b*) the perceived desirability of outcomes that may result from performance (20, 27). Individual variation in need strengths is acknowledged in that not everyone values the same rewards equally. People attach different valences to outcomes and have different perceptions regarding the equity of the reward compared to others. The Goal-Setting Theory is similar to the Expectancy Theory but describes intentions or goals in addition to values as cognitive determinants of individual behavior. Goal setting appears to positively affect both performance levels and job satisfaction. The Equity or Social Comparison Theory builds on the previous cognitive theories and examines how an individual uses external or internal comparisons to determine the appropriateness of an attitude or opinion, behavioral act, or reinforcement. Figure 12.2 compares these three cognitive theories.

**Implications of cognitive theories for managers** include ensuring that highly valued organizational responses and performance behaviors are explicit and tied to reward through feedback and reinforcement. An individual may be seen as well rewarded in the organization, however, professional nurses, may not continue the behaviors or performance if their referent comparative others are perceived as better rewarded. Motivation is greatest when individuals believe that certain responses or behavior will lead to outcomes (performance-outcome expectancy), these outcomes have positive value for them (valence), and individuals believe that they are able to perform at the desired level (effort-performance expectancy). Rewards should be contingent upon successful performance of organizationally valued behavior (20).

A hospital plans to develop a clinical ladder as a retention strategy for professional nursing staff. Staff nurses representing each nursing unit, several clinical nurse specialists, and a clinical director are asked to participate on the task force charged with developing and implementing the program. The program is based on a nursing model and consists of the nursing process in the direct care of patients, quality assurance and research activities, professional education, and professional activities. As the program is designed to promote retaining clinical bedside practioners, there is a 65% weighting of the nursing process portion of the program, and the other practice components are equally weighted. Performance criteria for each section are described in the program, and the evaluation tools for each section are also included in the packet each nurse receives when applying for the program. The nurse has very explicitly defined performance behaviors described that will successfully satisfy each criterion in the program. Therefore, performance-outcome expectancy is built into the program.

The program is designed with three levels of recognition that build consecutively upon each other. Each level has significant financial and personal recognition rewards available upon successful completion of a level. Therefore, intrinsic and extrinsic rewards or valence are built into the program. As the program was developed by staff nurses and several nurses in the critical care unit, the critical care staff believe in their ability to perform at the desired level. Thus, the program has incorporated effort-performance expectancy in the program. Finally, the program is seen as increasingly credible as informal unit leaders begin to actively work to achieve all three levels.

Critical care staff enjoy the recognition and believe that their individual practice is strengthened, valued, and supported by hospital administration by implementation of the program. At the end of a 1-year evaluation period the program

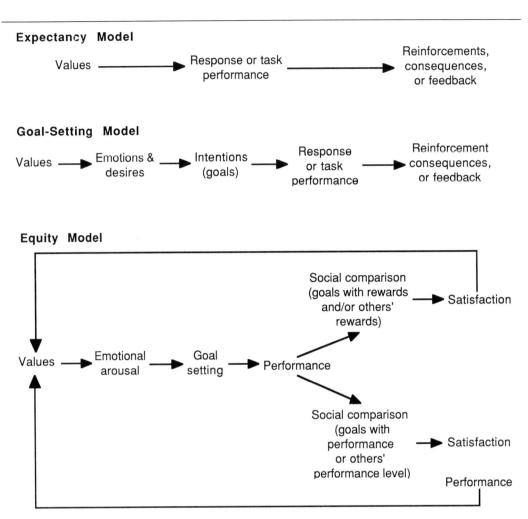

**Figure 12.2.** Cognitive theories of motivation.

was successful in that individuals believed they could work at their own pace to achieve different levels and could select elective criteria to achieve points in activities they enjoyed the most. Mandatory criteria were found to have strengthened nursing documentation, quality assurance, and professional education throughout the nursing departments. Retention of bedside clinical practitioners was evaluated and found to be a significant reason nurses chose to stay at the bedside rather than pursuing a management pathway or leaving their hospital staff nurse position.

### Reinforcement Theories of Motivation

B.F. Skinner (28) and Luthans and Kreitner (29) developed reinforcement and behavior modifica-

tion theories of motivation. Reinforcement theories assume that human behavior can be engineered, shaped, or altered by manipulating reward structures of various forms of behavior with positive reinforcement, as described by Skinner, or consequences (28, 29). Operant conditioning techniques are employed by the manager to obtain desired behavior (20).

**Implications of reinforcement theories for managers** are that the nurse manager must (20):

1. clearly inform staff which behaviors are desirable and will be rewarded;
2. not reward all staff equally;
3. clearly inform staff what they are doing wrong;

4. not punish the staff in front of others;
5. ensure that the consequences equal the behavior; and
6. remember that failure to respond to staff behaviors has reinforcing consequences in and of itself.

The reinforcement theories approach motivation with the idea that "behavior is a function of its consequences" (20). These theories have limited success in managing professional staff because individual differences, needs, and attitudes are not considered (20). According to Lancaster (19), "managers, in motivating environments, recognize that each individual is different and responds in a unique way to challenge, responsibility, praise, and punishment."

The Need, Cognitive, and Reinforcement theories of motivation all contribute to the nurse manager's understanding of the relationship between the professional staff nurse and the work environment. The theories are useful in assisting the nurse manager to manage professional staff more successfully by considering individual needs, ensuring that highly valued organizational responses and performance behaviors are explicit and tied to reward through feedback and reinforcement, and using positive reinforcement and counseling. The nurse manager can assist each staff nurse to respond to the work environment and view the staff nurse role as a professionally rewarding challenge (20).

## GETZELS-GUBA MODEL OF SOCIAL BEHAVIOR

The Getzels-Guba Model of Social Behavior integrates concepts from all of the major motivational theories with regard to individual dimensions of morale. It also provides the nurse manager with a helpful tool in understanding the relationship between professional nursing staff and their work environment (see Fig. 12.3) and 12.4 (30).

The model parallels the individual, personality, need dispositions, and goals with the institution, role, role expectations, and goals within the context of the social system. The extent to which an individual can identify personal goals with organizational goals has a direct relationship on individual productivity. The model describes belongingness as the individual's belief that he or she will be able to achieve satisfaction within the institutional structure because the required organizational role expectations serve personal needs. Rationality refers to the extent to which role expectations are perceived as appropriate to institutional goal achievement. Identification refers to the degree to which the goals of the organization are integrated with the individual's needs and concerns (30).

Congruence between roles, expectations, and goals of the institution with the individual's personality, needs, and goals is necessary to achieve high morale in the professional nurse (30). The extent to which the nurse manager is able to help professional nurses understand that in meeting organizational goals, they will also satisfy their own goal achievement determines individual motivation, satisfaction, and morale.

Some practical strategies for implementing the model in the clinical setting include:

1. familiarizing all staff with hospital, department, and unit philosophies and goals;
2. ensuring that unit objectives reflect hospital, department, and unit goals and have staff input;

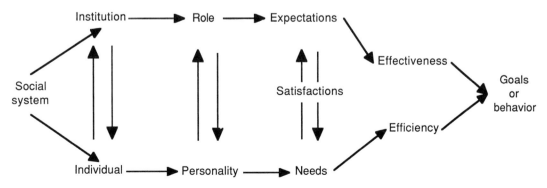

**Figure 12.3.** Getzels-Guba model of social behavior. Adapted from Moloney MM. Leadership in nursing—theory, strategies, action. St Louis: CV Mosby, 1979.

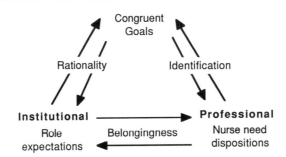

**Figure 12.4.** Dimensions of morale. Adapted from Moloney MM. Leadership in nursing—theory, strategies, action. St Louis: CV Mosby, 1979.

3. ensuring that the staff nurse job description is clear and includes professional role characteristics and expectations designed to motivate the professional nurse;
4. clarifying institutional expectations in regular meetings with individuals;
5. providing financial and recognition rewards when staff nurses meet these expectations and successfully achieve annually set individual goals;
6. developing a management care plan for each staff nurse that includes a brief history reflecting significant nursing and personal information;
7. identifying individual strengths and weaknesses or areas of improvement in conjunction with each nurse;
8. assisting the nurse to set measurable goals that provide a personal and professional challenge and encourage growth;
9. recognizing, reinforcing, and rewarding personal and professional excellence during daily exchanges with staff;
10. viewing oneself as a mentor and resource for staff, and ensuring regular informal and formal occasions for professional exchange.

The nurse manager can use these strategies to achieve congruence in organizational and individual goals. The congruence of organizational and individual goals contributes to the successful goal achievement in the delivery of effective and efficient nursing services for patients (2, 30).

## SUMMARY

By facilitating effective change, the nurse manager is able to achieve organizational goals and motivate professional nursing staff to achieve individual goals and realize their potential. Frank (31) observed that health care is rapidly changing the way we do business and the way we have always done business. The ability to successfully cope with constant change in our patients, nursing care, organization, and ourselves is critical (31).

Ask yourself whether Louis L'Amour (32) captured the importance of effective managed change in health care and nursing well when he observed: ''The one thing we know is that nothing remains the same. Things are forever changing, and one must understand the changes and change with them, or be lost by the way.''

REFERENCES

1. Arthur Andersen & Co, American College of Healthcare Executives. The future of healthcare: changes and choices. Chicago: Arthur Andersen & Co, 1987.
2. Rowland HS, Rowland BL. Nursing administration handbook. 2nd ed. Rockville, Maryland: Aspen Systems Corporation, 1985.
3. Mackenzie RA. The management process in 3D. Harvard Bus Rev, 1969;44:80–87.
4. Guralnik DB, ed. Webster's new world dictionary. 2nd college ed. Cleveland: William Collins Publishers, Inc, 1980.
5. Lewin K. Frontiers in group dynamics. Hum Relations 1947;1:5–41.
6. Workman RJ, Kenney MBA. The change experience. In: Pinkerton SE, Schroeder P, ed. Commitment to excellence: developing a professional nursing staff. Rockville, Maryland: Aspen Publishers, Inc, 1988.
7. Lewin K. Field theory in social science. New York: Harper & Row, 1951.
8. Spradley BW. Managing change creatively. J Nurs Admin 1980;10:32–37.
9. Haffer A. Facilitating change: choosing the appropriate strategy. J Nurs Admin 1986;16:18–22.
10. Chin R, Benne KD. General strategies for effecting change in human systems. In: Bennis WG, Benne KD, Chin R, eds. The planning of change. New York: Holt, Rinehart, & Winston, 1976.

11. Kosen S. The human side of organizations. New York: Harper & Row, 1978.

12. McConnell CR. Managing the health care professional. Rockville, Maryland: Aspen Systems Corporation, 1984.

13. Metzger N. The Healthcare supervisor's handbook. 2nd ed. Rockville, Maryland: Aspen Systems Corporation, 1982.

14. Bennis WG, Benne KD, Chin R, eds. The planning of change. New York: Holt, Rinehart, & Winston, 1964.

15. Beyers M. Getting on top of organizational change. J Nurs Admin 1984;14:32–39.

16. Greiner LE. Patterns of organizational change. Harvard Bus Rev 1967;36:119–122.

17. Tannenbaum R, Schmidt WH. How to choose a leadership pattern. Harvard Bus Rev 1958;36:95–101.

18. Sheridan DR, Bronstein JP, Walker DD. The new nurse manager. Rockville, Maryland: Aspen Systems Corporation, 1984.

19. Lancaster J. Motivation—creating the environment. Assoc Operat Rm Nurses 1986;43:202–208.

20. Steers RM, Porter LW. Motivation and work behavior. New York: McGraw-Hill, 1983.

21. Dunnette MD, Kircher WK. Psychology applied to industry. New York: Appleton-Century-Crofts, 1965.

22. Maslow AH. A theory of human motivation. Psychol Rev 1943;50:370–396.

23. Maslow AH. Motivation and personality. New York: Harper & Row, 1954.

24. Alderfer CP. Existence, relatedness, and growth. New York: Free Press, 1972.

25. Murray HA. Explorations in personality. New York: Oxford University Press, 1967.

26. Herzberg F. The motivation to work. New York: John Wiley & Sons, Inc, 1969.

27. Vroom V. Work and motivation. New York: John Wiley & Sons, Inc, 1964.

28. Skinner BF. Science and human behavior. New York: Free Press, 1953.

29. Luthans F, Kreitner K. Organizational behavior modification. Glenview, Illinois: Scott, Foresmann, 1975.

30. Moloney MM. Leadership in nursing-theory, strategies, action. St Louis: CV Mosby, 1979.

31. Frank IC. When will it end? J Emerg Nurs 1986;12:3–4.

32. L'Amour L. The lonesome gods. New York: Bantam Books, 1983.

# Chapter 13

# Negotiating

CATHY RODGERS WARD

Negotiation is a process inherent within the role of the critical care nurse manager, and negotiation skills are necessary for survival in this position. The need for these skills arises in everyday life in multiple situations ranging from negotiating with your spouse about the grocery shopping to bargaining with a vendor when shopping in a foreign country. The consequences of the outcomes of negotiating in a professional setting may be more important, however, and for critical care nursing this generally means ultimately an effect on patient care. The effectiveness of the nurse manager at negotiating issues for her unit and for the nursing staff of that unit may affect the quality of patient care and the morale and therefore the retention of critical care nurses. This chapter will outline the principles of the negotiation process, delineate the role of the nurse manager as negotiator within a health care organization, and provide specific examples of successful negotiation tactics.

## DEFINING THE TERMS

The word "negotiation" has connotations of the formal process of a union bargaining with management over a compensation and benefits package (see Chapter 18) or a large company bargaining with a supplier for a contract. Although this formal type of negotiation may occur in the nurse manager's role on specific occasions, the more informal, yet principled, process of negotiation as described in this chapter is an ongoing one with the need for the nurse manager to exercise these skills on a daily basis with multiple parties. This type of negotiation is a process in which two or more parties are interdependent upon each other and must rely on the other party to achieve their own objectives. Other definitions of negotiation include:

- a basic means of getting what you want from others (1);
- an interaction that occurs when two or more

parties attempt to agree on a mutually acceptable outcome in a situation in which their preferences for outcomes are negatively related (2);
- the use of information and power to affect the other party's behavior within a web of tension (3);
- the process of conferring with another so as to arrive at the settlement of some matter (4);
- the barter system applied to the business of improving productivity, work quality, and work attitude (5).

The concepts of change, influence, perception, motivation, dispute resolution, dissent, and conflict resolution are related to the concept of negotiation in that they may be considered as antecedents or consequences of the negotiation process. For example, a critical care nurse manager may want to change the staff's behavior to increase their documentation of a particular nursing diagnosis. The staff may feel they do not have the time to document any more patient problems and yet the nurse manager feels it would enhance the patient's care plan. By understanding the staff's perception of the conflict, the nurse manager may understand what motivation is needed to achieve this goal. Negotiation is that process that needs to occur between the nurse manager and the nursing staff to avoid further dissent, conflict, and dispute between the two parties. The nurse manager may then negotiate with the staff to create a way to meet both parties' needs (short amount of time required versus adequate documentation) by offering a standardized form of charting the diagnosis, which would require little time to individualize for each patient. This approach to problem solving seeks mutual gains for both negotiating groups.

## DEFINING THE PROCESS

Fisher and Ury (1) developed the method of *principled negotiation* for the Harvard Negotiation

**Table 13.1**  Principles of Negotiation[a]

1. Don't bargain over positions.
2. Focus on interests, not positions.
3. Invent options for mutual gain.
4. Separate the people from the problem.
5. Insist on using objective criteria.
6. Develop the best alternative to a negotiated agreement.
7. Use negotiation jujitsu.
8. Tame the hard bargainer.

[a]Adapted from Fisher RJ, Ury W. Getting to yes: Negotiating agreement without giving in. New York: Penguin Books, 1984.

Project. This research project works on negotiation problems and develops and disseminates improved methods and theories of negotiation that have been implemented in mediations such as the Camp David Middle East peace negotiations in 1978. These principles (Table 13.1) are applicable to all negotiating situations, and each principle will be addressed in the following discussions as they apply to the negotiations of the critical care nurse manager.

## DO NOT BARGAIN OVER POSITIONS

When two negotiating parties state their positions, there is a tendency for both parties to defend those positions and become increasingly more committed to them. Egos become identified with each negotiator's respective position and therefore the interest of both parties is to preserve their stand on the issue, rather than to reconcile the parties' original interests. Consider, for example, the intensive care unit (ICU) where the patients' scheduled medications are consistently not available from the pharmacy in a timely fashion. The ICU nurse manager schedules a meeting with the pharmacy director to discuss this problem. The nurse manager may take the stand that the lack of available medications is due to his or her observation that the pharmacy is disorganized and poorly managed. The pharmacy director may take the stand that the ICU nurses are at fault for not delivering the orders to the pharmacy in a timely manner. The remainder of the meeting is spent with each party defending its position, providing support data to back its claims, and trying to convince the other party to accept its position. No agreement is likely to be reached in such a situation. A more experienced nurse manager would avoid the pitfalls of stating positions, recognizing that positions obscure the real interest of both parties, which in this case was the timely administration of medications for patients.

## FOCUS ON INTERESTS, NOT POSITIONS

Positions may be easier for negotiators to identify than interests and therefore tend to surface early in the negotiation process. Positions are likely to be concrete and tangible while interests may be abstract and intangible. The critical care nurse manager who has identified the need to have an arterial blood gas analyzer located in the ICU rather than in a centralized laboratory may negotiate with the director of the clinical laboratory to fulfill her request. The historical reaction by the laboratory director may be to take the position that traditionally the policy of the clinical laboratory has been to stay centralized and provide equal service to all areas of the hospital. Instead of outlining his or her position of wanting the equipment for the ICU, the nurse manager should outline his or her interests in this situation and help the other party to identify their interests. It is unlikely that the laboratory director would identify maintenance of tradition as his or her motivation in approaching this problem although both parties might be mutually interested in obtaining laboratory results quickly in the interest of patient care. The nurse manager should then be prepared to present data that laboratory results are not being returned in a timely fashion and lead the discussion as to how this objective could be achieved in a collaborative manner. Several options may be explored, and the ideal outcome in this negotiation would be that the laboratory director may suggest the addition of an arterial blood gas analyzer in the ICU as his or her own idea. Realizing the unimportance of ownership of the idea, the shrewd nurse manager has achieved his or her goal and a successful, "win-win" outcome for both parties.

## INVENT OPTIONS FOR MUTUAL GAIN

In the preceding example both parties were able to identify mutual interests, but another consideration is what both parties can hope to gain. In solving the problem, the nurse manager gains improved patient care without any expense to the unit. What are the gains for the other party? Although the laboratory director may be interested in quality patient care, he or she is also interested in controlling the budget. The nurse manager will need to explore possible increased revenue generation and/or an opportunity for potential enhancement of the departmental budget of the laboratory in order to promote awareness of potential gains under these circumstances. Negotiated outcomes should have identifiable mutual gains for both parties.

With further discussions the laboratory director and ICU nurse manager may explore another option of decreasing the transportation time of specimens delivered to the laboratory and therefore still achieving the same objective of receiving laboratory results in a timely fashion. The nurse manager must be firm in his or her objective, yet flexible in methods and options in achieving that objective.

## SEPARATE THE PEOPLE FROM THE PROBLEM

It is important to remember that all negotiators possess human emotions, differing values, and various backgrounds and perspectives. It is possible for the negotiating parties to observe the same events or behaviors and arrive at completely different conclusions about what occurred (6). Discrepancies in self-perceptions versus others' perceptions create multiple realities that may complicate the negotiation process. A study of hospital administrators' self-perceptions of their performance demonstrated a more favorable perception of their performance than the perceptions of their supervisors (7). McCloskey and McCain (8) studied staff nurse versus nurse manager perceptions of staff nurse performance. Staff nurses perceived that they were better at leadership than their nurse managers thought they were, an important finding for the nurse manager interested in negotiating with critical care staff nurses to increase their leadership potential. Other nursing studies have reported significant, although not high, correlations between staff and nurse manager ratings of performance, indicating a need for nurse managers to assess congruency of perceptions with staff before initiating negotiations (9–12).

The substance of the negotiation may become confused with the relationships of the negotiation parties if caution is not exercised. The critical care nurse manager in a negotiating situation should avoid use of the word "you" in an attempt to separate the people from the problem. An assistant director who says "*You* are over budget this month and I want to know what *you* are going to do about it" to a nurse manager is likely to provoke a sense of personal attack rather than mutual problem solving. It would be more persuasive and positive to say, "More money was spent in the ICU last month than was budgeted. Let's explore possible reasons and solutions to avoid this happening next month."

Speaking about one's self rather than the other party is a good tactic and is difficult to challenge. For example, the nurse manager who was promised more nursing positions by the director or assistant director in the new fiscal year budget but did not receive them, may say, "I'm very disappointed and feel let down." This method describes the indisputable impact of the problem upon the nurse manager, whereas a statement such as "You promised me those positions" or "You misled me" is disputable and likely to inflict anger in both parties. Participants in any negotiation process should perceive themselves as working with each other to solve the problem, not as two parties in conflict who attack each other personally.

## INSIST ON USING OBJECTIVE CRITERIA

It is important to prepare in advance for a pending negotiation and to examine standards or objective criteria both parties can agree upon. For example, as an entering nurse manager negotiating a salary for the position, it would be important to establish criteria as to how the salary will be decided and to have outlined beforehand how you relate to those criteria. For example, the nurse manager is quoted a salary range of $38,000 to $48,000 a year and believes he or she deserves to start toward the top of the range as this was the salary in a previous position. The nurse manager has also learned that other local hospitals' salaries for nurse managers start at that level. Before entering into a discussion about dollar figures with the person offering the salary, there must first be an agreement as to how the salary will be decided. Such criteria may include years of total experience, years of management experience, and educational preparation. If the nurse manager can negotiate to include previous salary history and comparable starting rates of local hospitals as objective criteria upon which to reach a final dollar figure, it is likely that a desired outcome will be reached and both parties will feel that the salary was negotiated fairly. Agreement upon objective criteria for the process of the negotiation facilitates the win-win desired outcome of the process. Table 13.2 lists other rules for negotiating salary as developed by Lax and Sebenius (13).

## DEVELOP THE BEST ALTERNATIVE TO A NEGOTIATED AGREEMENT

Some negotiations are not successful in spite of utilizing principled methods of negotiation. The

**Table 13.2** Rules for Negotiating the Best Deals[a]

1. Ask (ye may receive).
2. Find out what the job usually pays.
3. Think total compensation, not salary.
4. Negotiate for the things you need to be successful.
5. Make a rational case for your requests.
6. Timing is all.
7. Don't sulk if you don't get the compensation you asked for and you take the job anyway.
8. Remember not to gloat if you do cut the deal of your life.

[a]Adapted From Lax DA, Sebenius JK. The manager as negotiator: bargaining for cooperation and competitive gain. New York: Free Press, 1986.

other party may be more powerful and have more resources within the institution than the nurse manager. It is wise to recognize this fact as a negotiator and to always enter into a negotiation with an alternative solution. In negotiating for salary, for example, instead of determining a ''bottom line'' figure at which he or she will walk away from a desired position, the nurse manager may develop an alternative proposal that may mean negotiating for other forms of compensation, e.g., benefits, relocation expenses, office location.

Vice presidents, directors, and assistant directors of nursing in hierarchical organizations are generally more powerful within the institution than the unit level nurse manager and therefore may refuse to negotiate certain matters. Suppose the ICU nurse manager has identified the need for an ICU technician to assist the critical care nurse by performing nonnursing tasks. A proposal is developed by the nurse manager including national and local data regarding the position, job description, fiscal impact, and evaluation criteria. The nurse manager presents the proposal to the director focusing on mutual interests of nurse retention, improved patient care, and minimal fiscal impact. The director reviews the proposal but indicates that it is not possible to add new positions to the nursing budget due to fiscal constraints of the hospital. The nurse manager offers a counterproposal to be allowed to pilot the position with the stipulation that the ICU not go overbudget during the pilot period and that the fiscal impact will be carefully scrutinized. This approach focuses on the merits of obtaining the position rather than responding to rejection. Remaining positive about accepting alternative solutions may assist the nurse manager in future negotiations with powerful parties.

## USE NEGOTIATION JUJITSU

Jujitsu is the Japanese art of defending oneself by grasping or striking an opponent so that his own strength and weight are used against him. Negotiation jujitsu, as described by Fisher and Ury (1), avoids opposing an opponent's strength directly, but rather encourages stepping aside and turning that strength to one's advantage. This involves not accepting or rejecting the other party's position, but rather to treat their position as one possible option.

Criticism should be invited and channeled into advice. If the nurse manager develops and presents a proposal for a nurse fellowship experience for master's-prepared staff nurses and the proposal receives criticism, the criticism could be turned into advice by asking, ''What ideas do you have for improving this proposal?''

When one party personally attacks the other party, the temptation to retaliate the attack should be avoided. Allow the attacker to ventilate and listen attentively to what is being said. When the opposing party is finished, try to redirect the personal attack to the problem. The use of silence may also be an effective tool in making the attacker feel uncomfortable and compelled to break the silence, perhaps offering other solutions to the problem.

## TAME THE HARD BARGAINER

Opponents in the negotiation process may utilize unfair tactics to obtain desired outcomes. These maneuvers may include imposing deliberate deception, presenting false information, or introducing threats. A critical care nurse manager may encounter a physician who insists that a staff nurse be fired because the physician has experienced a conflict situation with this nurse. The physician further threatens to take this request to higher hospital authorities if the nurse manager does not comply. The nurse manager may choose to ignore the threat or try to offer alternative solutions depending on his or her assessment of the physician's intentions to carry out the threat and the perceived consequences if the physician does go to the nurse manager's superiors with the problem.

If deceptive tactics are suspected, the issue should be raised so that the process of negotiation is agreed upon. For example a common ''dirty trick'' is for one opponent to seat the other negotiating party facing the sun so that he or she is physically uncomfortable and distracted. An astute negotiator will recognize this tactic and announce a move to another seat so that the negotiation process may proceed in an equitable manner. The negotiator should be aware of the physical setting in which negotiation will occur and to be aware of any conditions such as noise, temperature of the room, or seating arrangements that may induce stress. Raising such issues forthright forces both parties to address the process of negotiation, which facilitates positive solutions for both parties.

## COOPERATIVE VERSUS COMPETITIVE NEGOTIATION

Greenberger et al. (14) have described two types of negotiation strategies that are cooperative (win-win) and competitive (win-lose) bargaining. Cooperative negotiation seeks joint problem solving and solutions that meet the needs of both sides. Also referred to as integrative bargaining, cooperative negotiation is implemented when both parties want to work together to achieve the best possible mutual agreement and when each party believes the other party is trustworthy (15). Cooperative negotiation occurs when both parties have clear goals, believe a cooperative settlement is possible, and there are sufficient resources available for both parties to achieve their goals.

Competitive negotiation, also called the win-lose or distributive bargaining strategy, is utilized when parties believe resources are limited and both parties cannot achieve their goals (15). One party maximizes its own objectives at the expense of the other party and there is usually distrust or hostility between the negotiating parties. This leads to motivation to defeat the other party rather than to work with it (14).

Not all negotiations are strictly cooperative or competitive. Table 13.3 outlines the phases of each type of bargaining and questions to ask to determine what type of strategies to use. Nurse managers entering into any type of negotiation should consider which type of negotiation is likely to occur and develop a strategy accordingly.

## PLAYERS IN THE GAME

At least two parties or individuals are necessary for the negotiation process to occur. The critical care nurse manager interacts with multitudes of people on a daily basis, entering into the negotiation process with many of them. Nurses negotiate with patients frequently for them to be compliant with their prescribed regimen, e.g., negotiating with hypertensive patients to take their antihyper-

tensive medication. Critical care nurses negotiate with patients to get them to do deep breathing and coughing or with an agitated patient to be cooperative. Critical care nurse managers may have to negotiate with patients who request that certain nurses not take care of them.

Critical care nurse managers also negotiate with family members of patients. Family members may have special requests such as ''Would it be okay if I brought our cat in to see my husband?'' or ''My husband's nurse is spending more time with her other patient than with my husband. Could you speak with her?'' The nurse manager will need to negotiate with the family members regarding these requests.

Negotiating with the critical care nurses and support staff under his or her supervision is a continuous process for the critical care nurse manager in order to improve the quality of patient care and promote staff performance and productivity (5). Individual differences and staff personality characteristics may influence the negotiation strategy selected by the nurse manager. Some recent research has suggested that different cultures respond differently to varying styles of dispute processing (16).

The nurse manager's superiors within the organization, including nursing and hospital administrators, are important and frequent players in the negotiation arena. Certainly nurse managers negotiate with each other, for example, the ICU nurse manager may be asked to accept an older pediatric patient when the pediatric ICU has no available beds for that patient.

Interdepartmental negotiation is a common practice for the critical care nurse manager including housekeeping, radiology, pharmacy, respiratory therapy, clinical laboratory, personnel, payroll, clinical engineering, social service, physical therapy. Nurses and physicians work interdependently in critical care, which provides many opportunities for negotiation between these two parties. ICU joint practice committees may provide a forum for cooperative nurse-physician bargaining to take place (see Chapter 8).

Nurse managers must first recognize these interactions with others as a negotiation process in achieving goals for him- or herself, the ICU, and the nursing staff. Employing the process of principled negotiation will facilitate the nurse manager's comfort level in problem solving and managing conflict.

**Table 13.3** Differences between Cooperation and Competitive Bargaining[a]

| Phase | Competitive Bargaining | Cooperative Bargaining | Key Strategic Questions |
|---|---|---|---|
| Preparation | Set specific goals, bottom lines, and opening bids. Develop firm "positions" and competitive tactics to attain those goals at the expense of the other. | Develop general goals and broad objectives. Cultivate good options. Cultivate good relations of trust and openness with opponent to promote effective problem solving. | Is this going to be a fundamentally competitive or cooperative negotiation? How broadly or narrowly should I state my goals? Should I prepare competitive or cooperative tactics? |
| Entry-problem identification | State the problem in terms of one's own preferred solution. Publicly disguise or misrepresent own needs and goals; don't let the other side know what's really important. | State the problem in terms of the underlying needs of all parties. Represent own needs accurately to the other party; listen carefully to understand their needs. | How can I state the problem as broadly as possible while still protecting my own interests and preferences? |
| Elaboration/education | Disclose only that information necessary to support our position and have the other side understand it. Hide possible vulnerabilities and weaknesses. | Disclose all information that may be pertinent to a problem, regardless of whose position it supports. Expose vulnerabilities in order to protect them in the joint solution. | How much information should I disclose? What should be the "timing" of this sharing process? How can I present a complete case, as opposed to only the "most positive" case. |
| Bargaining | Include false issues, "dummy" options, or issues and options of low personal priority in order to trade them away for what you want. Make an early public commitment and stick to it. | Minimize the inclusion of false or "dummy" issues and stick to the major problems and concerns. Avoid early and public commitments to preferred alternatives in order to give all options full consideration. | Do I confine the definition of the problem and issues to only those things that I am most concerned about, or that we are both concerned for? How hard should I stick to, and fight for, the solution that I think is best? |
| Closure | Maximize own utilities while not caring about the other's. Overvalue concessions to other; undervalue gains one achieves. "Nibbling" strategy of taking issues off the table as one achieves a favorable settlement. | Maximize solutions that have joint utility; be honest and candid in disclosing preferences. "Nothing is ever final until all issues are settled" strategy. | How fully do I disclose what are my true priorities and preferences and what I stand to gain by particular outcomes? Should I try to negotiate issues one at a time or strive for a joint package? |

[a]Reprinted with permission from Greenberger D, Strasser S, Lewicki RJ, et al. Perception, motivation, and negotiation. In: Health Care Management: a text in organization theory and behavior. Shortell S, Kaluzny A, eds. New York: John Wiley & Sons, 1988:81–141.

## CONCLUSION

Negotiation is a new term to nursing although the process is encountered on a daily basis by nurses and nurse managers. Most nursing management books do not address the concept, and the subject heading is not found in nursing reference indices. In a review of nursing management journals in the last 4 years, only one article title included the word negotiation (17). Nurse managers must recognize the negotiation process, learn the principles of negotiation, and exercise them. As nurse managers are increasingly recognized as powerful resource coordinators within the health care organization, the need for increased participation in the decision-making of an organization becomes evident (18). The critical care nurse manager must be equipped with the tools to participate at that level to achieve objectives for nursing. Learning the art of principled negotiation is one essential skill to facilitate the nurse manager's success in this endeavor.

REFERENCES

1. Fisher R, Ury W. Getting to yes: negotiating agreement without giving in. New York: Penguin Books, 1984.
2. Rubin J, Brown B. The social psychology of bargaining and negotiation. New York: Academic Press, 1975.
3. Cohen H. You can negotiate anything. Secaucus, New Jersey: Lyle Stuart, 1980.
4. Webster's ninth new collegiate dictionary. Springfield: Merriam Webster, Inc., 1983.
5. Kennedy MM. Negotiation for cooperation and support. Hosp Manager, 1984;14(6):1–2.
6. Valloone RP, Ross L, Lepper MR. The hostile media phenomenon: biased perception and perceptions of media bias in coverage of the Beirut massacre. J Pers Soc Psychol, 1985;49(3):577–585.
7. Shapiro G, Dessler G. A comparison of self and superior performance ratings. Paper presented at the National Academy of Management Meetings, Division of Health Care Administration, New York, 1982.
8. McCloskey JC, McCain B. Nurse performance: strengths and weaknesses. Nurs Res, 1988;37(5):308–312.
9. McCloskey JC. Nursing education and job effectiveness. Nur Res, 1983;32:53–58.
10. McCloskey JC. Toward an educational model of nursing effectiveness. Ann Arbor, Michigan: UMI Research Press, 1983.
11. Schwirian PM. Evaluating the performance of nurses: a multidimensional approach. Nurs Res, 1978;27:347–351.
12. Schwirian PM. Prediction of successful nursing performance, parts III and IV. (DHEW Publication No. HRA 79-15). Washington, DC: United States Government Printing Office, 1979.
13. Lax DA, Sebenius JK. The manager as negotiator: bargaining for cooperation and competitive gain. New York: Free Press, 1986.
14. Greenberger D, Strasser S, Lewicki RJ, et al. Perception, motivation, and negotiation. In: Health care management: a text in organization theory and behavior. Shortell S, Kaluzny A, eds. New York: John Wiley & Sons, 1988:81–141.
15. Lewicki RJ, Litterer J. Negotiation. Homewood, Illinois: Richard D Irwin, 1985.
16. Leung K. Some determinants of reactions to procedural models for conflict resolution: a cross-sectional study. J Pers Soc Psychol, 1987;53(5):898–908.
17. Rambaud R. Negotiation through justification. Nurs Management, 1987;18(7):79–80.
18. Kaluzny AD, Shortell SM. Creating and managing the future. In: Health care management: a text in organization theory and behavior. Shortell SM, Kaluzny AD, eds. New York: John Wiley & Sons, 1988:492–522.

# Part IV

## EVALUATING
### AND
## CONTROLLING

# Chapter 14

# Evaluating Critical Care Staff

RITA M. BARDEN

Performance appraisals are an integral component of the critical care nurse manager's responsibilities. Appraisals serve to evaluate performance and develop individuals (1, 2). Performance is determined by the individual's ability and motivation. Ability includes intrinsic aptitude as well as scope of knowledge that is influenced by learning and experience. Motivation is characterized by an individual's desire to achieve a goal or goals and a willingness to work. Systematic ongoing performance appraisals can optimize performance and motivation.

This chapter will examine the purpose of performance appraisals, evaluation standards, methods of performance appraisals with special emphasis on peer review, and evaluation tools. Mechanisms for effective delivery of performance appraisals and potential problems related to the evaluation process will also be highlighted.

## PURPOSE OF PERFORMANCE APPRAISALS

Employee evaluations provide data for a number of personnel decisions. These include decisions to promote, transfer, or terminate an individual, as well as to provide guidelines for wage and salary determinations. Appraisals provide feedback to employees about their performance, recognizing accomplishments as well as indicating areas of deficit that may require additional training and development (1–4). The goal of any appraisal system is to motivate the employee to maintain acceptable standards of care and/or improve their performance. Although the formal appraisal may be rendered on an annual basis, the critical care nurse manager is continually assessing the employees' performance. This input allows the nurse manager to distribute the necessary work and provide counseling, guidance, and career development (2). Knowledge of the employee's strengths and weaknesses allows the nurse manager to match the most critically ill patients with the highest skilled practitioner. Institutional-wide systems for evaluating employees enable management to assess the talent that is available and provide consistency and equity in evaluating employees' performance. For these reasons the value of systematic, ongoing, formal, and informal performance appraisals cannot be underestimated.

## STANDARDS FOR EVALUATION

Employees are evaluated on predetermined performance standards that are outlined in a job description. The Joint Commission on Accreditation of Health Care Organizations (JCAHO) requires all job classifications to have a detailed description of the duties and responsibilities expected of the employee. JCAHO also requires job descriptions to be criteria based. Webster (5) defines criterion as ''. . . means of judging a standard, rule, or test by which something can be judged: measure of value.''

Standards for nursing performance should be based on professional standards of practice as outlined by the American Nurses Association (ANA) and more specifically by the American Association of Critical-Care Nurses (AACN). Standards of practice for disease processes that commonly occur in the intensive care setting are outlined in *AACN Procedure Manual for Critical Care* (6). Criteria or standards are developed to reflect consistency with nursing standards of practice and medical practice within a hospital. Development of these standards by staff in the intensive care area fosters professional growth and commitment to achieve these standards in the day-to-day performance of nursing care. Identification and communication of the criteria on which an employee is evaluated are imperative. One way to communicate the performance standards is to provide the critical care nurse with the job description/evaluation tool and standards of care upon employment. Incorporating the standards into the preceptor program serves to reinforce the criteria on which an employee is evaluated. This may be an effective method to ensure knowledge and understanding of the expectations required to maintain an optimal level of performance.

Some institutions combine the job description with the evaluation tool. In institutions in which a clinical ladder or levels exist that delineate varying levels of expertise, separate job descriptions/evaluation tools may exist for every level. Each level of the clinical ladder builds on the previous one to delineate behaviors specific to a clinical or administrative position. Areas of performance that are typically evaluated include clinical practice, patient/family teaching, leadership and coordination, professional and staff development, and a research/quality assurance component (Table 14.1).

Illustration of this idea may better explain the delineation in criteria needed to develop separate job descriptions/evaluation tools for each level of a clinical ladder. In the area of clinical practice the clinical nurse 1 (entry level position) is expected to perform initial assessment, collect accurate, complete, and pertinent data, and through continuous assessment maintain awareness of the status of each patient. The clinical nurse 1 in the intensive care area would obtain a thorough physical assessment, obtain results of procedures and laboratory tests, and be able to determine abnormal values. The nurse at this level is usually assigned the uncomplicated heart surgery patients, chronically ventilated individuals, or patients receiving stable intravenous medication.

The clinical nurse 2 is expected to comply with the previously mentioned behaviors in addition to planning and implementing nonstandardized nursing interventions and planning for discharge or transfer of patients. The critical care nurse at this level needs to perform rapid observational assessments to determine changing priorities. The clinical nurse 2 would be expected to rapidly and accurately assess changing clinical status in a patient, be knowledgeable enough to handle unstable surgical and medical patients, and be able to integrate the laboratory and radiologic findings into the nursing care plan. The nurse's understanding of the ''whole'' patient presentation allows him or her to predict possible outcomes for the individual.

The clinical nurse 2 has a broad enough knowledge base to order laboratory tests.

The performance expectation of the clinical nurse 3 (clinical expert) is that he or she expertly perform a comprehensive physical and psychosocial assessment and incorporate this data into clinical practice. The nurse at this level is also expected to utilize an interdisciplinary approach in evaluating patient and family care. Additional clinical practice components of the clinical nurse 3 role may include acting as a resource to patients, family, and colleagues, and as a consultant to other health care team members. This nurse is aware of minute changes in the patient's status, and he or she uses the radiologic and laboratory findings to predict several possible scenarios and to begin interventions that mitigate negative outcomes. This expert nurse's knowledge base is so extensive that other health care providers seek this nurse's assistance to problem solve patient issues (see Chapter 7).

## PERFORMANCE APPRAISAL METHODS

Numerous methods for performance appraisal exist, and selecting the format that accurately documents an individual's performance may be difficult (7). Production outputs as a mechanism of evaluating performance are common in industrial settings. This method is objective and allows no room for rater bias. Another form of appraisal consists of graphic rating scales that list characteristics and qualities necessary for satisfactory job performance that are then evaluated on a continuum or scale. This method allows for recognition of the employee for superior performance in all or certain areas.

Rank ordering is yet another method of appraisal. Based on specified criteria, all employees are ranked according to their performance with only one individual per ranking. If a manager has forty employees, every person would be placed in one of the forty positions with number one being the most effective and valuable employee. The advantage of this type of evaluation is that not only is performance considered, but potential value to the institution is also determined. The forced distribution method plots the appraisals on a normal frequency distribution.

Another method of evaluation consists of a checklist of behaviors necessary to perform a job that the rater utilizes to check off those behaviors

**Table 14.1.**   Performance Appraisal: Clinical Nurse 2 Job Description and Evaluation

Employee: _____ Date: _____

Title: _____ Department: _____

Period Covering: _____

Statement: The LEVEL 2 performs all behaviors of the LEVEL 1. In addition, the LEVEL 2 demonstrates increased knowledge and an expanded base of clinical expertise by demonstrating the following behaviors:

| *Clinical Practice* | 0 | 1 | 2 | 3 |
|---|---|---|---|---|
| 1.  UTILIZES NURSING PROCESS | | | | |
| 1.1 Consistently demonstrates the ability to assess, plan, implement, and evaluate nursing care of the trauma, general surgery, cardiothoracic, and head injury patient | | | | |
| 1.2 Plans and implements nonstandardized nursing interventions | | | | |
| 1.3 Plans for disposition of the patient; continually assesses need for intensive care; is proactive in working with health care providers to ensure timely disposition | | | | |
| 2.  COLLECTS DATA IN A COMPREHENSIVE MANNER | | | | |
| 2.1 Augments initial nursing assessment data with experiential knowledge to refine patient care plan | | | | |
| 2.2 Integrates verbal and nonverbal behaviors exhibited by patient and significant others to make nursing decisions | | | | |
| 2.3 Compiles, interprets, and incorporates laboratory data into the plan of care for the patient | | | | |
| 2.4 Performs rapid observational assessment to determine changing priorities<br>MEETS:          Needs colleagial assistance to determine patient status<br>EXCEEDS:       Immediately aware of patient clinical status, requires assistance to intervene<br>FAR EXCEEDS: Immediately aware of patient status and intervenes to mitigate negative outcomes | | | | |
| 2.5 Obtains pertinent information from patient/families, coworkers, anesthesia, and other health care providers resources to enhance patient care | | | | |
| 3.  DEMONSTRATES EXCELLENCE IN CLINICAL PRACTICE | | | | |
| 3.1 Functions independently with more complex treatments, procedures, and equipment:<br>Intraaortic balloon pump<br>Hemodynamic pressure lines and monitors<br>Intracranial pressure devices<br>Ventilators<br>Open chest procedures<br>Cardiopulmonary arrest | | | | |
| 3.2 Demonstrates expanded knowledge base as documented on skills inventory (includes all skills/procedures that require a certification process) | | | | |
| 3.3 Coordinates physical, psychological, social, and spiritual needs of patients with other health team members | | | | |
| 3.4 Shares expertise in clinical skills with other team members (documented educational sessions, instruction on new equipment or procedure, consulting on problem patients, nursing rounds, and formal patient care conferences) | | | | |
| 4.  UTILIZES MULTIDISCIPLINARY APPROACH TO PATIENT CARE | | | | |
| 4.1 Recognizes and utilizes the knowledge and expertise of colleagues | | | | |
| 4.2 Identifies available resources for patients and initiates referrals as appropriate | | | | |
| 4.4 Communicates patient outcomes to other health team members; informs physicians of changes in patients' clinical status in a timely manner; aware of patients' limitations to procedures and treatments | | | | |

**Table 14.1** *Continued.*

| | 0 | 1 | 2 | 3 |
|---|---|---|---|---|
| 5. PARTICIPATES IN NURSING STANDARD PRACTICE DEVELOPMENT | | | | |
| 5.1 Formulates and evaluates nursing standards of practice to reflect trends in critical care | | | | |
| MEETS: Recognizes changes in practice that require a standard practice be developed | | | | |
| EXCEEDS: Recognizes and participates in the development of the standard of practice | | | | |
| FAR EXCEEDS: Develops standard of practice and channels through appropriate committees for approval | | | | |
| 6. ANTICIPATES AND RESPONDS EFFECTIVELY TO CRITICAL SITUATIONS | | | | |
| 6.1 Proactive nursing interventions reflect assessment skills that minimize negative outcomes | | | | |
| 6.2 Follows advanced cardiac life support protocols in emergency situations | | | | |
| 6.3 Coordinates resources for effective response in the emergent situation, i.e., anesthesia intubation, equipment, x-ray, defibrillation | | | | |
| 6.3 Evaluates nursing interventions in relationship to patient outcomes and recommends appropriate change | | | | |
| 7. PROMOTES AND PROVIDES HEALTH CARE TEACHING | | | | |
| 7.1 Demonstrates effective teaching skills with colleagues, physicians, other health care providers, patients/families | | | | |
| 7.2 Evaluates the effectiveness of teaching and revises appropriately | | | | |
| 7.3 Documents all teaching, including patient's/family's response | | | | |
| *Professional and Staff Development* | | | | |
| 8. PARTICIPATES IN CLINICAL SUPERVISION | | | | |
| 8.1 Familiar with the objectives and expected competencies of orientees and students | | | | |
| 8.2 Serves as a positive role model | | | | |
| 8.3 Reviews with the orientee and student the outcomes of nursing intervention | | | | |
| 9. SERVES AS A CLINICAL RESOURCE PERSON | | | | |
| 9.1 Participates in the formal/informal teaching and guidance of other staff (documentation required) | | | | |
| 9.2 Precepts the level 1 RN after completing a preceptorship program | | | | |
| 10. PARTICIPATES ON COMMITTEES | | | | |
| 10.1 Initiates participation in unit and/or hospital committees | | | | |
| 10.2 Solicits the input of peers | | | | |
| 10.3 Provides feedback to colleagues of committee activity | | | | |
| 11. INITIATES AND CONDUCTS PATIENT CARE CONFERENCES | | | | |
| 11.1 Collects pertinent and useful information for patient care conferences | | | | |
| 11.3 Involves other health care members in patient care conferences or nursing rounds and coordinates health care providers for the conferences | | | | |
| 11.4 Assists level 1 RN in preparing patient care conferences | | | | |
| 12. PARTICIPATES IN EDUCATIONAL OPPORTUNITIES | | | | |
| 12.1 Presents educational programs for staff development | | | | |
| MEETS: 1 per year | | | | |
| EXCEEDS: 3 per year | | | | |
| FAR EXCEEDS: 5 per year | | | | |
| 12.2 Attends education programs in the unit | | | | |
| MEETS: 7 per year | | | | |
| EXCEEDS: 9 per year | | | | |
| FAR EXCEEDS: 11 per year | | | | |

**Table 14.1**  *Continued.*

| | 0 | 1 | 2 | 3 |
|---|---|---|---|---|
| 12.3 Maintains required certifications: | | | | |
| Every other year: Cardiopulmonary (CPR) | | | | |
| Advanced cardiac life support (ACLS) | | | | |
| Venipunctures | | | | |
| Arterial blood gases (manual) | | | | |
| Blood administration | | | | |
| Every year: Defibrillation | | | | |
| Cardioversion | | | | |
| Epidural injections | | | | |
| Dysrhythmia recognition | | | | |
| 12.4 Identifies needs and suggests programs for education | | | | |
| 12.4 Attends educational programs at the hospital and in the community | | | | |
| MEETS:           7 per year | | | | |
| EXCEEDS:        9 per year | | | | |
| FAR EXCEEDS:  11 per year | | | | |
| 12.5 Maintains own record of continuing education unit (CEU) information and makes this available upon request of the manager | | | | |
| 12.6 Develops educational programs based on information gleaned from attendance at educational offerings | | | | |
| *Leadership-Coordination* | | | | |
| 13.   UNIT GOALS AND OBJECTIVES | | | | |
| 13.1 Demonstrates awareness of short- and long-range goals | | | | |
| 13.2 Incorporates goals and objectives in clinical practice | | | | |
| 13.3 Provides input for goal and objective development | | | | |
| 14.   COORDINATES UNIT ACTIVITIES FOR A GIVEN SHIFT | | | | |
| 14.1 Serves as a charge nurse when assigned by manager | | | | |
| 14.2 When in charge, works toward an effectively coordinated shift (i.e., completes patient assignment, works toward an effective productivity standard, delegates additional responsibilities to staff as patient needs warrant, able to match patient acuity with skill level or learning needs of staff, schedules educational opportunities, knowledgeable about resources/equipment available to meet patients needs) | | | | |
| 14.3 Identifies and solves unit problems | | | | |
| 14.4 Presents a positive unit and nursing image when communicating with other departments, nursing units, and physicians | | | | |
| 15.   PARTICIPATES IN QUALITY ASSURANCE | | | | |
| 15.1 Assimilates quality assurance data reflective of nursing standards into clinical practice | | | | |
| 15.2 Participates in monitoring quality assurance issues | | | | |
| 16.   PARTICIPATES IN PLANNING AND IMPLEMENTING CHANGE | | | | |
| 16.1 Identifies unsafe patient care practices and initiates interventions | | | | |
| 17.   SHIFT ACCOUNTABILITY | | | | |
| 17.1 Handles problems in a positive, mature, reasonable, and professional manner | | | | |
| 17.2 Uses established lines of communication for problems and interpersonal conflict | | | | |
| 17.3 Seeks guidance when appropriate | | | | |
| 18.   DEMONSTRATES AN AWARENESS OF COST-EFFECTIVENESS | | | | |
| 18.1 Demonstrates awareness of unit and patient charges | | | | |
| 18.3 Utilizes supplies and equipment judiciously | | | | |
| 18.4 Recognizes and suggests cost-effective measures | | | | |

**Table 14.1  *Continued*.**

| | 0 | 1 | 2 | 3 |
|---|---|---|---|---|
| *Research* | | | | |
| 19.  IDENTIFIES NURSING RESEARCH PROBLEMS OR QUALITY ASSURANCE ISSUES | | | | |
| 19.1 Participates in unit research projects | | | | |
| 19.2 Incorporates findings from nursing research/nursing science into clinical practice | | | | |

1.  Comments if performance exceeds standard

2.  Comments if performance does not meet standard

3.  Goals (include time frame for completion)

4.  Manager's comments

5.  Employee's comments

demonstrated by the employee. Free form essays can be used as a method of performance appraisal, although this exclusive format is problematic as it provides no common criteria for evaluation and may be dependent on the evaluator's literary skills (2).

Critical incidents or anecdotal review is another type of performance appraisal. This method requires major effort to maintain adequate numbers of incidents and lacks common criteria for assessment of performance. If used without other methods, this format may be subject to rater bias. It is not uncommon in a variety of institutions to combine the checklist and free form essay methods to arrive at an objective rating.

Management by objectives (MBO) performance appraisals require the employer and employee to develop agreed-upon goals, a time frame for completion, and a means of measuring goal achievement. The manager and employee meet periodically to determine whether the goals are progressing toward completion (8).

Performance appraisals may use a multiple rater technique as another method of evaluation. Stokes and Stinson (9) found that job responsibilities that are multidimensional, such as technical staff and administrative personnel, lend themselves to the multiple rater format. The critical care nurse's responsibilities are multidimensional as they include knowledge of numerous technical skills and procedures, coordination of other health care providers, and the ability to intervene rapidly in the patient's behalf and to mobilize the effective response of other members of the health care team. The critical care nurse's role has an administrative component in that he or she must effectively manage patient, family, physicians, other health care

providers, support services, and the administration of the organization. An accurate evaluation of the performance of the critical care nurse is extremely difficult if there is one evaluator or several evaluators who are all in an administrative capacity. The rater or raters may not have adequate exposure to all areas of the nurse's performance to evaluate the individual fairly. Peer review may alleviate this difficulty by having an administrative rater and several peer raters whose assessment is derived from numerous interactions with the employee (10, 11).

## PEER REVIEW

Peer review is emphasized in this chapter as it is an expectation of professional practice. A profession is accountable for and answerable to society for the quality of the services provided. Peer review assists in the definition of standards and assurance that those standards are practiced. Peer review provides one mechanism to ensure nursing's standing among other respected profession (12–14).

The American Nurse's Association in its publication entitled *Peer Review Process* writes that "Peer review is nursing's value system made visible. The collegial process can be carried on with security in the knowledge that quality of care, however extensive, costs of care, however contained, lose meaning unless the quality of that care is professionally affirmed" (12).

In addition to the compelling argument of professionalism, there are other reasons for establishing a peer review method in the performance appraisal process. Collegial evaluations can assist to define standards of care, identify the individual's performance in a more objective manner, and provide a comprehensive assessment of the actual performance. The ANA notes that peer review also assists in identifying areas of practice deficit that can guide development of standards to ensure clinical competency, increase nurses control over their own practice, and provide the practitioner with specifics to improve documentation, communication, and clinical expertise.

JCAHO requires documentation of a peer review process for medical staff, that reviews credentials of physicians seeking appointment to a health care institution and monitors performance after admission to the medical staff. In the past it was only the manager's prerogative to evaluate an employee's performance. Peer review uses a mutiple rater format to assess performance of the nurse.

Porter-O'Grady and Finnegan (15) in their book *Shared Governance* outlines a professional practice model that includes a quality assurance committee that annually reviews the credentials and the evaluation of employees' performance. The evaluation includes data from the employee, manager, assistant manager, and several colleagues in determining reappointment to practice in that institution.

Hinshaw and Field (17) in their research on psychological effects of peer evaluations suggest that this process has favorable effects on nurses' self-esteem. Perceptions that the manager's evaluations are unfair and/or biased are common complaints of employees (16, 17). Rapid changes in the health care arena with reorganization, downsizing, and flattening of the hierarchical structures in bureaucratic organizations have resulted in the reduction of the supervisory ranks and increased the responsibilities of the nurse manager. The manager may be left with less time to observe and objectively evaluate the employee's performance.

Implementation of this process requires staff acceptance and an environment of trust and mutual support to be successful (3). Involving staff in the development of the peer review process not only promotes acceptance but also provides an opportunity for growth and development. The ANA guidelines recommend the development of a temporary committee that through research, planning, and discussion would develop a standardized method for the peer review process (12). Representation on this committee should reflect an adequate sampling of the individuals affected by the peer review process. Some institutions would hold elections for this ad hoc committee, voting on a representative

from each shift and from each of the intensive care units. It is recommended that the manager from each of the units be involved in the initial planning committee. Peer review alters the traditional role of the manager and may be perceived as a threat to their control and power. The commitment and understanding of the process by management and administration are vital to success of peer review.

The first responsibility of the planning committee needs to be thorough research of the literature on peer review and performance appraisals. The development of standards of practice is the next area of responsibility for the committee members, and finally the establishment of the procedure for determining achievement of those standards completes the development of the peer review process. After the peer review process has been outlined, the next and possibly the most important step is informing and soliciting feedback from the committee members' colleagues.

Institutions that have adopted a peer review process found that some staff voiced concerns about feeling uncomfortable and believed that this evaluation process may not adequately assess their clinical expertise or may reflect rater bias. Assurance that the manager's and the individual's own evaluations are continued components of the data collection may allay some of the nurses fear. The assistance of the human resource department may be necessary to develop a series of lectures on performance appraisals to assist the staff in accurately assessing their colleagues' performance.

Adoption of the peer review process in institutions varies (13, 17). Peer review may be voluntary and utilized in addition to a separate evaluation performed by the nurse manager, or it may be mandatory for all staff and incorporated into the performance appraisal system of the institution. A formal established system for determining the evaluators of the individual decreases subjectivity and rater bias that may plague the peer review process. A random process of selection of the raters diminishes the possibility of favoritism. The number of peer reviews completed on an individual is a matter of preference, but caution is advised in requiring numerous peer evaluations as the process may become too cumbersome. The use of two to three peer evaluators provides an adequate review of the individual's performance without being too time consuming.

Consideration needs to be given to the length

of employment of the raters. Insufficient exposure to the individual who is being evaluated will result in the dissemination of inaccurate information. The availability of the option to refuse to evaluate a peer because of insufficient exposure to their clinical practice decreases inaccuracy and promotes an atmosphere of collegiality. Administration of the information obtained in the peer review process can be done verbally between peers or by the manager allowing for anonymity (14, 17). In certain institutions a panel of the employee's peers presents the findings that have already been summarized in writing. This particular format allows the nurse being evaluated to question and clarify the report of his or her peers. Review of clinical practice is based on direct observation and review of the nurse's documentation (3). Mechanism of chart audit can be random or the nurse may select and submit for review a predetermined number of charts. Documentation review by peers is related to criteria that have been preestablished. Institutions implementing the peer review process may discover the need to revise and/or develop a more appropriate evaluation tool.

The steps involved in the implementation of a peer review process are as follows:

1. Develop a committee comprised of staff nurses and management.
2. This committee reviews the literature on peer review and performance appraisals.
3. Review, revise, or develop existing standards of practice, as appropriate.
4. Examine the existing evaluating tool to determine whether it measures standards of care required to perform adequately. Revise or develop a new tool.
5. Develop guidelines for peer review as follows:
   a. Employees should be notified of an evaluation, given an evaluation tool to complete, and required to obtain three nursing care plans, admission resumes, and nursing documentation. They must submit evidence of continuing education attendance, and authorship of a Nursing Standard Practice (NSP) presented lecture, publications, certifications, or research.
   b. The employee's packet is submitted to the manager or designee, and three peers are randomly selected to review the packet of information compiled by the employee. (Peer reviewers must have a minimum of one year

of exposure to the individual being evaluated.) Two peers should be selected from the shift the employee works and one from the opposite shift. Peer reviewers document the evaluation and submit it to the manager or designee.
   c. The manager/assistant manager completes an evaluation.
   d. A meeting is arranged to deliver and review the evaluation.
   e. Provide a program for education of staff regarding evaluations and the peer review process.
   f. Encourage feedback on process resolution of issues that may evolve.

## EVALUATION TOOLS

Characteristics of an effective evaluation tool include development of criteria that are specific, relevant, practical, measurable, and unbiased (19). Behaviors being measured need to be based on the job characteristics and not on the personality of the individual being evaluated (1, 7, 18). Examples such as "able to function well in stressful situations" or "helpful to colleagues" are not specific enough to ensure consistency in evaluation. Several raters may evaluate the same employee very differently. A statement such as "demonstrates ability to make effective decisions during an emergency situation reflecting judgment and validity" is measurable and diminishes rater bias (Table 14.1).

Employee performance of characteristics and behaviors required of the job may be evaluated using a rating scale. These scales require clear definitions as to their meaning to be effectively used (Table 14.2). Advantages of a rating scale for each criterion is that it is easy to use and readily demonstrates areas of exception and deficit in the employee's performance. A disadvantage in the use of rater scales is that the mechanism will not provide indepth information (2). Requiring essay documentation of specific examples of the employee's substandard or exceptional performance may provide more in-depth information.

Maintaining ongoing documentation of the employee's performance presents a time management dilemma for the critical care nurse manager, especially when the nurse manager is responsible for evaluating a large number of employees. Computerization of files that objectively document the employee's performance can greatly reduce the time

**Table 14.2**   Rating Scale for Performance Appraisal

| | |
|---|---|
| 0. DOES NOT MEET: | Does not meet expectations of majority of critical areas of position; demonstrates less initiative and/or requires more supervision than is consistent with job description |
| 1. MEETS: | Meets expectations in majority of critical areas of position; demonstrates initiative in completion of tasks; requires a moderate amount of supervision |
| 2. EXCEEDS: | Exceeds expectations in majority of critical areas of position; demonstrates additional initiative; requires minimal supervision; considered a role model for this position |
| 3. FAR EXCEEDS: | Exceeds expectations in all critical areas of position and consistently demonstrates significant additional initiative; requires little or no supervision; extraordinarily high level of performance |

involved in maintaining and gathering information pertaining to an employee's evaluation. Annual attendance at staff meetings can be located in one computer file or on a single sheet of paper to quickly determine the number of meetings the individual has attended. Computerized scheduling can sort the number of absences an employee has had in the past year. JCAHO requires documentation of communication pertaining to new or revised NSP requirements. Forms with all of the employees listed by unit on the horizontal axis and the new or revised NSP requirements listed vertically can assist in rapid recognition of the employees who have maintained their professional responsibility by reviewing the new standards and signing the form. As with any form of documentation, absence of a signature indicates that the employee has not reviewed the policy and/or procedure. Although this mechanism does not ensure compliance with the standard, it does indicate professional commitment. Certifications such as basic life support (BLS), advance life support (ALS), critical care (CCRN), mobile intensive care nurse (MICN), certified emergency nurse (CEN), operating room nurse (AORN), or other national certifications can be maintained in a central file that allows for rapid data collection.

The nurse manager may decide that maintenance of documentation of professional activities is the responsibility of the individual employee. At the time of the annual evaluation, the nurse manager may request that the person provide evidence of professional activities, to include certifications, continuing education classes, lectures given, publications, patient care conferences held, nursing audits performed, NSP requirements authored by the employee, and documentation of involvement in hospital or unit-specific activities.

Whatever standards are determined must be communicated to the employees and applied to all

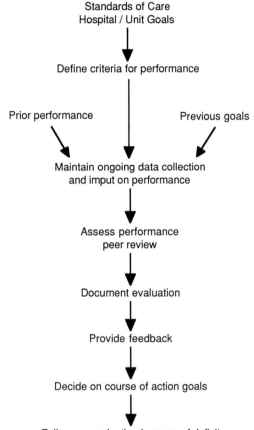

**FIGURE 14.1**   Performance appraisal process.

individuals being evaluated (Fig. 14.1). To decrease subjectivity, every employee must be evaluated on all elements in the evaluation tool. Selectively applying criteria diminishes the effect of the appraisal process in identifying strengths and weaknesses and in motivating the employee to achieve a high level of performance.

## DELIVERY OF PERFORMANCE APPRAISAL

Care in delivering the performance appraisal is essential to maximize the positive effects of the feedback. Advance notice of the evaluation process is necessary to provide the employee with an opportunity to prepare for the appraisal. Supplying the individual with the tool for their self-evaluation can provide the employee with the stimulus to review his or her past performance and future goals. Instruction on self-assessment, the evaluation tool itself, and goal development may be necessary.

Preparation of the evaluation by the critical care nurse manager is a step that is often underestimated, which can lead to undesirable consequences (4). The valuable opportunity to provide appropriate feedback to the employee regarding his or her performance and reinforce standards of care and expectations of superior performance may be lost. Poor preparation may result in demoralizing the individual and an unwillingness by the employee to share strengths, weaknesses, goals, and aspirations. Understanding the employee's work habits, interests, and prior achievements is vital in developing strategies to motivate the individual to peak performance (Fig. 14.2).

Delegation of evaluation is dependent on the structure of the institution. It is appropriate for the assistant manager, charge nurse, and/or supervisor to prepare and deliver the performance appraisal. To ensure the consistency, objectivity, and equitable delivery the nurse manager reviews and attends the evaluation interview. The manager has the responsibility to establish the measurable, objective standards and educate those he or she delegates this task. The evaluators must be able to observe the employee regularly to obtain an ongoing assessment of their performance.

Accurate information regarding clinical practice, committee work, community endeavors that are related to nursing, absenteeism, and peer evaluations need to be obtained and documented on the evaluation tool. Clinical nurse specialists (CNSs), if available in the institution, provide valuable input into the evaluation. Their unique role in a staff position affords the CNS the opportunity to observe the staff nurse's clinical skills, adherence to standards of practice, documentation, and patterns of communication with colleagues, physicians, and families.

Formal peer evaluations may be delivered as they are, if anonymity has not been specified in the program guidelines developed to implement

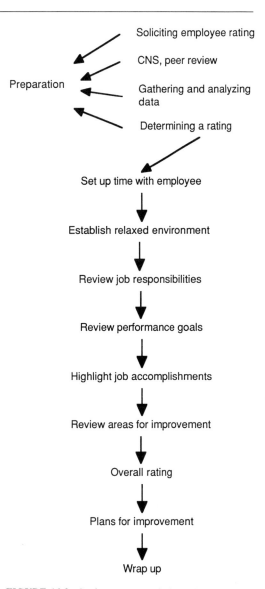

**FIGURE 14.2**  Performance appraisal administration.

peer review. Goals may be written by the evaluator or the employee, or they may be mutually developed at the time of the appraisal. Another part of the preparation is developing a logical rationale that results in the employee rating. The overall rating needs to be based on the performance of the previous year, not on recent events or on the individual's personality (4).

With the advent of merit raises or pay for performance programs in health care settings, assigning a rating for the employee presents a unique challenge for the nurse manager. The nurse manager, CNS, and staff nurse need to develop specific criteria for achievement of each rating level. With pay for performance programs it is imperative that each criterion be as specific as possible. Criteria that can be quantified should be assigned a value. For example, "attending educational programs" is subject to different interpretations. Therefore, "meets" attending educational programs may be defined by the group involved as seven programs per year, "exceeds" as nine programs per year, and "far exceeds" as 11 programs per year. It is advisable to discuss the caliber of programs that are acceptable for inclusion in achieving this goal and make the specifics known to the staff. Delineating behaviors required of each criterion decreases the dissent that may result from some staff members receiving higher merit raises than others. Employees will know in advance what they need to accomplish to achieve each of the ranges in the merit system. Clarification of the performance standard can eliminate the perception of inequity by the staff.

After the nurse manager's preparation of the evaluation is complete, the next step is creating the right time and environment for the performance appraisal. Asking the person to set a time for the evaluation during an emergency with his or her patient or after an extremely busy shift might make the employee feel less positive toward the process. Allowing the employee some control over the time for the appraisal creates a more positive perception.

Once the time has been established, the setting for the environment must be considered. to give feedback formally or informally in a public arena diminishes the impact and seriousness of the information and may be a source of humiliation for the employee. A quiet, private environment without interruptions demonstrates to employees the importance of the evaluation process and of their contribution to the institution. Allow sufficient time for discussion and questions, usually one to three hours.

Once the time and environment are established, the evaluation can be administered. Casual conversation may assist in relaxing employees and encouraging them to participate in the evaluation process. Reviewing with employees the process of evaluation, including sources of information obtained and job responsibilities, may allow for easy transition into the assessment of the nurse's performance. Reflective questioning can reveal the employees' perception of their performance. Questions such as "In what areas do you think you are most effective?" or "What aspect of your job has interested you most?" encourage the employee to articulate their accomplishments. "How might we use your talents and time more effectively?" highlights the employees' perception of their talents and provides input into the goal-setting process (2). After employees have identified their strengths and accomplishments, the critical care nurse manager can validate the nurse's views and provide additional insight into employees' contributions.

Discussion regarding weaknesses or areas of deficit is frequently the most difficult aspect of administering the performance appraisal (2, 4). Often employees are aware of their deficits and by asking questions about the areas most frustrating for them or areas in which they think they are least effective, those weaknesses can be identified by the manager and/or their peers. Olson (4) recommends dealing with one negative area at a time, stating the deficit in behavioral terms related to the job responsibilities. Avoid any reference to personality issues. Encourage the employee to discuss the issue and to provide possible explanations. Express understanding and develop a mutual plan to correct the area of weak performance. Ending on a positive success-oriented note can assist the employee in remedying the areas of concern.

Despite the critical care nurse manager's best efforts, a nurse may react in a hostile manner. Anticipating this eventuality, especially with employees who have difficulty accepting criticism, may be the manager's best strategy. Listen to the employee's perception of the issues, focus on the area of disagreement, and negotiate with the employee for a mutually agreeable resolution (see Chapter 13). If this refocusing technique is ineffective, reschedule the appraisal to allow the employee time to reflect and gain control. Follow-through on the disagreement provides further clarity and imparts a message to the employee that the manager is serious and concerned about this area of weakness (19). If there is improvement in the employee's behavior, immediate feedback to the employee rather than waiting until the next evaluation session is the most effective method to ensure continued improvement (20).

Goal setting provides the nurse manager with an opportunity to learn more about the employee's aspirations and motivations. Asking open-ended questions about areas of interest and plans for the future can assist in defining goals. Reconciling the employee's goal with the goals of the institution may result in the development of talents that can be utilized for the benefit of both the employee and the institution (8).

The final component in the delivery of a performance appraisal is the summary of the evaluation. Feedback from the individual regarding his or her perceptions of the evaluation and the process can be valuable for the nurse manager. The employee's participation and involvement throughout the evaluation is critical to motivating the individual to an optimal level of achievement.

## PROBLEMS ASSOCIATED WITH PERFORMANCE APPRAISALS

The critical care nurse manager's understanding of common problems associated with the appraisal process is essential in effectively evaluating employees. Problems can be related to the system within an institution or result from errors of the evaluator in arriving at a rating. System or method difficulties will diminish the purpose and benefit of the appraisal (21, 22).

Systems problems include inaccurate job descriptions or evaluation tools. Some institutions use the same evaluation tool for all levels of employees, professional as well as technical. Development of an adjunct evaluation specific to the critical care setting and nursing in general is advised. This may be in addition to or may be incorporated in the tool required by the human resource department. Appraisals that are specific for the requirements of a critical care nurse will be more meaningful (Table 14.1). Some hospitals have a generic evaluation tool for all nurses that requires modification to reflect the responsibilities required on a specific nursing unit (23). Involvement of staff in the development of a tool specific for their area promotes professional growth and development and encourages commitment to achieve a high standard of practice.

Another system concern relates to preparation of evaluators. Frequently nurse managers are promoted due to their clinical expertise. Education in management responsibilities may be limited or expected to develop while in the role. This lack of knowledge diminishes the positive effect of properly completed and administered appraisals. The new critical care nurse manager needs to assess his or her own values and standards and determine if they are reasonable

and attainable. Staff involvement in this process provides the nurses with the opportunity to incorporate these values and standards as their own. Researching the available literature on performance appraisals and taking educational courses in evaluating performance can assist new managers and revitalize veteran managers in effectively completing and administering appraisals.

Education and awareness of problems associated with performance appraisals can alleviate errors in the method of completion of the evaluation. These rater errors if uncorrected can promote demoralizing behaviors in employees and create inequity in the rewards administered and the promotions that occur within the institution (24).

The bias effect toward leniency protects the weak performer because the manager believes an accurate evaluation will damage the nurse's self-concept. This fear of providing negative feedback in actuality promotes substandard performance. The employee is rewarded for minimal performance despite the effort on the part of the manager to encourage improvement (1). Weak performers who "get away with it" are demoralizing to coworkers and potentially dangerous to patients.

Nurse managers can also err by rating their employees harshly or too critically. This bias toward strictness may lower performance. Standards set that are unattainable or performance that is never quite "good enough" serve to frustrate employees and create negative attitudes toward their jobs (24, 25).

The halo effect can be equally as detrimental in evaluating an employee. This rater error is due to observation of only one aspect of the individual's performance and the assumption that this applies to all aspects of the person's performance. Appraisals that indicate exceptional performance in all areas are suspicious and are usually due to the halo effect.

Errors of central tendency can be the result of lack of sufficient observation of the employee's performance so that all aspects of the performance appraisal are rated as average. The nurse manager has no factual information to substantiate the employee's performance so he or she is forced to guess, usually resulting in average scores. Another reason for this bias error can be fear on the part of the nurse manager of creating discontent among employees because of variations in ratings between employees. By not distinguishing between individuals who excel and those whose performance is minimal or substandard, the evaluator may be encouraging mediocrity.

The performance appraisal reflects behavior over a period of time, usually 6 months to a year. If the critical care nurse manager allows positive or negative events just before the completion of the evaluation to bias the entire appraisal he or she has committed a rater error of recency. An employee, knowing that an evaluation is imminent may improve performance, then lapse after the evaluation into minimal levels of achievement. Maintaining documentation of year-round performance enhances the nurse manager's accuracy in evaluating the employee.

## SUMMARY

Performance appraisals evaluate and develop the employee. Accurate, comprehensive evaluations document and recognize the individual's accomplishments and deficits. Identified areas of weakness direct the training and development needs of the employee. Primary components of the role of the critical care nurse manager are the assurance of competency and the professional development of his or her employees. Development of standards of practice and awareness of the nurse manager's expectations are the foundation for any evaluation tool. Standards of practice must be consistent with the standards established by professional nursing organizations and the specific institution. Criteria-based evaluation tools are recommended by JCAHO and provide consistency in the behaviors rated and expected of every employee.

Professions are mandated authority, responsibility, and accountability related to the development of a specialized body of knowledge and the provision of a service to society. Peer review, which ensures appropriate standards of care by evaluation of individuals delivering that care, enhances the professional status of nursing. Peer review as a mechanism of evaluation of a colleague's performance promotes development of standards of practice and ensures clinical competency. Therefore, peer review allows nurses greater control of nursing.

Proper preparation and administration of the evaluation are essential to obtain a positive and motivating result. Encouraging involvement in the evaluation process with self-assessments and employee participation during the evaluation meeting can be a learning experience for both the nurse manager and the employee. Evaluating

the critical care nurse's individual talents and desires is beneficial for the nurse and the institution.

*Special thanks to Barbara Nastari, R.N., B.S.N., and Mary Ellen Dellefield, R.N., M.N., for their assistance in the preparation of this manuscript.*

REFERENCES

1. Nauright L. Toward a comprehensive personnel system: performance appraisal—part 4. Nurs Management 1987;18:67–77.
2. Sikula A, McKenna J. The management of human resources; personnel text and current issues. New York: John Wiley and Sons, 1984:251–266.
3. O'Loughlin EL, Kaulback D. Peer review: a perspective for performance appraisal. J Nurs Adm 1981;September:22–26.
4. Olson R. Performance appraisal: a guide to greater productivity. New York: John Wiley and Sons, 1981:12–35.
5. Gove PB, ed. Webster's third new international dictionary. Springfield: G and C Merriam, 1976:538.
6. Millar S, Sampson L, Soukup M, eds. AACN procedure manual for critical care. Philadelphia: WB Saunders, 1985.
7. Mandelenbaum L. Periodic competency review: an assessment and policy model. Eval Health Prof 1987;10:342–358.
8. Clark M. Performance appraisal. Nurs Management 1982;13:27–29.
9. Stokes J, Stinson J. Breathing fresh air into the performance appraisal system: the use of multiple raters. Hum Res Planning 1981;4:1–10.
10. Dombeck M. Faculty peer review in a group setting. Nurs Outlook 1986;34:188–192.
11. Bennett M. Effective credentialing and peer review of nursing personnel. Crit Care Nurse 1985;5:104.
12. American Nurses Association. Peer review guidelines. Kansas City: The Association, 1988:14.
13. Maas M, Specht J, Jacox A. Nurse autonomy: reality not rhetoric. Am J Nurs 1975;75:2201–2208.
14. Boyar D, Avery J. Peer review: change and growth. Nurs Adm Q 1981;5:59–66.
15. Porter-O'Grady T, Finnigan S. Shared governance for nursing. Rockville: Aspen Publications, 1984:79–105.
16. Mio S, Speros D, Mayfield A. The effect of peer review evaluations upon critical care nurses. Nurs Management 1985;16:42A–H.
17. Hinshaw A, Field M. An investigation of variables that underlie colleagial evaluation. Nurs Res 1974;23:292–300.
18. Selfridge J. Criteria based performance evaluations using the ENA standards of emergency nursing practice. J Emerg Nurs 1987;13:91–95.
19. Cox S. Peer and self-assessment. Nurs Times 1987;83:62–64.
20. Dickson B. Maintaining anonymity in peer evaluation. Supervisor Nurse 1979;5:21–29.
21. Anderson P, Davis S. Nursing peer review: developmental process. Nurs Management 1987;18:46–48.

22. Pelle D, Greenhalgh L. Developing the performance appraisal system. Nurs Management 1987;18:37–44.
23. Nadzam D. Documentation evaluation system: streamlining quality of care and personnel evaluations. Nurs Management 1987;18:38–42.
24. Bernadin JH, Beatty R. Performance appraisal: assessing human behavior at work. Boston: Kent Publishing, 1984:71–94.
25. Bray K. Performance appraisal of staff nurse. Part 1. Crit Care Nurse 1982;10:7, 8, 13.

# Chapter 15

# Competency-Based Managing

REBECCA KATZ

Competency-based education (CBE) has received much attention recently as a method for orientation in critical care. But CBE is much more than orientation. It is a method for management to evaluate all competencies in critical care nursing and it is a tool for management to ensure quality and effective nursing care. This chapter provides the nurse manager with the specific steps for instituting competency-based education, a specific method for guaranteeing that each employee has the same level of knowledge and skill level, as well as a way of developing the nursing staff professionally. CBE assists the nurse manager in developing a professional spirit of caring and a reward system, whether the hospital has a career ladder or not. This chapter will address CBE in the critical care setting although it is applicable to the entire nursing division.

One of the most penetrating criticisms of nursing education is that no one can identify which competencies or skills are directly related to effective critical care nursing practice (1). Competency-based education is a tool for management that evaluates whether a nurse can do certain skills, apply clinical knowledge, and maintain a professional demeanor in a specific clinical setting (2, 3). Although the competency may describe the behaviors or skills, it becomes a statement that describes the demonstration of a "composite of the specific skills" (4, p. 29). Therefore, competency-based education involves more than an individual sitting in class. It involves someone observing the student and critiquing the performance. CBE teaches the information needed in the clinical environment. It promotes the "need to know" information, as opposed to the "nice to know" information. CBE involves a total commitment by the hospital. Even if one nursing unit is utilizing this method, risk management, personnel, administration, and education must be involved and committed to the success of CBE.

Competency-based education has various labels: "performance-based education, mastery learning, individualized instruction, criterion-referenced evaluation, and self-instruction modules" (5, p. 197). Most of these labels refer to elements of CBE.

Before progressing, it is important to understand the meaning of competency. Webster's dictionary defines competency as "capacity equal to requirements: adequate fitness or ability: the state of being competent. . . ." Competent is defined as "answering all requirements. . .2. having ability or capacity: duly qualified. . ." (6).

Competencies are defined according to the many activities or practices of each profession. The literature is replete with references to banking, physical therapy, health education, pharmacy, medicine, and occupational therapy developing competencies for their professions (7–14). A competent practitioner is one who can perform these activities under certain conditions with a demonstrated degree of mastery (14, 15). Therefore, competencies are the expectations the manager has of the staff nurse. These competencies are the composite of performance skills, along with the integration of knowledge and affective behaviors. In critical care nursing, these competencies entail a growth process from the beginning practitioner to the expert level. The emphasis in CBE, or competency-based managing, is on competencies, on the ability to demonstrate a total performance building. Competency-based training involves deciding which competencies the critical care nurse must have in order to do his or her job, designing an educational program to ensure that he or she possesses these competencies, and evaluating whether the nurse can perform these competencies in the clinical arena.

CBE is learner centered. The outcomes specified describe what the learner must do to demonstrate competency. It holds the learner accountable for meeting explicit performance criteria or outcome statements. The new orientee can assume this role as quickly as he or she is capable of learning the necessary skills or while displaying the required knowledge.

Because the new employee can proceed at his or her own pace, the potential for decreased training costs exists. Two of the programs that costed out orientation programs are Maryland General Hospital, Baltimore, Maryland (16), and Presbyterian Hospital, New York, New York (17). Both hospitals reported a savings with the competency-based model for orientation when compared with the traditional model. No literature was found comparing costs of a totally designed CBE program, using various levels of practice, with the classroom style method.

The competency-based education approach has its origins in the philosophy of education known as "experimentalism" (18). CBE defines what constitutes competency in a given field. In CBE, time needed to achieve the competencies may vary, but achievement is held constant and the learner cannot proceed forward until certain predetermined criteria are met. A beginning nurse may be having difficulty demonstrating competency with basic arrhythmias. However, he or she has achieved mastery of other competencies. The manager might choose to provide the nurse with a self-paced ECG program or utilize a computer review program. However, the manager would not have him or her advance to the next level or the succeeding plateau until all competencies for the beginning level had been met.

In the late 1960s, CBE began to succeed when nurses in the clinical setting related to nursing educators that staff nurses were unable to perform in the clinical setting what they had been taught in nursing programs. CBE became an educational approach that emphasized the learner's ability to demonstrate proficiencies that are of central importance to a given nursing task or nursing activity (1, 19).

In the past, traditional nursing education has emphasized what a nurse should know at the end of an educational program. In contrast, CBE is primarily concerned with ensuring that the nurse can perform in the clinical setting. Therefore, CBE shifts the emphasis from what is to be taught to what is to be learned (20). It places responsibility on the instructor to teach the skills, knowledge,

and behaviors needed in the clinical setting by the nurse. It deemphasizes the needs of the instructor to teach the areas about which he or she knows the most and challenges the instructor to improve the variety of teaching methods used.

Several authors have written about CBE, giving more meaning to competencies. Berner and Bender (20) suggest that competencies are the knowledge and skills a professional needs to perform adequately. Hinojosa (14) suggests that being competent involves doing something, in a specific environment, in accordance with a specified standard. This implies that one who is competent demonstrates the ability to perform a set activity skillfully. Klemp (21) defined competence as a "generic knowledge, skill, trait, self-schema, or motive of a person that is causally related to effective behavior referenced to external performance criteria."

Competencies are the expectations of a practitioner who has achieved a certain level of experience and knowledge (20). There can be different sets of competencies in critical care nursing, based on the knowledge and skills needed to meet the complexity of patients in the clinical setting. In determining competencies, the technology, patient population, medical standard of care, nursing education, and support services need to be taken into account.

However, competencies are just one part of competency-based education.

CBE is a process of not just describing the expectations of nursing for the critical care staff, but it also necessitates a change in the educational structure as well as the evaluation process (22).

Many authors have described the characteristics of CBE (2, 3, 5, 23). These characteristics include competency statements developed by expert practitioners specific for a clinical setting. It has been described as learner centered, and specific outcomes are identified with measurable criteria. The competency-based curriculum is designed to contribute to the learner attaining the competencies for a broad area such as "provide care for the patient undergoing major abdominal surgery classified at risk for cardiovascular and respiratory complications." The curriculum must be designed so the learner can demonstrate prior acquisition or mastery of learning. For example, if a nurse manager hires an experienced critical care nurse, it would not be economically feasible to send this nurse to classes designed for a beginning critical care person if he or she has already mastered the content. Yet, as a nurse manager there is an obligation to assure that the nurse has met these expectation. One way to achieve this is to develop specific competencies for each level of nursing practice. These specific competencies will then be used to assure that the nurse demonstrates the same level of knowledge.

There are many parts to designing a CBE program for management of a unit. CBE is founded on clearly articulated competency statements (2, 23, 24). These competency statements are developed by the experienced staff nurses. Competency statements define the overall expectations, or skills and behaviors, that the nurse manager looks for in the well-developed staff nurse. There is a difference between competencies, behavioral objectives, and goals. Competencies are not independent of goals and objectives. Goals are the broadest statements that can be made about the outcomes of a CBE program (4). An objective is a very specific formal statement made about expected learning outcomes. The competency statement lies midrange between goals and objectives. The size or number of competencies is determined by how broad the goal is. For each competency, there will be a number of subcompetencies as these are more specific than competencies (2). Examples of a goal, competency, subcompetencies, and objectives are in Table 15.1.

The next step is to formulate levels of nursing practices. Once the stages of nursing practices for the given unit are decided, the competencies that are realistic for that level of nursing practice are agreed upon by a committee. Then the competencies are subdivided into subcompetency statements and, finally, criterion-referenced evaluation state-

ments that can be used to judge whether a nurse has met the subcompetency statements that have been developed.

CBE is based on the clinical practice of critical care nursing practice. The competency statements and CBE programs originate from the experience, observation, and validation of what real performance of competent practitioners in that role actually comprises.

The competencies are highly specific for a given field or discipline and level of practice. Levels of critical care nursing practice must be decided for a given critical care nursing unit. These include not only the cognitive or knowledge expectations, but also the psychomotor or skill and affective or behavior capabilities. The competencies must be specific for the critical care unit.

Competencies must be developed by expert practitioners. The nurse manager should not decide the competencies by sitting in an office. Expert staff nurses, with the assistance of the clinical nurse specialist, nurse manager, education specialists, and other specialists, must identify and validate the elements that comprise the broad expectations.

The competencies must be centered on practice/performance outcomes. Each level of practitioner must demonstrate an ability to perform all essential aspects of a role. He or she must be able to show suitable performance. The criterion reference statements evaluate whether a nurse has achieved the competencies and demonstrate whether or not the learner can act upon what he or she has learned. One tenet of CBE is mastery learning. This process states that given enough time and opportunity, the learner can achieve performance criteria. For example, a new critical care nurse might be experiencing difficulty achieving competency in

**Table 15.1**    Examples of Competency Statements

Goal: The nurse will provide care to the patient with complex cardiovascular problems.
  Competency: Provides care for the patient with actual or potential cardiac dysfunction
    Subcompetency: Provides care for the patient with an arterial line
      Criteria Statements
      1. Balances and calibrates the arterial line after zeroing it at the phlebostatic axis
      2. Assesses and documents peripheral pulses and circulation to appropriate extremity
      3. Changes solutions, arterial line setup, stopcock, and sterile dressing according to procedure
    Subcompetency: Provides care for the patient with a Swan-Ganz catheter.
      Objectives
      1. List four indications for arterial line placement
      2. Identify the normal ranges for intravascular pressure readings
      3. Describe the abnormal intravascular pressure readings in terms of the pathophysiology that produces them
      4. Identify the necessary intervention for specific abnormal intravascular pressure readings

hemodynamic monitoring. Perhaps he or she has mastered the skill of balancing and calibrating an arterial line and a thermodilution but cannot interpret data that relate to the patient's physiologic problem. The preceptor might assign three patients for 3 consecutive days as well as provide a self-instructional program to the orientee. After a mutually agreed upon time frame by the preceptor and the new employee, the orientee is reevaluated.

CBE publicizes the expectations of the learner. Once the levels of nursing practice and the competency statements for each level have been developed, they should be used in the hiring process. The expectations for the nursing unit should be clear to the potential new nurse. Everything expected of the possible new employee should be clearly detailed in writing before hire.

CBE adheres to flexibility in means of instruction. The traditional method of classroom lecture is not necessarily the best method of instruction for each nurse. Because CBE focuses on the ends rather than on the means of instruction, the education department in the hospital or employing agency must be flexible in developing different methods of instruction. Self-instructional packets, computer-assisted programs, videotapes, and demonstration laboratories are just some of the methods that can enhance learning.

The entire evaluation process changes with CBE. CBE uses criterion-referenced evaluation instead of the traditional evaluation tool that employs such elements as nursing process, attendance, and professionalism. This type of evaluation judges a nurse's performance against a set of criteria that are specified as standards for that performance. By comparing the performance of the nurse against these criteria, the evaluator makes a "yes/no" type of judgment on the adequacy of that performance. The critical care nurse must document mastery of the specific criteria deemed necessary to demonstrate competency. Specific detailed criteria must be determined for each set of criteria. For example, the competency for hemodynamic monitoring might be: provides care for the patient with hemodynamic monitoring. One of the subcompetencies could be: provides care for a patient with a thermodilution catheter. Some of the criteria statements could include:

1. balances and calibrates thermodilution catheter;
2. states normal parameters for patient based on pathophysiology.

Criteria statements provide the preceptor or evaluator with objective criteria against which the nurse can be evaluated. The statements can be answered with a yes or no and can be validated by any number of evaluators.

CBE provides for "recycling" of learners. For example, if the learner has not accomplished a certain competency, he or she should be able to have further remedial instruction and be evaluated on this competency at a later date. The nurse manager must decide a reasonable time frame within which the competencies should be achieved. If the competency has not been achieved, the employee becomes a liability to the unit. Perhaps a nurse hired for an open-heart recovery unit is experiencing difficulty with the competency, "provides care for the patient with an intraaortic balloon pump" (IABP). The nurse manager might say to the nurse that this competency must be mastered within 2 weeks. Obviously, if the new nurse cannot master this competency and a high percentage of open-heart patients come from surgery with the IABP, this nurse could become a liability to the patient as well as the unit.

The next step in implementing competency-based management is to explore the level of commitment that must be displayed by various departments at the institution.

## ADMINISTRATION

When implementing CBE programs, the hospital administration will need to be informed regarding the purpose and intent of CBE. Often, the administration may understand the concept of competency, but they may not be familiar with the way the term relates to CBE or they may believe the development of competencies is a solitary program goal. They may lack the education about the developmental process and need to be convinced that competency differentiation is part of the phenomenon, not merely a means to an end. They need to understand that the development of competencies, subcompetencies, and criterion-referenced statements can require 2–3 years, if the expert staff nurses meet on a regular basis and validity and reliability of the tool are established. To hurry through the competency statements produces a product wrought with problems for the nurse manager. To develop an effective CBE program the administration must support giving the staff nurses time off the unit on a regular basis for the purposes of developing competency statements and the evaluation tool. In order to implement a CBE program, one individual who is extremely motivated and well educated with regard to CBE needs to serve as the project leader. A project leader can also assist the various units in getting started with the launching of a CBE program and ensure that a common format and process are used throughout the institution.

## HUMAN RESOURCE DEPARTMENT

The human resource department needs to understand the concept of criterion-referenced evaluation. The human resource department needs to support the concept of showing the potential candidate the competency list on the initial interview. The entire process must be explained to the prospective critical care nursing candidate. The various levels of nursing practice, the competencies for each level, and the evaluation tool need to be shared with the prospective employee. If this department cannot change the use of the generic evaluation tool, then attach the criterion-referenced evaluation tool to the generic evaluation. Employment departments need to be educated about the concept of levels of nursing practice and if no clinical ladder is used, they need to value the rewards you have attached to each level as a unit-based reward.

## NURSING OR HOSPITAL EDUCATION

CBE focuses on the ends rather than on the means of instruction, therefore the education department must be flexible in developing various methods of instruction (16). The learners must determine the sequence, methods, and pace that are best suited to their needs and preferences. In order to accomplish this, the institution must be committed to developing or providing self-learning packets, self-assessment tools, or perhaps computer-based training. They must be committed to more than the lecture style.

## RISK MANAGEMENT

Some of the questions that need to be addressed when developing a CBE program are:

1. What will be the consequences of a nurse not meeting the competencies after being afforded ample opportunities?
2. How long will tenured nurses have to achieve the competencies when the system is implemented?
3. Will tenured staff nurses be grandfathered in at a certain level or will they need to work through each competency level?
4. How long will a nurse transferring from one unit to another have to achieve the competencies of the new unit?
5. Will the hospital support voluntary or mandatory accomplishment of competencies?
6. What is the fiscal impact of this type of program?

Thinking through these questions ahead of time will reduce and/or prevent problems as the program moves from the developmental phase into the implementation phase.

## PRECEPTORS

Preceptors are frequently chosen for a unit-based competency committee because they have been identified as "experts" by nursing management.

However, as the competencies for each level of nursing practice are developed, this process may become a real threat to the expert staff nurses' self-esteem as the expectations are being publicized. Some of the preceptors subconsciously have to admit they do not have the knowledge base they had been assumed to possess. Therefore they will need to expand their knowledge base. The nurse manager needs to be supportive of the preceptors and the CBE process.

Criteria for the preceptor must be developed (25). Table 15.2 shows sample criteria developed by the author for use in the intensive care unit of a major metropolitan hospital. Preceptors must write daily anecdotal notes and evaluate the performance of employees by using the criterion-referenced statements. The best time to do this is immediately after their normal shift while the day is still fresh in their mind.

Once the tools for evaluating the various levels of nursing practice have been developed, the preceptors need to learn how to use the instrument. The best person to assist the preceptors with the evaluation tool is the coordinator of the competency-based program. This ensures a consistent, quality approach to CBE.

Follow-up with the preceptors is required so that identified problems with using the tool may be solved. Common problems include lack of familiarity with the tool and problems in evaluating another individual's performance using the tool.

## HOW DO I START?

Now that the CBE program has been defined, you are ready to get started in designing your own

**Table 15.2**   Preceptor Criteria for Intensive Care Unit

Purpose: To establish measurable criteria that will aid in the identification of ICU[a] staff nurses to fulfill the role of preceptors for ICU orientees

Criteria

1. Critical care nursing experience
   12 months as ICU RN
          or
   6 months as ICU RN with previous 2 years of critical care experience.
2. Demonstrates teaching skills
   Presents 5-minute discussion on critical care-related topic such as patient care conference on nursing rounds
   Demonstrates ability to intervene appropriately when observing poor technique in simulated clinical situation
   Identifies resources available
   Has presented nursing rounds at least once in past year.
3. Demonstrates knowledge of use of ICU flowsheet in compliance with QA criteria
4. Demonstrates knowledge of ICU RN responsibilities by passing with 85% or greater in a quiz
5. Demonstrates role-modeling behaviors and attitude:
   Is flexible and adaptable with changes in ICU environment
   Demonstrates willingness to assist others
   Demonstrates strong organizational skills: work is completed in timely manner
   Interacts in positive manner with peers, house staff, and others in the ICU
   Absence of documentation on personnel record of poor work performance, poor attititude, use of ill time in excess
   Maintains certifications
6. Willing to attend preceptor workshop

[a]Abbreviations: ICU, intensive care unit; RN, registered nurse; QA, quality assurance.

CBE program. First, the hospital needs to make a decision as to whether CBE will be hospital wide or unit based. Some institutions may wish to pilot CBE in only one nursing section, such as the critical care division. If the decision is to implement a hospital-wide CBE program, then a steering committee with representation from each nursing unit needs to be selected. The mission of the committee is to develop competencies that are generic to each nurse in the hospital. From the basic generic competencies completed by the large hospital-wide steering committee, section competencies and finally unit competencies are completed. A hospital-wide committee prevents overlapping and duplication of work from one unit to another. The hospital-wide committee also provides uniformity and commonality rather than having individual units develop generic competencies with varying degrees of scope.

As well as a hospital-wide committee, each unit involved in the development of CBE needs to have its own committee. To form both the hospital and unit committees, the most expert nurses should be chosen by nursing management or voluntarily agree to serve on the committee. These experts are not necessarily the nurses who have tenure. They might

be newly employed nurses who bring years of nursing experience with them. In additional to the expert staff nurses, a successful committee needs to have someone from management (an assistant nurse manager or nurse manager), an educational representative, and a clinical nurse specialist. Each hospital or unit-based committee has an approach that works best for consistently meeting. Some institutions can regulate schedules so a weekly 1-hour meeting can be planned, while others need to schedule meetings off the unit for a block of time on a monthly basis, so that staff do not receive patient assignments. The committee meeting needs to be structured so that they meet on a consistent basis. Meeting on a consistent basis provides continuity to the project as well as increasing the awareness that the institution or unit is in the process of developing a CBE program.

One of the first decisions to be made by the committee is the number of levels of nursing practice in the hospital. There may be as many as four or five levels, or as few as three. A review of career ladders during 1986–1987 revealed either four or five levels, with a beginning level being referred to as zero. Therefore the competency committee may opt to follow national trends or they may chose fewer levels of nursing practice if they are following institutionally imposed time constraints or lack experience with the process.

Some questions the committee can ask when building levels of nursing practice are:

1. When is the staff nurse expected to be a preceptor?
2. Is the staff nurse expected to be in charge of the unit?
3. Are there certain numbers of units of continuing education expected?
4. Is there a building approach to skill and knowledge attainment?
5. Is the staff nurse expected to contribute to hospital-wide achievements such as committees of educational offerings?

Table 15.3 provides a framework that can be used to assist the committee in defining various levels of nursing practice. It includes some dimensions that the group might choose to place in various stages of growth for the employee. Figure 15.1 provides a model showing the progressive growth process of a critical care nurse, from one of technical orientation to one having complete synthesis, analysis, and application of knowledge.

Careful consideration must be given to the number of levels of nursing in a CBE program due to the fact that the CBE program may provide a blueprint for a nursing clinical ladder. It is obvious that one of the levels is a beginning and the highest level is expert, but what is in between?

Benner's (26) work, *From Novice to Expert*, provides a conceptual framework that may be used in developing a CBE program (see Chapter 7). Benner employs five levels: novice, advanced beginner, competent, proficient, and expert. The novice or beginning employee is just starting and when he or she completes orientation, there are certain expectations of this new employee. This novice nurse can be a new graduate, a critical care intern, or a nurse reentering the work force. He or she then requires an additional period of time to become an advanced beginner. This period may require anywhere from 6 to 12 months. Once this employee has basic skills and knowledge, you as the nurse manager are trying to motivate and challenge him or her to advance even further. There are certain courses that might be expected to be completed or certain certification examinations appropriate to the critical care area. The advanced beginner is the nurse transferring into critical care

**Table 15.3** Levels of Nursing Practice

*Beginning Level*
First 6–8 weeks of unit employment
Employees who fit in this category:
  In-house transfers without experience
  In-house transfers with experience
  External to hospital with experience
Knowledge concerned with:
  Physical environment, equipment
  Physical assessment skills
  Safety
  Becoming team member
  Basic nursing care

*Level One*
Validates knowledge with expert 50–60% of time
Is task oriented; self-centered
Collects data, but does not always know what to do with data
Takes questions to expert nurse
Does not always know what to question and asks "what" frequently
Utilizes in-services
Functions as code member in unit; BCLS[a] provider
Begins participation in hospital/unit-based committees
This level would be achieved maximally by end of 1-year employment.

*Level Two*
Rarely validates information, 20–30% of the time
Usually utilizes discrete data for decision making
Is consistent with intervention
Asks "why?"
Builds on knowledge base; seeks alternative educational methods
Becomes certified in specialty area
Integrates knowledge, but not consistently
Acts as unit-centered resource
Is ACLS provider
May serve as preceptor or substitute as preceptor
This level could take up to 2 years to achieve, after beginning employment.

*Level Three*
Anticipates and intervenes appropriately
Shares knowledge with others
Teaches in nonthreatening manner
Engaged in self-studies
Assimilates knowledge and continues to seek alternative educational opportunities
Participates in professional nursing organization
Acts as hospital-centered resource
Functions as preceptor
Participates in hospital/unit-based committees
Facilitates unit-based committees
Functions as expert communicator
Is instructor for BCLS and ACLS
Provides unit-based in-services

[a]Abbreviations: BCLS, basic cardiac life support; ACLS, advanced cardiac life support.

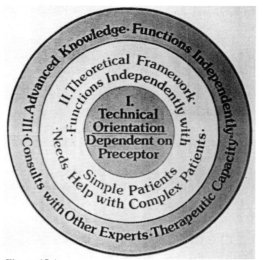

**Figure 15.1**

**Table 15.4** Simplistic Method of Development of Competencies and Subcompetencies for Committee Use

| Competency | Subcompetency |
| --- | --- |
| Ventilator | Suctioning |
| | Bagging |
| | Intubating |
| | Extubating |
| | Maintaining mean airway pressure |
| | Identifying chest x-ray |
| Charge nurse role | Making assignments |
| | Assisting others with clinical expertise |
| | Staffing for next shift |
| | Triaging patients |
| | Communicating with patients, families, and physicians |
| | Documenting quality assurance criteria |
| Caring for patient with ineffective airway exchange related to ARDS[a] | Using ventilators |
| | Suctioning |
| | Demonstrating knowledge about ARDS |
| | Interpreting chest x-rays |
| | SVO$_2$ monitoring |

[a]Abbreviations: ARDS, adult respiratory distress syndrome; SVO$_2$, mixed venous oxygen saturation.

from a high acuity medical-surgical unit who does not require as much time to orient as a new graduate. He or she has acquired skills of organization, knows some task, but is lacking in knowledge and skills specific to the critical care unit such as caring for a patient with adult respiratory distress syndrome (ARDS) on a ventilator. The competent nurse can take care of the patients in the "typical" environment of the critical care unit. If the critical care unit receives mostly postoperative patients and medical patients with chronic obstructive pulmonary disease (COPD), he or we might not be able to care for a cardiac surgery patient. The proficient nurse can care for any patient and would transfer this knowledge base from familiar patients to those whose care is not familiar. He or she serves as a resource to other nurses on the unit. The expert nurse provides care to patients and often functions as a case manager, providing care and consultation. He or she utilizes not only a physical, psychological, and holistic approach to the patient but deals with intuitive judgment in critical decision making. When developing a CBE program, one needs to think past the orientation period, past the next level where the nurse is competent, and decide how many different professional expectations there are for that unit or institution. The committee needs to determine the number of months or years in which these requirements should be completed.

The second step, after deciding on levels of nursing practice, is to explain what a competency is to the committee. The committee will be writing competency and subcompetency statements and criterion reference evaluation. Before delineating the competencies, subcompetencies, and criterion-referenced statements, they must determine the specific expectations of the unit.

To assist the competency committee in deciding the generic competencies, AACN Standards of Nursing Practice, the hospital policy and procedure manual, and job descriptions may serve as guidelines. The knowledge, tasks, and affective behaviors to use in the competencies need to be objectively determined. These can be organized according to nursing diagnoses format or according to body systems. Because a committee is not familiar with this process of defining competencies, the facilitator can encourage them by generating the skills, knowledge, assessment tools, and affective behaviors needed by the expert nurses. Table 15.4 provides the committee with a sample format to utilize when brainstorming the expected skills and knowledge of an expert nurse. It provides a different, simplistic approach to the development of competencies and subcompetencies with the appropriate wording to be completed at a later time. This provides a place for the committee to begin. The table demonstrates different approaches that can be used in determining competencies. Ventilators can be a competency by itself or it could be a subcompetency under the competency of a nursing diagnosis related to ARDS. This example illustrates the importance of choosing the framework for competencies before beginning.

delBueno (16) describes a priority matrix in which items can be checked as to risk and then frequency with which they are performed. Kieffer (27) used a modified priority matrix to define which psychomotor skills would be selected to teach new graduate nurses. Bayley (28) selected a priority matrix in developing a competency-based orientation for burn nursing. One of the ways to develop a priority matrix is to list all of the procedures, knowledge, and skills expected of a nurse. Assemble these in logical order, either by a systems or a nursing diagnosis approach. Next, make columns for the frequency with which the nurse might perform these items, such as daily, weekly, or monthly. Then, design columns for the risk to the patient if something is done incorrectly, such as high, medium, or low. This allows the committee to access information as to the procedures that are performed frequently and with greatest risk to the patient if the nurse does not perform them correctly. This information can become a starting point for the committee in developing competencies. Once the priority matrix is developed, it should be distributed to several staff nurses in the unit. Once completed, the competency committee will tabulate which are the high-risk, high-frequency procedures. The use of a priority matrix is one way of determining the competencies expected of an ideal critical care nurse. Table 15.5 demonstrates a priority matrix designed for use in a pediatric institution (29).

Another method that can be used to define competencies to be included in various levels is the critical incident technique. This tool was originally developed by John Flanager in 1941 to select, classify, and train air crews in the shortest time possible (30). In using the critical incident method, the person being interviewed describes a specific activity. Details of the setting in which the event took place, exactly what occurred, an account of the outcome, and why it was considered to be effective or ineffective practice are described (30, p. 209). This process can be time consuming as the interview can take 20–40 minutes, and many hours are spent compiling data and then constructing a list of competencies.

The Delphi technique was used by Kibbee (31) to determine which competencies would be used in an orientation program. This technique consists of developing group consensus. Samples of individuals are questioned via questionnaires and requestioned once the questionnaires are refined. Another way of defining the competencies for the ideal critical care nurse is to list all of the nursing diagnoses that apply to the unit and list those procedures and knowledge base that the nurse needs to implement them.

Ultimately the institution or unit needs to decide on what approach best suits their area and make this commitment before writing competency statements.

## WRITING COMPETENCY STATEMENTS

Once the committee has decided on the levels of nursing practice, the next step is determining competencies, subcompetencies, and criteria for evaluation. A competency statement must be specific, with an action verb, such as ". . .provides safe and competent nursing care for patients with actual or potential cardiovascular dysfunction. . . ." This statement gives the nurse an overall perspective of what the expectation is, but it is not specific as to its parts (32).

Submodular competency statements are then developed. An example of a submodular competency statement for the competency above is "obtains an accurate and complete assessment of a patient's cardiovascular status. . . ." This statement is more specific and outlines for the nurse a procedure that she must perform. Subsequent measurement of correct performance of the task comes from the use of criteria statements.

Criteria statements provide a yardstick by which to measure the performance of the subcompetency. Just as there are no "right or wrong" competency statements, there are no corrent or incorrect totals of criteria-referenced statements. There must be a sufficient number of statements provided to the evaluator so he or she can decide whether the employee has achieved the expectation desired by the manager.

Criteria statements for a submodular competency statement might be:

- identifies the location and evaluates the rate, rhythm, and volume of the following peripheral pulses: dorsalis pedalis, popliteal, femoral;
- describes heart sounds;

**Table 15.5** Priority Matrix

Unit _____

Person Completing _____

| Procedure/Task: Respiratory | Tracheostomy Tube | | | | | | | Nasopharyngeal or Endrotrachel Tube | | | | | | | Oropharyngeal Tube | | | | | | |
|---|---|---|---|---|---|---|---|---|---|---|---|---|---|---|---|---|---|---|---|---|---|
| | Frequency | | | | Importance[a] | | | Frequency | | | | Importance | | | Frequency | | | | Importance | | |
| | Daily | Weekly | Monthly | Yearly | 1 Very Import. | 2 | 3 Not as Import. | Daily | Weekly | Monthly | Yearly | 1 Very Import. | 2 | 3 Not as Import. | Daily | Weekly | Monthly | Yearly | 1 Very Import. | 2 | 3 Not as Import. |
| I. Airway maintenance | | | | | | | | | | | | | | | | | | | | | |
| A. Intubation—preparation for—nurses do not intubate | | | | | | | | | | | | | | | | | | | | | |
| B. Suctioning | | | | | | | | | | | | | | | | | | | | | |
| C. Taping | | | | | | | | | | | | | | | | | | | | | |
| D. Logan Bow Tape | | | | | | | | | | | | | | | | | | | | | |
| E. Determination of proper tube placement | | | | | | | | | | | | | | | | | | | | | |
| 1. Auscultation breath sounds | | | | | | | | | | | | | | | | | | | | | |
| 2. Portable CXR | | | | | | | | | | | | | | | | | | | | | |
| F. Bag Breathing | | | | | | | | | | | | | | | | | | | | | |
| G. Collection Sputum specimen | | | | | | | | | | | | | | | | | | | | | |
| H. Determining Patency of airway | | | | | | | | | | | | | | | | | | | | | |
| I. Monitoring Function Ability of Cuff | | | | | | | | | | | | | | | | | | | | | |
| J. Restraints | | | | | | | | | | | | | | | | | | | | | |
| K. Extubation | | | | | | | | | | | | | | | | | | | | | |
| L. Charting | | | | | | | | | | | | | | | | | | | | | |

[a]Importance means if procedure or task not done correctly, the patient will be placed in jeopardy.

- evaluates skin color and capillary refill of central and peripheral cyanosis;
- determines the presence, location, and degree of edema.

There is no specific number of criteria statements that need to be developed. The key is to have enough statements so that each person who is evaluating the individual will be able to state whether the nurse can perform the submodular competency. The key elements for performing the skill need to be included as well as any elements that might be particularly troublesome to the unit. For example, if you are experiencing a difficult time with everyone using petroleum gauze around chest tubes, you might encourage the committee to include this element as a criteria statement. Table 15.6 shows a section with competency, subcompetency, and criteria statements developed for use at a pediatric hospital (29).

Once the competency, subcompetency, and criteria statements are developed, the committee will need to decide the tool for measurement of the criterion-referenced statements. Testing or evaluation of the criterion-referenced statements is the area about which the least amount has been written (1, 33). Benner identified several reasons why there are problems in developing competency-based tools in nursing. They are: (*a*) Nursing outcomes are difficult to identify as well as research. (*b*) Confusion exists as to what a competency statement is. (*c*) "Predictive validity of tests relaying to clinical judgment and problem-solving is a problem. . ." (33, p. 305). (*d*) Affective domains of behaviors are difficult to test. (*e*) "With a task list approach, unending classifications are generated with no method of guidelines for determining which are important" (33, p. 305). (*f*) Task analysis is difficult because unlimited lists can be produced.

The difficulty inherent in developing an evaluation of criterion-referenced statements has led many programs to utilize skills checklists. Most of these allow the orientee to classify his or her own knowledge or skills. Subjectivity by the new nurse can be a potential problem if he or she is permitted to independently evaluate his or herself. The individual who is collaborating that the orientee can correctly identify wheezing or proper suctioning should be the individual appropriately evaluating the employee.

A better method of evaluation that gives more feedback about possible strengths and weaknesses

the nurse is exhibiting is an evaluation tool using degrees of expectations adapted from the work of Kersick (34). Table 15.7 provides a sample of this evaluation tool developed for the beginning critical care staff nurse (29). This table takes some of the criteria statements from Table 15.6, but it shows not only whether the nurse is meeting the competencies, but also whether he or she is exceeding or performing at a substandard level. This differentiation allows the nurse manager to decide not only whether the individual is progressing satisfactorily, but whether he or she is excelling, needs additional assistance, or perhaps needs to be counseled about several poor performances. The nurse is evaluated on whether he or she has achieved the expectations. For example, if the competency is "assumes charge nurse responsibility; appropriately carries out job responsibilities," this is the expected performance or 0 level. Less than expected performance or $-1$ performance is "assumes charge nurse role but needs continuous guidance in fulfilling job responsibilities" while the worst possible outcome or $-2$ performance is "refuses charge nurse responsibility." With this evaluation tool, not only is less than competent performance identified, but above competent accomplishments are also demonstrated. This tool assists in the identification of the growth process of the employee. It validates assumptions a nurse manager might have about an employee's nursing process and provides an objective tool for discussion between the nurse manager and the employee. If an individual had several $-2$ outcomes, this nurse would be someone who needs counseling, might be placed back on probation, or might even be discharged, while a nurse receiving several $-1$ scores would be identified as someone who needs more assistance. You might be willing to put much time and effort into someone who has five of fifty $-1$ scores, but you might decide that it is not worth the time, energy, and resources to assist someone who has received five of fifty $-2$ scores. On the other hand, if the nurse has received several $+1$ or $+2$ scores, this individual is demonstrating more rapid progression than the average employee.

The hospital needs to support the competency committee as it might take 6 months to 1 year to develop the various competency and subcompetency statements and criterion-referenced evaluation for one level of the CBE program.

After the competencies for the "novice" nurse

**Table 15.6.**  Cardiovascular Clinical Evaluation of the Beginning Nurse in Pediatric Critical Care[a]

| Cardiovascular Module | Done Date/Signature | Comments Date/Signature | Self-assessment |
|---|---|---|---|
| **Competency** | | | |
| Provides safe and competent nursing care for patients with actual or potential cardiovascular dysfunction | | | |
| 1.  Submodular Competency | | | |
| Obtains an accurate and complete assessment of a patient's cardiovascular status | | | |
| Criteria Statements | | | |
| a.  Identifies the location and evaluates the rate, rhythm, and volume of the following peripheral pulses: | | | |
| 1.  Carotid | | | |
| 2.  Femoral | | | |
| 3.  Brachial | | | |
| 4.  Radial | | | |
| 5.  Apical | | | |
| 6.  Dorsalis pedis | | | |
| 7.  Posterior tibialis | | | |
| b.  Describes heart sounds | | | |
| c.  Evaluates skin color and capillary refill of central and peripheral cyanosis | | | |
| d.  Determines the presence, location, and degree of edema | | | |
| e.  States abnormal values and their clinical manifestations for hemoglobin and hematocrit | | | |
| 2.  Submodular Competency | | | |
| Provides care for the patient with use of the following ECG monitors: | | | |
| Datascope | | | |
| Hewlett Packard | | | |
| Criteria Statement | | | |
| a.  Demonstrates operations of the bedside monitor: | | | |
| 1.  Sets alarm limits correctly for patient's age and condition | | | |
| 2.  Specifies the locations for placement of electrodes to monitor standard lead II | | | |
| b.  Demonstrates operation of the central monitor: | | | |
| 1.  Runs printout on specified patient | | | |
| 2.  Changes monitor paper | | | |
| c.  Using a monitor strip from five different patients recognizes: | | | |
| 1.  atrial rate | | | |
| 2.  ventricular rate | | | |
| 3.  P-R interval | | | |
| 4.  QRS duration | | | |
| 5.  Interprets rhythm | | | |
| 6.  States normal, P-R, QRS, and rate considering patient's age and condition | | | |
| d.  Provides for correct documentation of cardiac strip: | | | |
| 1.  Labels strip with name, date, time, and lead | | | |
| 2.  Documents rate, PR, QRS interval, and interpretation | | | |

**Table 15.6 Continued.**

e. Demonstrates use of Dinamapp:
   1. Chooses correct cuff sizes _____
   2. Calibrates machine _____
   3. Alternates extremities in continuous use _____

3. Submodular Competency

Criteria Statements

a. Describes/demonstrates how to assist with insertion and removal of the following lines:
   1. Systemic arterial _____
   2. UAC _____
   3. CVP _____

b. Describes/demonstrates how to monitor systematic arterial, UAC, CVP lines.
   1. Balances and calibrates _____
   2. Sets alarm limits (high/low) appropriately _____
   3. Maintains patency and sterility _____

c. Describes the complications of deep lines and preventive interventions _____

d. Obtains blood samples from arterial lines _____

e. Provides an accurate running blood drawing total in nurse's notes _____

f. Demonstrates/describes steps to be taken to correct the following problems with any waveform;
   1. Dampened tracing _____
   2. Inappropriate high/low reading _____
   3. No tracing _____

4. Submodular Competency

   Demonstrates/describes how to administer drugs that affect cardiovascular system functioning _____

Criteria Statements

a. States the action, side effects, indications, and dosage for the cardiac drugs most frequently used:
   1. Atropine _____
   2. Sodium bicarbonate _____
   3. Epinephrine _____
   4. Calcium _____
   5. Dextrose 25% _____
   6. Dopamine _____
   7. Lasix _____

b. Demonstrates use of IMED/IVAC pump:
   1. Sets up the pump _____
   2. Identifies potential problems with the IMED pump _____
   3. Describes/demonstrates corrective actions to be taken for problems with the pump _____

5. Submodular Competency

   Provides/describes nursing care for patients with cardiac arrhythmia. _____

Criteria Statements

a. Identifies normal sinus rhythm and correlates the ECG waveform with electrical and mechanical events occurring in the heart _____

**Table 15.6  *Continued.***

b. Identifies the following rhythms and states three
   nursing interventions for each:

1. Bradycardia _____

2. Tachycardia _____

3. 60-cycle interference _____

4. Artifact _____

5. PVCs _____

6. Submodular Competency

Provides nursing care for patients with abnormal coagulation studies _____

[a]Modified from Competency Committee, Children's Hospital, Columbus, Ohio, 1985.
[b]Abbreviation: ECG, electrocardiogram; UAC, umbilical artery catheter; CVP, central venous pressure; PVC, premature ventricular
contraction.

have been completed, field testing needs to occur so validity and realiability are established. Validity is established by having a group of staff nurses evaluate the content of the competency, subcompetency, and criterion-referenced assertions and corroborating the substance of these expectations. Each nurse reviewing the statements needs to agree with their content. Reliability is established by having these statements used in the clinical setting. Each nurse using the competency, subcompetency, and criterion-referenced evaluation tool would apply it in the same manner as he or she evaluates another nurse yielding the same result.

In order to field test the competency statements, preceptors require extensive training. The concept of competency-based education, along with competency statements and how to use this new evaluation tool, must be presented to this group. Usually preceptors are accustomed to using a subjective tool and the switch from the "old" way to the new CBE objective tool must be valued by them. If some of the preceptors have been on the committee, this change will be facilitated.

One individual must be committed to the process so each preceptor uses the tool in a standard method. Therefore, the development of a procedure for using the CBE tool needs to be established. New orientees also need education about the trial format. The one individual who is coordinating the process needs to track any problems, changes, or additions the preceptors or new orientees suggest. An evaluation form for both the new orientee and the preceptor should be developed so formal feedback can be gathered for the committee. A sample of both preceptors and new orientees should be

determined so validity and reliability can be achieved. At the same time, risk management needs to be involved so that they can investigate any potential legal problems with the tool.

At the same time the beginning levels are being field tested for reliability and validity, the competency committee should be working on the next level of practice. This procedure should be repeated until all levels in the CBE program have been delineated.

At some point, the issue of peer evaluation will need discussion (see Chapter 14). If the committee has decided on four levels, probably after the beginning and competent level evaluation tools have been determined, the reality of who will evaluate nurses at higher levels will surface. If you are in an institution where there are few nurses at higher levels, peer review might be an alternative. For example, two or three fellow nurses might be chosen, one by management and two by the nurse being evaluated. The tool developed for evaluating beginning and competent nurses could be used with higher levels of nurses. However, as the committee develops the competencies for the more expert nurse, the numbers of statements specific to nursing tasks are fewer and more of the statements will deal with professional activities. The nurse at a higher level is already expected to be an expert care giver. He or she has additional responsibilities such as being in charge, orienting new employees, and attending codes on the general nursing units. The issue of evaluation for the more advanced nurse may be achieved by having the nurse identify 10 patients' charts for review of quality care, including documentation, outcome, and care planning by his or her peers. Another method is to have this individual

**Table 15.7** Cardiovascular Clinical Evaluation for the Beginning Nurse[a]

+2
Best optimal outcome
   Recognizes, inteprets, reports changes in PMI[b]
   Auscultates apical pulse, identifies normal/abnormal heart sounds, rate, rhythm, as appropriate for growth
      and development parameters and condition
   Identifies and interprets abnormal dysrhythmias and reports changes
   Assesses peripheral pulses and distinguishes between normal, thready, and bounding
   Recognizes significance of color changes, i.e., pink, pallor, cyanosis, and gray, and reports changes
   Grades peripheral edema

+1
Better than expected
   Identifies and marks area of PMI
   Identifies life-threatening dysrhythmias and reports
   Determines posterior tibial peripheral pulses

0
Expected
   Identifies usual area of PMI
   Identifies and ausculates apical pulse
   Knows normal rate and rhythm for age and condition
   Meets expected criteria for evaluation of ECG
   Determines presence/absence of peripheral pulses (radials, femorals, brachials, and pedals)
   Assesses color and recognizes abnormalities, reports, and documents
   Assesses capillary refill and states normal/abnormal
   Identifies peripheral edema, documents, and reports changes

−1
Less than expected
   Is unable to locate usual area of PMI
   Recognizes normal/abnormal but does not document
   Cannot identify landmarks or peripheral pulses
   Recognizes normal/abnormal skin color but does not document
   Does not document capillary refill
   Documents incompletely (specify)

−2
Worst possible outcome
   Does not know what PMI is
   Is unable to recognize normal/abnormal rhythms
   Is unable to recognize normal/abnormal skin color
   Is unable to recognize normal/abnormal capillary refill
   Is unable to recognize peripheral edema

[a]Modified from Competency Committee, Children's Hospital, Columbus, Ohio, 1985.
[b]Abbreviations, PMI, point of maximal impulse; ECG, electrocardiogram.

present at the hospital nursing grand rounds program on one of the patients for whom he or she has cared. As the committee is close to finishing the project, human resources should be included.

## SUMMARY

Designing and implementing a CBE program is a long and sometimes arduous task. The rewards to both the staff and institution can be great if the units and institution are supportive of each other. This chapter has presented a definition of CBE and suggested a format for the development of CBE for an individual unit or institution. Methods for evaluation have been discussed. The effectiveness

of CBE is dependent on many disciplines: administration, human resources, risk management, education, and committee structure. When the departments are committed, CBE provides a good working environment for the nurse manager and the staff nurse in which a professional, caring environment exists.

REFERENCES

1. Thurman GK, Sanders K. Competency-based education versus traditional education: a comparison of effectiveness. Radiol Technol 59(2):164–169.
2. Alspach J. Designing a competency-based orientation

for critical care nurses. Heart & Lung 1984;13:655–662.

3. delBueno D. Implementing a competency-based orientation program. Nurse Educ 1980;May–June:16–20.

4. Hall G. Identifying competencies, goals and objectives in competency-based education: a process for the improvement of education. Englewood Cliffs, New Jersey: Prentice-Hall, 1976;26–58.

5. Stein KZ. Nursing assistants learn through the competency-based approach. Geriatr Nurs July/August 1986;197–200.

6. Webster's new twentieth century dictionary. New York: World Publishing, 1970.

7. Aston-McCrimmon, E. Analysis of the ratings of competencies used in physical therapy practice. Phys Ther 1986;66(6):954–960.

8. Taub, A. A curriculum framework for preparing health educators. HYGIE 1986;5(1):16–19.

9. Scruggs R, White V, Sams D. Competency assessment and remediation in dental auxiliary teacher education. J Dental Educ 1986;50(6):316–318.

10. Drewry S, Fiene MA. Cost-effective curriculum planning in health education. J Allied Health 1985;2:109–117.

11. Gaskins SE, Badger LW, Gehlbach SH, et al. Family practice residents' evaluation of a competency-based psychiatry curriculum. J Med Educ 1987;62(1):41–46.

12. Moncur C. Physical therapy competencies in rheumatology. Phys Ther 1985;65(9):1365–1371.

13. Dunn WR, Hamilton D, Harden R. Techniques of identifying competencies needed of doctors. Med Teacher 1985;7(1):15–25.

14. Hinojosa J. Implications for occupational therapy of a competency-based orientation. Am J Occup Ther 1985;39:539–541.

15. Porter SF. Ensuring competency: toward a competency-based orientation format. Crit Care Q 1984;6:42–52.

16. delBueno D. Competency based education. Nurse Educ 1978;3:10–14.

17. Boyer C. Performance-based staff development: the cost-effective alternative. Nurse Educ 1981;September–October;12–15.

18. Klingstedt JL. Philosophical basis for competency-based education: an introduction. In: Burns RW, Klingstedt JL, eds. Competency-based education: an introduction. Englewood Cliffs, New Jersey: Education Technology Publications, 1973:7–19.

19. Broderick M. Developing competency-based instruction in health fields: rationale and process. In: Peterson CJ, Broderick M, Demarest L, et al, eds. Competency-based curriculum instruction. New York: NLN, 1979.

20. Berner ES, Bender KJ. Determining how to begin. In: Evaluating clinical competence in the health professions. St Louis: Mosby, 1978:3–10.

21. Klemp GO. Identifying, measuring, and integrating competence. In: Pottinger PS, Goldsmith J, eds. Defining and measuring competence. San Francisco: Jossey-Bass Inc, Publishers, 1979:41–52.

22. Peterson C. Competency-based instruction: evolution of a new perspective. In: Peterson CJ, Broderick M, Demarest L, et al, eds. Competency-based curriculum instruction. New York: NLN, 1979.

23. May J. Competency-based education: general concepts. J AMRA 1983;6:21–26.

24. Spady W. Competency based education: a bandwagon in search of a definition. Educ Res 1977;6(1):9–14.

25. Neumark A, Flabertz M, Girard F. Individualized orientation in critical care. Focus Crit Care 1987;14(5):34–44.

26. Benner P. From novice to expert: promoting excellence and career development in clinical nursing practice. Chicago, National Commission on Nursing, 1983.

27. Kieffer J. Selecting technical skills to teach for competency. J Nurs Educ 1984;23(5):198–203.

28. Bayley E. Development of competency-based orientation for burn nursing. JBCR 1983;4(1):January–February:36–55.

29. Competency Committee, Children's Hospital, Columbus, Ohio, 1985.

30. Dunn W, Hamilton D. The critical incident technique—a brief guide. Med Teacher 1986;8(3):207–215.

31. Kibbee P. Developing a model for implementation of an evaluation component in an orientation program. J Contin Educ Nurs 1980;11(5):25–29.

32. Beare P. The clinical contract—an approach to competency-based clinical learning and evaluation. J Nurs Educ 1985;24(2):75–77.

33. Benner P. Issues in competency-based testing. Nurs Outlook 1982;5:303–309.

34. Kersick, C. Antedoctal notes from lecture series, 1985–1987.

# Chapter 16

# Evaluating Chemical Dependency in Critical Care Nurses

DONNA KEMP

In the past 100 years, we have witnessed a remarkable change in our lifestyles as a result of the rapid growth of scientific technology. In this short time span we have gone from the horse and buggy to the space shuttle, from the abacus to the digital computer, and from the telegraph to the telecommunication satellite. Along with this host of marvels, technology has brought us face to face with many philosophical, moral, and social issues. What is consciousness? How should we define death? When shall life support systems be removed from the terminally ill or brain dead? Is chemical dependency a disease, a lack of moral fiber, a genetic defect, or a chosen lifestyle? Does a colleague deserve more, less, or the same compassion that our patients receive?

These questions are only a small sample of what today's policy makers MUST confront. In the critical care settings the policy makers are the nurse managers. As such, we must recognize that chemical dependency in our colleagues is a reality. Chemical dependency has an impact on the institutions, working units, and the profession of nursing while destroying competent and valuable human beings.

Alcohol abuse is currently endemic to American society. Drug abuse is a recent phenomenon receiving widespread attention by the news media, legislature, and now the health care industry.

The history of alcoholism and drug dependency in nursing is well presented by Church (1) who has used a vivid description by Charles Dickens in his novel *Martin Chuzzlewit*. The characters of Sarah Gamp and Betsy Prig, professional nurses, were portrayed as opportunistic mercenaries who sought work that provided accessibility to alcohol. Sarah was further described as having a fragrance that indicated she had consumed wine.

The decade of the 1960s produced the beginnings of media and public awareness of hallucinogenic drug use by the "love generation" in the Haight-Ashbury district in San Francisco, California. The majority of Americans believed these people were the aberrant minority of society and another fad. In fact, they were the tip of the iceberg. Madison Avenue began to commercialize the selling of the little blue pill Compose, perpetuating the concept that it is acceptable to take drugs to help relieve everyday tension. Although it was medication, it was never identified as such. The media innocently did a disservice to society.

The 1970s became an escalation of society's use of harmless "recreational drugs" to cope with the ever-increasing stressors of daily living. The end of the unpopular Vietnam conflict, Watergate, the oil embargo, and runaway inflation with dual family incomes necessary to provide for the same standard of living, were just a few of the stressors which society had to face.

The 1980s ushered in double-digit inflation, double-digit unemployment, and increasing alcohol/drug misuse and abuse as the equal opportunity addictors for all of American society. The "health care professions" did worse than the lay public because of opportunity, accessibility, and the belief that their education shielded them from the addiction. The health care industry began offering a variety of inpatient and outpatient substance abuse programs for the lay people. Employers wrestled with the costs associated with inadequate reimbursement by the insurance companies for substance abuse programs. Mandatory drug screening for job applicants became media headlines. The legislature issued laws that mandated punitive sentences for those involved in all aspects of drug abuse, without regard for treatment or even recognition that there was a disease state involved. They wanted to cure the "drug problem."

## STATISTICS

American women have a 5% alcoholism rate. Of all nurses, 2–3% are estimated to be addicted to drugs (2). Substance or alcohol abuse affects 10–20% of health care workers, or about 128,000 nurses (3). Chemically dependent nurses whose licenses are affected may be 70% (4). Chemical dependency in the general American population is estimated to be 10% with nurses showing a dependency 50% higher than nonnurses (5). Chemical or alcohol dependency is 8–10% as estimated by the American Nurses' Association (ANA), while rehabilitation programs estimated the dependency to be 20% for health care professionals (6).

From September 1980 to August 1981 971 actions were brought against nurses' licenses, with 649 for chemical dependency, based on statistics by the National Council of State Boards of Nursing (2). During 1985 and 1986, the Florida State Board of Nursing reported 60% of disciplinary cases were for chemical dependency (7).

In 1985 drug misuse or abuse claimed $36.3 billion in lost productivity, medical expenses, and theft to American industry. Alcohol-related problems used 8 times more medical care, 2.5 times more absenteeism, and 3.6 times on and off the job accidents (8). The cost to the hospital for a chemically dependent employee amounts to $50,000 to $75,000 per year excluding salary. These figures include the decreased productivity, unnecessary overtime, absenteeism, overuse of health insurance claims, possible workers' compensation claims from on the job injuries, and the retraining and payment of replacement personnel (9).

Perhaps the most encouraging statistics concern the nurses who have undergone rehabilitation. The recovery rate after treatment is 90% (4). The importance of support, assistance, and guidance toward rehabilitation gives nurses with problems of substance misuse or abuse hope for their future personal and professional life.

The previously mentioned statistics taken from the literature show how difficult it is to determine the exact numbers or costs for this dynamic problem. Nor do they address how many nurses were merely ignored, encouraged to resign, or terminated to avoid reporting to the state boards. They indicate that within the American society and the health care industry we have a complex problem. We have the opportunity to utilize a variety of resource experts from the legislative, judicial, organizational, research, medical, and third party payors to tackle this negative problem. These experts would be responsible for obtaining accurate statistics, costs, and methods to punish "pushers" or treat those consumed by the disease.

## DEFINITIONS

Numerous terms are used to describe alcohol/chemical dependency, such as drug abuse, substance abuse, chemical abuse, alcohol abuse, addiction syndromes, and drug or chemical dependencies. Somehow these descriptors seem inadequate as there are both chemical abuse and misuse by both health care professionals and the general layperson. The use of prescription chemicals, street chemicals, and over-the-counter chemicals alone or in combination encompasses the broader picture of chemical/alcohol dependency/addiction. Substance misuse and abuse will be used in order to eliminate some of the prejudices and preconceptions attached to the aforementioned list of terms.

Gaskin (10) points out that the World Health Organization used the term drug dependent to indicate a state of psychic and/or physical dependence on a drug that is used on a periodic or continuous basis to produce pleasure or avoid discomfort. Abbott (19) defines chemical dependency as the "use of drugs or alcohol that causes problems in an individual's life" (10).

According to Smith et al. (11) the primary symptom of the disease is compulsion, defined as the "illogical, irrational, irresponsible, continued, repeated use of the drug as it becomes destructive to the individual's life." He further explains that "alcoholism and drug dependence are not related to volume, dose, duration, or degree of intoxication."

Levine (12) suggests there is no single agreed-upon definition of alcoholism or drug addiction in the current literature. He points out key phases in several definitions as follows: compulsion, need, desire, loss of control, craving, tendency to increase the dosage, obtain it by any means, psychological and occasionally physical dependence.

It is important to remember that substance misuse and abuse include the addiction or compulsive urge that is progressive and self-destructive to the person's physical, psychosocial, and spiritual being.

The disease is treatable. The diseased person's main defense against treatment is DENIAL, self-deceptions and rationalizations to cover up their profound feelings of powerfulness to control the quality and perhaps the quantity of their life. The first step to effectively managing substance misuse and abuse by the critical care nurse is identification by the critical care nurse manager.

## IDENTIFICATION

The philosophy, mission, and policies of the institution and the nursing department are key components that must be in the nurse manager's repertoire. In addition, there are federal statutes that must be observed. Each state has its own statutes that influence the rules and regulations by which the Board of Registered Nursing operates, along with the Joint Commission on Accreditation of Health Care Organizations (JCAHO) guidelines, and ANA and American Association of Critical-Care Nurses (AACN) standards.

Every institution has methods of dealing with the employee who is identified as having a substance misuse or abuse problem. The disciplinary process implemented depends on the commitment and sophistication of the administrators in determining the coordination of the organizational needs/ constraints with those of the employee. Several approaches have been identified in the literature and are described below (5, 13–15).

The first approach is to ignore that this problem exists. This ostrich approach results in termination or forced resignation for a variety of job performance deficiencies. In either case the Board of Registered Nursing is not notified of any question of substance misuse or abuse. This eliminates the institution from an association with the problem but does nothing to help the nurse or protect future patients' safety in another institution.

The second approach is the punitive administrative process. Substance misuse or abuse is not tolerated and results in immediate termination, involvement in the legal process, and notification of the Board of Registered Nursing of the violation. This process attempts to remove the cancerous growth before it infects others by osmosis. This is the situation in which the nurse is slapped in handcuffs and led off to jail and the great unknown. We have all heard and fear this tale of reality. This method is a dehumanizing process and may totally destroy the nurse's career. The punitive approach assists most of the employees in continuing the conspiracy of silence in an effort to protect peers from ruination by them.

The third approach has been referred to as cooperative. Administrators recognize a potential problem and act to protect the patient's safety as well as offer/provide assistance to the employee. They have developed a program of notification of the proper authorities while providing assistance with the legal system and treatment programs available.

Ideally, the fourth approach should be the proactive or enlightened process in which the administrators recognize that it has a dual role or responsibility. First and foremost is the provision of safe, quality patient care based on policies established, federal and state mandates, and professional standards. The second responsibility is the promotion of a positive, professional, and caring relationship and environment with the employee based on a belief in the value of the human being. Each employee's potential need for assistance at one time or another to deal effectively with various life stressors is recognized. An example of such an approach is demonstrated by policies related to medical leave of absence, insurance benefits that provide for both inpatient and outpatient services, and compensation during the period of rehabilitation. An employee assistance program (EAP), in-house consultant, and peer assistance or support programs may be utilized to assist the employee as indicated.

This proactive method focuses on recognition, prevention, and assistance for the employee with personal problems as well as actual substance misuse or abuse. The pivotal points in this process are communication and educational growth for all employees.

Education of employees from the bedside nurse to the nurse manager greatly assists in the identification and reentry/recovery process of the nurse. Several authors (2, 15–18) have suggested the following training and education:

1. The foundation for the formal communication is the policy explaining how an employee is to be handled when substance misuse or abuse is encountered.
2. The employees should be made aware that the substance misuse or abuse problem is a disease process. Discuss the myths and misconceptions

that are associated with this disease. Point out the stressors associated with the health care industry, such as working weekends and holidays, 12-hour shifts, night shifts, rotational shifts, dealing with critical life and death situations requiring accurate monitoring and critical judgment or action, demanding physicians and families, and inability to take breaks due to the deterioration of a patient. Examine how stress is handled or relieved in the unit. Discuss the coping mechanisms utilized to cope with daily stress or life crisis situations as a unit and/or on an individual basis. Learn relaxation and/or quick tension relievers. Discuss the chemicals that may be involved in misuse or abuse (Table 16.1). Discuss the signs and symptoms that many indicate substance misuse or abuse (Table 16.2). Look at the feelings that may be involved when a peer is suspected of substance misuse or abuse. Examine and role-play how to intervene appropriately with a peer to inform him or her of changes in behavior and/or job performance in a factual and constructive manner. Help each person examine and openly discuss feelings of anger, mistrust, and fear of this disease. Explain and encourage use of the in-house consultant, voluntary self-referral to the employee assistance program, or peer assistance program if available. Examine how the unit would handle the reentry process for the recovering nurse after he or she has received treatment for the disease. Determine how the unit would respond to the reentry of one of their own versus a new employee or outsider. Identify an employee who would be interested in becoming a buddy for the reentry nurse. Create a separate educational program based on the commonly used preceptor concept for newly hired nurses.

3. Nurse managers should have specific administrative action plans or guidelines created. The initial interview begins the process (see Table 16.3). Unsatisfactory job performance ratings are indicators for suspected substance misuse and abuse, and proper documentation of these indicators is necessary. The following considerations must be addressed by the nurse manager: utilization of the proper disciplinary based on presentation of the problem and in accordance with policy for the specific institution; techniques to be used to constructively confront the employee and anticipate expected reactions

from the employee; proper use of voluntary or mandatory referral to the employee assistance program; maintenance of confidentiality; the reentry process for the recovering nurse; construction of a contract between the nurse and the manager (see Table 16.4); ongoing evaluation and contract adjustment; determination of what support systems are available for the nurse manager before and after the confrontation situation.

The other important link for the nurse manager is to understand each nurse's unique personal viewpoint, belief system, usual coping mechanism, and professional standard. Dealing with a nurse who has a substance misuse or abuse problem is a very stressful occasion that pushes the nurse manager outside his or her comfort zone. This "push" can be a positive growth development as long as the situation is appropriately identified and openly discussed in an unemotional and constructive manner. The nurse manager should be prepared to deal with the gradual downhill situation and the unexpected crisis. In either situation the goal should be a win-win solution for the nurse who has a substance misuse or abuse problem. When successful, the nurse, the profession, the health care industry, and humanity become the winners.

## ASSESSMENT

How does one recognize the chemical dependent nurse?

Various authors (5, 19, 20) have described some general characteristics as follows: Usually he or she graduates at the top one-third of the class, holds advanced degress, is an achiever and a supernurse, acquires technical skills easily, holds responsible positions, is well liked by peers, and has outstanding job performance. This description sounds like a nurse all critical care nurse managers would like to have working in their units. As long as these traits predominate and performance is consistent, there is generally little concern or suspicion of substance misuse or abuse. However, when job performance deteriorates, the nurse manager should remember that the former stellar performer may have a bigger problem than one suspects. Behavioral and job performance changes that may be observed are listed below as presented by various authors (2, 5, 11, 17, 19–22). Remember when an employee appears to have many of the traits or characteristics listed, substance misuse or abuse

**Table 16.1.** Categories of Substances Misused or Abused[a]

Narcotics
    Codeine
    Diphenoxylate (Lomotil)
    Heroin
    Hydromorphone (Dilaudid)
    Meperidine (Demerol)
    Methadone (Dolophine)

    Morphine
    Oxycodone (Percocet and Percodan)
    Paregoric (camphorated tincture of opium—Paregoric)
    Pentazocine (Talwin)
    Propoxyphene (Darvon and Darvocet-N)
    Fetanyl (Sublimaze, Innovar)

Cocaine

Depressants: barbituates, sedatives, tranquilizers
    Alprazolam (Xanax)
    Clorazepate (Tranxene)
    Chlordiazepoxide (Librium)
    Diazepam (Valium)
    Amobarbital (Amytal)
    Chlorpromazine (Thorazine)
    Fluphenazine (Prolixin, Permitil)
    Flurazepam (Dalmane)
    Haloperidol (Haldol)
    Meprobamate (Equanil)
    Midazolam (Versed)
    Molindone (Moban)

    Halazepam (Paxipam)
    Lorazepam (Ativan)
    Oxazepam (Serax)
    Prazepam (Centrax)
    Pentobarbital (Nembutal)
    Perphenazine (Trilafon)
    Quazepam (Dormalin)
    Temazepam (Restoril)
    Thiothixene (Navane)
    Thioridazine (Mellaril)
    Triazolam (Halcion)
    Trifluoperazine (Stelazine)

Antidepressants
    Amitriptyline (Elavil)
    Amoxapine (Asendin)
    Desipramine (Norpramin)
    Doxepin (Sinequan)
    Maprotiline (Ludiomil)

    Nortriptyline (Aventyl, Pamelor)
    Protriptyline (Vivactil)
    Trazodone (Desyrel)
    Trimipramine (Surmontil)

Stimulants
    Alka-Seltzer
    Allerest
    A.R.M.
    Bronkaid
    Comtrex
    Contac
    Actifed
    Benzedrex Inhaler
    Drixoral
    Fedahist

    Dexatrim
    Dimetapp
    Marax
    Nyquil
    Sine-Aid
    Sudafed
    Midol
    Novahistine
    Tedral
    Vicks Inhaler

Hallucinogens
    Phencyclidine (PCP)

    Lysergic acid diethylamide (LSD)

Alcohol

Several of the substances above fall into more than one category depending on their dose and combination with alcohol.

[a]This is not to be considered as a complete list of substances misused or abused, but a reminder of the numerous drugs available to the health care professional. *Physician's Desk Reference* is another excellent reminder of the numerous temptations we face daily.

may NOT be the problem. The employee could be pointing out an isolated personal problem or crisis. These are only building blocks of a profile and the data must not be used surreptitiously. Additional data collection will be necessary for verification and appropriate intervention. If there is a change in performance, ask the following questions and identify characteristics as listed:

1. Is the nurse complying with the posted work schedule? Is there evidence of:
   - multiple instances of unauthorized leave;
   - excessive sick leave with or without medical confirmation;
   - frequent Monday and/or Friday absences;
   - absence patterns associated with days off or payday;

**Table 16.2.**    Signs and Symptoms of Substance Misuse and Abuse[a]

Narcotics
    Dilated pupils
    Runny Nose
    Yawning
    Drowsiness
    Nausea
    Watery Eyes
    Anorexia
    Restlessness

    Insomnia
    Tachypnea
    Elevated or lowered blood pressure
    Hyperactive bowel sounds
    Euphoria
    Insensitivity to pain
    Cold moist skin
    Piloerection

Cocaine
    Feeling of well-being followed by depression
    Brief intense euphoria
    Excitement
    Restlessness

    Increased heart rate and blood pressure
    Runny nose
    Dry sniffles

Depressants
    Sedation
    Drowsiness
    Dizziness
    Dry mouth
    Increased or decreased heart rate
    Dilated pupils

    Depressed breathing
    Uncoordinated movements
    Confused behavior
    Difficulty in operating some of the equipment in
      the unit

Stimulants
    Decreased fatigue
    Alertness
    Increased initiative
    Talkativeness
    Wakefulness
    Mood elevation
    Tachypnea
    Tremors
    Vasomotor center stimulation
    Loss of appetite

    Weight loss
    Increased gastrointestinal motility
    Increased heart rate and blood pressure
    Pale and diaphoretic skin
    Restlessness
    Dizziness
    Tremors
    Hyperactivity
    Confusion

Hallucinogens
    Nystagmus
    Hypertension
    Tachycardia
    Bizarre behavior
    Agitation
    Hallucinations

    Delusions
    Altered mood and perceptions
    Detail focused
    Anxiety attacks
    Can be violent without apparent cause

Alcohol
    Slurred speech
    Impaired coordination
    Slowed reflexes
    Unsteady gait
    Relaxed inhibition

    Alcohol smell on breath
    Glazed eyes
    Frequently used in combination with depressants,
      antidepressants, and stimulants

[a]This list is based on the categories found in Table 16.1. These are general signs and symptoms and the list is not inclusive. Mixture of substances may also present differently.

- excessive tardiness at the beginning of a shift, returning from breaks, or lunch;
- frequent early departures before the end of a shift or during a shift with a variety of improbable excuses;
- excessive early arrival when scheduled;
- frequent requests for overtime at the end of a shift;
- frequent trips out of the unit (e.g., water fountain, restroom, pick up supplies, deliver tests to other departments);
- confusion with work schedule (i.e., comes

**Table 16.3.** Interview Tips[a]

The following interview tips are specific for recovering nurses and/or detection of a new employee who has been in a voluntary treatment program and who decided not to return to a previous employer:

1. Examine the application carefully for gaps in employment, registry or agency employers, per diem or float status, length of employment, geographic jumping about the country.
2. Observe handwriting.
3. Ask if there is anything that might prevent the nurse from meeting the job performance criteria. This gives the nurse the opportunity to discuss his or her disease and treatment program.
4. Ask for validation if the nurse admits to a disease.
5. Ask what the stressors were at his or her last job.
6. Ask if there are any stressors in the new job that would cause difficulty.
7. Ask about outside activities.

This gives the recovering nurse ample opportunity to discuss his or her disease and treatment plan. If there is admission of a disease, refer to Table 16.4 for the work contract. If there is no admission of a disease but the nurse manager's "alert system" senses a problem, it is appropriate to ask the nurse to submit to a drug and/or alcohol urine and blood screen done by the hiring institution. Refer to the policy established by your institution.

[a]Data from Abbott CA. The impaired nurse. Part II: Management strategies. Assoc Rn Nurses 1987;46(6): 1104–1115; and Robbins CE. A monitored treatment program for impaired health care professionals. J Nurs Admin 1987;17(2):17–21.

to work when unscheduled or does not show when scheduled);
- changing shifts with peers on the spur of the moment;
- volunteering to work on weekends or nights due to personal reasons (e.g., babysitting problems, car problems, or school schedule);
- volunteering to work extra shifts when previously unwilling;
- unexplained absence during shift?

2. Is there a change in the work pattern of the nurse? Does he or she:
- consistently request the acutely ill or most stable patient;

**Table 16.4.** Work Contract Between Employer and Recovering Nurse[a]

Key points to be considered in the contract are:

1. identification of disease state of substance misuse/abuse or alcoholism;
2. documentation indicating the nurse has received treatment for his or her disease by inpatient and/or out-patient program;
3. documentation indicating the nurse is currently continuing to participate in AA or NA meetings and/or peer support group;
4. permission for random, weekly urine and/or blood tests as requested and assumption of test costs;
5. documentation of continued evaluation by employee assistance program or appropriate health care profession every 6 to 8 weeks;
6. yearly physical examinations by personal physician who is aware of disease state with documentation of health status;
7. abstinence from all alcohol or mood-altering substances during employment;
8. inclusion of the date when the nurse will return to work;
9. identification of the specific shift in which the nurse will work;
10. type and time of orientation to unit;
11. agreement to work with a "buddy" on the unit.
12. analysis of when nurse may have access to narcotics or controlled substances. This includes actually giving the medication to the patient as well as carrying the narcotic keys and participating in the narcotic shift counts.
13. adhere to Nurse Practice Act for whatever state he or she practices;
14. agreement to sign a waiver of confidentiality so the nurse manager can receive treatment progress reports;
15. identification of administrator and file location of confidential information;
16. frequency of contract review;
17. inclusion of signatures of both the nurse and the nurse manager.

[a]Data from Penny JT. Spotlight on support for impaired nurses. AM J Nurs 1986;86(6):689–691; O'Connor P, Robinson R, Ferrara E. On the scene: the troubled nurse at the University of Cincinnati Hospital. Nurs Admin Q 1985;9(2):31–57; Jefferson LV, Ensor BE. Help for the helper confronting a chemically impaired colleague. Am J Nurs 1982;82(4):572–577; and Abbott CA. The impaired nurse. Part II: Management strategies. AORN J 1987;46(6):1104–1115.

- seem eager to administer pain or sedative medications for other nurses who are busy;
- demonstrate excessive concern for patient comfort, especially when PRN medications are involved as necessary;
- volunteer to do narcotic counts before and at the end of a shift;
- manipulate possession of keys to controlled substances;
- become too busy to help another nurse when assistance is requested;
- seem overly anxious to assist another nurse when assistance has not been requested;
- submit expected projects late (e.g., quality assurance monitoring sheets, chart audit, peer or self-evaluatons, required unit or institutional certifications);
- request a change in patient assignment during a shift;
- provide incomplete documentation in the clinical record (e.g., generalizations instead of details, failure to report risk occurrences, missing medication entries);
- alternate periods of low and high productivity;
- resign from or decrease assigned committee participation?

3. Is there a change in concentration or attention? Is there evidence of:

- inattention to details;
- inability to follow simple instructions;
- increased difficulty in handling or understanding complex statements or assignments;
- difficulty in following specific verbal instructions;
- taking more time to complete tasks;
- taking greater effort with work, requesting assistance from peers inappropriately;
- inconsistency between statements and actions;
- difficulty in recalling own mistakes;
- demonstrating cognitive impairment in assessing patient's condition;
- simple mathematical errors;
- memory lapses;
- questionable judgment decisions?

4. Is there a change in the nurse's attitude or interaction with others? Does he or she:

- find fault and complain about the policy or regulations of the institution without identified reason or cause;

- demonstrate reduced enthusiasm or enjoyment of work;
- act negatively about work and personal life;
- voice general complaints about peers and patients;
- demonstrate a tendency to project blame on others;
- show wide swings in mood (happy to sad, depressed to anxious, withdrawn and quiet to sociable and talkative);
- overreact to real or imagined criticism;
- demonstrate overly aggressive behavior;
- have unexpected blowups at peers without reason;
- carry seemingly unreasonable resentments;
- have outbursts of crying inappropriate to current situation;
- demonstrate increased irritability;
- voice general negative comments regarding personal problems with family, social contacts, or lifestyle;
- increase conversation concerning methods to relax (having several drinks to unwind, pills to decrease stress, pills for various vague physical ailments);
- seem argumentative;
- act defensively;
- borrow money and not pay back;
- seem always short of money but able to pay back regularly after payday;
- act overly positive;
- deny having a problem when approached;
- act unconcerned with peer's problems;
- avoid the nurse manager
- elicit complaints from healthcare team members, patients, or families?

5. Does the nurse seem to have a high accident rate? Is there evidence of:

- increased breaking of equipment;
- frequently dropped objects;
- above average on-the-job incidences (e.g., needle sticks, slipping, falling, losing patient's personal items, improper disposal of waste, inattention to own safety);
- workers' compensaton claims from normal preventable causes;
- numerous off the job injuries or accidents?

6. Has there been a change in the nurse's general or physical appearance? Does he or she appear with:

- a wrinkled or dirty uniform;

- inappropriate clothing for climate and/or working environment (e.g., sweater in summer, long-sleeved uniforms or jackets worn at all times);
- a change in uniforms from dresses to pants or from short sleeves to long sleeves;
- deterioration in general personal grooming (e.g., fingernails dirty or in disrepair, makeup not quite right, hair dirty and unkept looking, general untidiness);
- sudden weight gain or loss;
- a tired look (e.g., frequently yawning, nodding off after lunch, sitting whenever possible);
- bruises over general body (from bumping into furniture or unaware causes);
- slow and slurred speech;
- pupils dilated;
- pupils constricted;
- tinted glasses or sunglasses (to cover pupil response);
- breathmints or mouthwash (to cover alcohol odor);
- runny nose or dry sniffles (blamed on allergies, flu, cold);
- diaphoresis;
- undescribable body odor (due to inhalants)?

Do the traits or characteristics from the six questions above indicate a change in job performance? If the answer is yes, begin to assemble additional documentation.

## ASSEMBLING DATA

Deteriorating job performance usually is a gradual process that occurs over 6 months to 1 year. Suggestions for additional documentation are listed below:

1. Write down the characteristics or trait answers to the previously listed six questions.
2. Perform a current evaluation of performance. Compare it to the previous evaluation of performance and note the changes.
3. Does the employee file contain informal or formal counselings? Is there a pattern in the counselings?
4. Actively begin to observe the nurse and document your observations accordingly.
5. Review the patient care assignments to determine whether there is indeed a pattern of preferred acuities.
6. Check the narcotic records to determine whether

there is a pattern showing the nurse cosigning the narcotic count or carrying the narcotic keys more than usual.
Have there been inaccurate counts when the nurse is on duty?
Does the nurse cosign for frequent drug wastage or broken tubex containers?
Have there been any reported irregularities in the package seals?
Have there been any situations in which analysis of injectables has been needed to identify the substance and strength?
Have there been large changes in the locked inventory, especially early or late in the shift?
Contact the pharmacy for any information they can contribute.

7. Identify several past patients the nurse has cared for and have medical records pull the charts for review.
Check the medication administration record and compare it to the physician's orders to determine whether the orders are being carried out properly.
Examine the nursing notes for PRN medication administration for accuracy in medication given, dose, time, site, and charted patient response after administration.
Observe the handwriting during the shift for consistency.
Is the charting documentation consistent and detailed?
Are the physician's orders signed off according to policy?

8. Talk to patients and families currently under the nurse's care for their input. Review their charts in the same manner used for no. 7 above.
9. Obtain input from other staff nurses concerning any changes in mood, attitude, or general behavior.
10. Review the work schedule for the past year to see whether there are any patterns identified.
11. Talk with the physicians to determine their viewpoint on the performance of the nurse.

Evaluate the data collected. Does it indicate a change in job performance related to potential substance misuse or abuse in your mind? If the answer is yes, seek a peer with whom to share the data. Request the peer nurse manager to assist in evaluating the data and to make suggestions for improvements or additional data. This provides the opportunity to "hear" the case and evaluate it for objectivity. If there is agreement that substance misuse or abuse is strongly suspected, a plan of action is indicated..

## CONFRONTATION

The nurse manager will find confrontation to be the most uncomfortable aspect of this entire process. Remember the purpose of confronting the nurse is to get the individual into treatment. Keeping his or her job is a strong motivator for the nurse to accept the treatment approach.

The defensive behaviors and reactions by the nurse must be anticipated in order to keep the meeting constructive. The expected defensive behaviors are denial, anger, and hostility (11). The nurse has taken several months and/or years to build and reinforce a profound denial and rationalization coping mechanism. Breaking this defense system requires a tremendous amount of focused energy and concentration by the nurse manager.

The use of two member interveners is recommended (11, 20). The nurse manager's supervisor, employee assistance program representative, in-house consultant, and human resource representative are excellent resources available. This two-member approach assists in predicting the response and the appropriate intervention. Practice or role-play the expected reaction of the nurse who has gradual unsatisfactory job performance based on personal problems and/or suspicion of substance misuse and abuse. Practice for the "crisis" situation in which the nurse is actually caught "using" or "stealing" drugs, requiring immediate action.

The following recommendations for the practice session have been made in the literature (9, 11, 20, 21):

- Have the meeting preset, without interruptions, selecting a room away from the unit.
- Keep responses unemotional, factual, and focused on the problem behavior.
- Offer a clear, concise presentation of the performance deficiencies.
- Present firm expectations for improvement.
- Include a specific time frame for improvement.
- Rehearse an intervention/action plan as outlined below.
- Document an action plan to be signed by both the nurse and nurse manager.
- Schedule another meeting.
- Use a calm, even voice, remaining unemotional, restating, and focusing on the performance when

the nurse's reaction is anger at you or other persons.
- Use open-ended questions or statements requiring verbal responses when the nurse's reaction is silence.
- Practice being silent as this situation often makes the interveners uncomfortable and talkative to break the silence.
- When the nurse is incapacitated, present the above but add a mandatory laboratory drug analysis of urine and blood.
- Schedule another meeting within 24 hours to discuss the situation and put it in writing as the nurse may not recall the verbal instructions.
- Examine transport alternatives for the nurse to keep him or her from driving under the influence of alcohol/drugs.

The role and function of the employee assistance program (13, 19) is listed below:

1. Assist the nurse in examining his or her decreased job performance in a confidential setting usually outside of the institution.
2. Provide referrals for inpatient or outpatient treatment programs if indicated.
3. Provide referrals to peer assistance programs, Alcoholics or Narcotics Anonymous programs, financial assistance programs, and legal assistance programs.
4. Obtain information on financing available within the institution and on the benefits provided and the costs of various programs.
5. Maintain confidential conversations with the nurse.
6. Provide the nurse manager, Board of Registered Nursing, and legal agencies required progress reports. Assist in the medical/personal leave policy documentation.
7. Assist in the work contract between the nurse and the institution when the nurse reenters the work setting.
8. Assume responsibility for total case management including relapse.

## ACTION PLAN AND INTERVENTION

The *first plan* is based on probable suspicion that a personal problem or substance misuse or abuse accounts for the decline in job performance. There is no conclusive data, such as positive drug tests, actual observations of drug usage by the nurse while on duty, or deviations in the narcotic records. The two interveners will follow the practice sessons outlined above when confronting the nurse. The interveners will focus on the nurse's explanations, perceptions, and defensive behaviors. Observe the body language. Suggest voluntary referral for personal problems. Schedule another meeting to discuss improvements in job performance. The nurse manager and nurse should sign the action plan with each having a copy.

Evaluation of the plan will include the following:

1. Show improvement requiring routine follow-up.
2. If there has not been any contact with the nurse manager from the referral and there is no improvement in job performance, refer to the second action plan.

The *second action plan* is based on the entry into the disciplinary process according to the policy of the institution (see Chapter 17). As described in the practice session above, meet the nurse to reinforce the failure in job performance improvements as outlined in the first meeting. Explain the consequences of continued unsatisfactory job performance. Again suggest voluntary referral. Schedule the third meeting. Document this meeting and sign accordingly with each party having a copy.

Evaluation of the plan will include the following:

1. Show improvement requiring routine follow-up.
2. Improvement and notification by the referral agency will indicate the nurse is in voluntary counseling. Continue to meet with the nurse as scheduled. Plan for on-going meetings until the job performance is acceptable and consistent.
3. If there is no improvement in job performance or notification from the referral agency, refer to the third action plan.

The *third action plan* is based on continuation of the disciplinary process. This meeting will again present the continuing unsatisfactory job performance and expectations for immediate improvement. Make a mandatory referral for counseling. Outline the negative consequences of noncompliance as a condition of continued employment.

Evaluation of the plan will include the following:

1. Show improvement in some areas and notifi-

cation by the referral agency that the nurse is in mandatory counseling. The referral agency usually will send reports of progress. Continue to hold on-going meetings at 2-week intervals to review performance.
2. If there is no improvement in job performance but notification by the referral agency that the nurse is in mandatory counseling, hold weekly meetings with the nurse to review performance. Document accordingly.
3. There is no improvement in job performance or attendance in the mandatory counseling, refer to the fourth action plan.

The *fourth action plan* continues the disciplinary process. This meeting will consist of termination of the nurse for noncompliance with the mandatory counseling referral related to unsatisfactory job performance. The action plans have all been based on probable suspicion and not conclusive data that the nurse had a substance misuse or abuse disease and/or personal problem. The nurse may be offered voluntary resignation with no opportunity for rehiring by the institution. This action plan is also appropriate for the nurse who does not have continued improvement in job performance while receiving mandatory on-going counseling.

The *fifth action plan* occurs when the referral representative informs the nurse manager that the nurse wants to enter an inpatient substance misuse/abuse program immediately. Follow policies for personal/medical leave. Refer to the secton describing the reentry/recovery phase in this chapter.

The *sixth action plan* is the crisis situation. In this situation there is evidence that the nurse is:

- actually caught stealing drugs from the unit and/or patient;
- altering seals on a narcotic package during the shift;
- observed, by peers, tampering with the controlled substance seals or solutions;
- implicated in a laboratory analysis of a questionable controlled substance (tubex syringe) that indicated tampering, such as, adding water or normal saline to decrease the concentration of narcotic;
- altering the volume in tubex syringe or bottles;
- caught injecting or consuming controlled substances/alcohol;
- found incapacitated;
- tested positive in a laboratory drug analysis of urine and blood for chemical or alcohol content.

Remove the nurse from the unit and take him or her to another area. Using two interveners, explain briefly, clearly, and concisely what behaviors were observed. State that the behaviors are unacceptable and place the patient at risk for harm. Place the nurse on investigatory leave, suspend, or terminate immediately. How this crisis is handled depends on the policy of your institution as discussed in the previous identification section.

If the institution is "proactive" or "cooperative," document the crisis meeting and schedule another meeting within 24 hours. Give the written documentation to the nurse. Send the nurse home in a taxi or have a family member or friend provide transportaton. Do not allow the nurse to drive under the influence of drugs or alcohol.

The next day's meeting should focus on the previous day's events and behaviors. Explain the choices of:

1. immediate mandatory counseling referral for evaluation as a condition for employment with notification of the appropriate enforcement agencies and Board of Registered Nursing;
2. immediate inpatient care with notification of the indicated enforcement agencies and the Board of Registered Nursing;
3. reinforcement of the proper law enforcement agencies and notification of the Board of Registered Nursing in the event that the nurse resigns.

Termination and reporting to the appropriate enforcement agencies and the Board of Registered Nursing are appropriate in about 15% of employees. This job loss and legal involvement may be the last method possible to break the wall of DENIAL (15).

## RECOVERY

Successful recovery depends on treatment and careful follow-up (16) (see Table 16.4). Inpatient treatment is highly recommended with peer group therapy to deal with the unique problems that influence health care professionals. Structured outpatient care associated with Alcoholics Anonymous (AA) and/or Narcotics Anonymous (NA) support systems are critical after inpatient care. This takes 2 to 4 months to complete.

The reentry phase is a gradual process of rehabilitation that occurs over 1 to 2 years. It should be noted that the recovering nurse may be capable of fulfilling entire job performance expectations within the first year. This includes administration of controlled drugs to the patients as well as the responsibility for handling the controlled drug keys and counts. Thus, monitoring is essential with contract adjustments made based on progress shown by the nurse. Lifelong continuous participation in AA or NA is believed to be necessary to maintain sobriety (3, 11, 19).

Smith et al. (11) define recovery as: "complete abstinence from mood-altering chemicals in addition to serenity, job, freedom, happiness, and a sense of personal accountability".

*The author acknowledges the assistance of Joe Draskovich and the recovering nurses known to the author for their assistance and encouragement in this project.*

REFERENCES

1. Church OM. Sairey Gamp revisited: a historical inquiry into alcoholism and drug dependency. Nurse Admin Q Winter 1985;9(2):10–21.
2. Green PL. The impaired nurse: chemical dependency. J Emerg Nurs 1984;10(1):23–26.
3. Cross L. Chemical dependency in our ranks: managing a nurse in crisis. Nurs Management 1985;16(11):15–16.
4. Curtin LL. Throw away nurses? Nurs Management 1987;18(7):7–8.
5. Creighton H. Legal implication of the impaired nurse—Part I. Nurs Management, 1988;19(1):21–24.
6. Naegle MA. Drug and alcohol abuse in nursing: an occupational hazard? Nurs Life 1988; 42–52.
7. Hutchinson SA. Chemically dependent nurses: implications for nurse executives J Nurs Admin 1987;17(9):23–39.
8. Cherskov M. Substance abuse in the workplace. Hosptials 1987;6:68–73.
9. O'Connor P, Robinson RS. Managing impaired nurses Nurs Admin Q 1985;9(2):1–9.
10. Gaskin J. Nurses in trouble. Can Nurse 1986;82(4):31–34.
11. Smith HE, Talbott GD, Morrison MA. Chemical abuse and dependence: an occupational hazard for health professionals. Topics Emerg Med 1985;7(3):69–78.
12. Levine HG. The discovery of addiction changing concepts of habitual drunkenness in America. J Studies Alcohol 1978;39(1):143–174.
13. Penny JT. Spotlight on support for impaired nurses. Am J Nurs 1986;86(6):689–691.
14. O'Connor P., Robinson R, Ferrara E, et al. On the scene: the troubled nurse at the University of Cincinnati Hospital. Nurs Admin Q 1985;9(2):31–57.
15. Kabb GM. Chemical dependency helping your staff. J Nurs Admin 1984;13(11):18–23.
16. Caroselli-Karinja MF, Zboray SD. The impaired nurse J Psych Nurs 1986;24(6):14–19.
17. Isler C. The alcoholic nurse what we try to deny. RN 1978;41(7):48–55.

18. Veatch D. When is the recovering impaired nurse ready to work? A job interview guide. J Nurs Admin 1987;17(2):14–16.

19. Abbott CA. The impaired nurse. Part I: a description of chemical dependency. AORN J 1987;46(5):870–876.

20. Jefferson LV, Ensor BE. Help for the helper confronting a chemically-impaired colleague. Am J Nurs 1982;82(4):572–577.

21. Baldwin LJ, Ramos NB, Baldwin LE. Developing an alternative disciplinary process for the troubled nurse. Nurs Admin Q 1985;9(2):77–87.

22. Halsey J. The moderately troubled nurse: a not-so-uncommon entity. Nurs Admin Q 1985;9(2):69–76.

23. Abbott CA. The impaired nurse. Part II: management strategies.. Assoc Operat Rm Nurses 1987;46(6):1104–1115.

24. Robbins CE. A monitored treatment program for impaired health care professionals. J Nurs Admin 1987;17(2):17–21.

# Chapter 17

# Counseling and Disciplining Staff

LYNNETTE M. HOLDER

The word "discipline" is used in many connections and understood in several different ways. When one hears the word discipline used in the workplace, one is often inclined to think of the use of authority or force. To many managers, discipline connotes rule violations, confrontations with the violators, and the need for punishment with a swift imposition of penalties. This negative, punitive, or autocratic definition of discipline generates a "big stick" approach by managers, whereby the threat of punishment is employed to keep employees in line. The autocratic disciplinary approach generally achieves only the minimal employee performance necessary to avoid punishment or punitive responses. With a negative approach to discipline, the power of the manager to suspend or discharge is ever present in the minds of employees. Employees spend their energies on avoiding punishment, not on cooperating and working toward group or institutional goals.

However, the root word of discipline is "disciple," defined as "to learn" (1). The first meaning of discipline in the dictionary is "training that corrects, molds, strengthens or perfects (2). Thus in its optimal sense and best usage, discipline is a state of self-regulation that results from a high level of commitment and motivation within a work group.

In the work place, discipline is the process of building and maintaining a sense of personal commitment to achieving organizational objectives and goals through compliance with established procedures and rules. It is an essential function of the critical care nurse manager's role to promote a sense of personal responsibility and self-discipline in each employee, and to create an environment that fosters the commitment of the individual. This can be accomplished through positive support and reinforcement for approved actions, coupled with penalties for improper behavior, carried out in a supportive, constructive manner. With a constructive discipline approach, employees adhere to desired work standards because they understand, believe in, and support them. Employees thus develop a willingness to obey and abide by institutional rules and regulations because they want to, not because they fear a punitive consequence.

Although most employees demonstrate a considerable degree of self-discipline, there are always a few in every large organization who occasionally fail to observe established rules and standards, even after having been informed of them. They simply will not, or have not learned to, accept the responsibility and benefits of self-discipline. As a supervisor, the critical care nurse manager cannot allow those few to "get away" with violations. Firm action is called for to correct the situation. Unless such action is taken, the morale of other employees in the work group will be seriously weakened. This is one time when the nurse manager has to rely on the authority inherent in his or her position. On such an occasion, the critical care nurse manager must clearly realize that he or she is in charge of the area and is therefore responsible for the discipline within it.

## PURPOSE OF DISCIPLINE

In the positive sense, discipline is more than the administration of selected punishments. Positive discipline is broader and more fundamental. It is the creation of a climate and attitudes wherein the employee willingly comforms to rules, regulations, and established norms of conduct. This is accomplished through sound leadership, efficient management, and the use of the principles of positive motivation.

Whereas traditional punitive discipline was achieved solely through the authority of the su-

To be treated fairly, with no favorites or biases
  To work in a healthy, safe environment
    To receive reasonable, competitive wages and benefits

To know what expectations are
  To know what consequences will be
    To know how well he or she is doing

To know what can be done to improve work performance
  To receive adequate training,
    Enabling him or her to perform the job well

To be treated as an individual
  With unique needs, skills, and aspirations
    To have his or her needs recognized

To be treated with courtesy, respect, and dignity
  To have interactions held in confidence
    To be critiqued in private

Figure 17.1    Employee rights.

pervisor, modern discipline is founded on the understanding that constructive and effective discipline involves employee self-control and a sense of personal responsibility for behavior and performance. With this approach to discipline, the emphasis of the critical care nurse manager is on assisting the employee in making a greater contribution to the organization by improving employee understanding of institutional objectives, how the objectives can be met, and the role played by the employee's workgroup. Self-control discipline is achieved through the influence of a common organizational frame of reference or rules that guide the actions of each individual.

The responsibility of the critical care nurse manager in the positive disciplinary environment is that of preserving the interests of the organization as a whole while protecting the rights of the individual employee (see Fig. 17.1) The nurse manager's focus should be on correcting employee behavior, thereby improving overall work performance. In all organizations some individuals will occasionally break the rules. Through the use of disciplinary sanctions, the critical care nurse manager can help these employees see the error of their ways and the need to improve their performance. Disciplinary sanctions are administered to correct and rehabilitate, not to injure, the employee. Their purpose is correction, with a clear warning as to what is required and the consequences of continued misconduct or noncompliance.

Discipline can be placed in its proper perspective and become a tool to be used for constructive

purposes if the critical care nurse manager remembers the following:

- Disciplinary action is taken against only those who cannot or will not exercise self-discipline
- Failure to maintain discipline in the workplace directly affects the morale of the majority (who play by the rules) and may affect patient care.
- Corrective action and prevention are the desired results of any disciplinary measure.

## PREVENTIVE DISCIPLINE

The most desirable approach to discipline is to create an environment that reduces the occurrence of situations that require corrective or disciplinary action. There are three key steps in reducing the need for disciplinary action: formulation of attainable policies and standards, dissemination of the rules to all employees, and consistent enforcement of all work rules.

Every person employed in the work area must know when hired what the management team and their immediate supervisor expects of them. There should be a focus on the positive behavior expected, not an emphasis on prohibitions. Standards must be fair, attainable with reasonable effort, and consistent from job to job. Work rules should be reasonable, clear, few in number, and clearly communicated in language that is understandable by the employee. During orientation and the probationary period there should be reviews of performance expectations and presentations (with reinforcement) of what help is available within the organization to achieve that performance. Principle standards of expected behavior should be reviewed, including at least attendance guidelines, notification of absence, punctuality, cooperation, morality and honesty, wastefulness, safety regulations, and courtesy (3).

Compliance with established policies and procedures will be enhanced if the critical care nurse manager reviews each work rule with the employee and explains its purpose. Staff members must know what the work rules are, understand them, and know why they are necessary. The nurse manager can make clear to the staff what behavior is acceptable, what is required, and what is unacceptable through simple communication. Staff must be instructed in the proper work practices and methods. Expectations should be explicit and reinforced consistently. In addition, employee awareness of policies and procedures should be updated at regular intervals. The critical care nurse manager who is knowledgeable of and compliant with work rules at all times will set a good example for the staff and foster constructive discipline in the work group. This, of course, requires that the nurse manager knows, understands, and abides by all policies and work rules.

Compliance will be further enhanced if the critical care nurse manager regularly and frequently evaluates and critiques the employee's behavior and performance. Criticism is the art of analyzing and comparing the quality of something against a standard. Critiques of staff members must include both positive and negative comparisons in order to be most helpful and fair to the employee. Constructive criticism in the form of employee counseling will help the employee mold his or her attitude, behavior, and performance to unit norms. In correcting errors in a timely fashion, the critical care nurse manager should:

- Review the standard or expectations with the employee;
- Point out the error;
- Indicate what must be done to correct the error and avoid its repetition.

When used constructively with nonthreatening feedback, criticism can guide the actions of the employee so that major infractions of work rules can be avoided.

The most crucial time for the critical care nurse manager to evaluate and critique an employee is during the employee's probationary period. The nurse manager should plan the employee's experiences in the probationary period so that at its completion there is enough evidence to decide on the adequacy of the employee's performance and behavior. Both the nurse manager and the institution have to live with the future consequences of a decision to keep a marginal employee. Thus, terminating the employment of a marginal probationary employee, although discomforting for the nurse manager, clears the way for the selection of an employee with greater personal responsibility and self-discipline.

An effective employee/manager relationship is key in supporting a constructive disciplinary environment. The critical care nurse manager's actions and decisions as a manager will be received in varying ways and have varying influence depending upon the general relationship the manager has established with the staff. This relationship is dependent on the unique interaction of elements that the nurse manager utilizes in his or her role as manager: management style, communication process, role definition, values, and knowledge and respect of employee rights (see Fig. 17.1). The critical care nurse manager should nurture his or her vital relationship with each staff member. This relationship should serve the unique needs of the individual while making the best use of the employee's capabilities. The most effective employee/manager relationship is one based on mutual dignity and respect.

The critical care nurse manager must know the employee. Some employees require regular contact and guidance, while others perform better when given more opportunity for self-control. There is no quick formula to use when dealing with employees. Each person is an individual and must be dealt with differently, yet all employees must be treated fairly and equally.

The critical care nurse manager typically supervises professional, technical, and skilled employees. Policies and work rules are to be applied equally to all employees regardless of their qualifications or classifications. Professional employees are as likely to be a source of disciplinary and behavioral problems as the technical or skilled employee. Professional employees should not be held to more rigid standards of behavior because of their professional status. On the other hand, infractions of professionals should not be overlooked because of their professional status either. It is essential that all employees receive equal treatment.

## ADMINISTRATIVE JUSTICE

Employers are subject to many restrictions and requirements in their relationships with employees. Because federal and state requirements extend to numerous aspects of the employee/manager relationship, the critical care nurse manager needs to develop a working knowledge of what the various laws require and how they affect supervisory decision making. The nurse manager should be acquainted with the basic concepts and "do/don'ts" of labor relations law (see Chapter 18), discrimination law, wage/hour law, and other statutes governing unemployment and termination at will (4).

Before 1964 the supervisor could hire, transfer, promote, discipline, or fire an employee for inherently unfair reasons as long as the supervisor did not violate the edicts of management or the policies of the organization. However, since 1964 a trend of protection of employees against discrimination and arbitrary treatment has emerged, and the employer has virtually lost the historical right to fire at will. Courts have found implied employment contracts in employee handbooks listing specific causes for termination of employment. Currently, if an aggrieved employee is a member of a recognized minority group, or of any group for which specific laws exist for protection of rights, the supervisor and the organization may have to deal with discrimination charges brought by any of several regulatory branches of the government. Even if the aggrieved employee is not clearly a member of a recognized minority group, the nurse manager may still have to deal with legal charges of unjust or unfair treatment (5). If the employer has documented job-related reasons for disciplinary action, the action will probably be upheld as long as similar actions in the organization have resulted in similar penalties in the past.

Numerous years of arbitration experience have generated a body of fairly well-accepted principles and procedural requirements for the administration of employee justice within the organization. These guidelines are based in the industrial code of common-law principles and precedents (3). Recognizing that management now bears the burden of proof in the disciplinary process to show both the fact of wrongdoing and the need for punishment, institutions are best served by following "due process" procedures:

- The employee must know beforehand that his or her conduct would lead to disciplinary action.
- The violated rule must be related to the efficient and safe operation of the hospital or patient care area. In other words, the offense must, in fact, call for some corrective action or penalty.
- Each individual to be disciplined must be provided with a written statement of the charges and reasons for penalty.
- Penalties should be reasonably related to the seriousness of the offense.
- There must be a fair and thorough investigation of allegations.
- It must be determined that the employee actually broke the rule.
- Disciplinary action must be applied consistently employee to employee, both within the work group and throughout the organization.
- Each individual must have a complete opportunity for self-defense and for full utilization of

a formal grievance procedure. Discipline and grievance procedures must interact because administered discipline is usually the root of later grievance actions.

Thus, management continues to have the right to discipline or discharge employees for "just cause," or for good and sufficient reason, using due process procedures. Critical care nurse managers must take care to administer discipline fairly and with concern for procedural safeguards that are designed to protect the rights of employees. Such managers are less likely to place the institution in the position of having to defend itself against charges of injustice or discrimination.

## PROGRESSIVE DISCIPLINE

In most organizations that support the concept of positive, corrective discipline, some type of verbal admonition is given for minor, first offenses. For the majority of employees, knowledge of error in behavior or performance is sufficient to prevent a repetition. If minor offenses continue to occur, penalties become increasingly severe. This is referred to as *progressive discipline*. The philosophical basis of progressive discipline is to:

- Attempt corrective action;
- Afford the employee reasonable opportunity to correct inappropriate behavior before it becomes serious enough to jeopardize employment;
- Make a reasonable effort to help the employee become a productive contributor to the organization.

The purpose of progressive discipline is to ensure that discipline is imposed consistently and equitably with an eye not toward punishment, but toward correcting deficient performance and securing compliance with work rules. Thus, with progressive discipline the employee is provided with the knowledge and the opportunity to meet established minimal standards of conduct and work performance and the knowledge of the consequence in failing to do so. At each step of progressive discipline, it is important for the critical care nurse manager to assure that the employee grasps the standards expected, identifies his or her error, understands how to avoid repetition, and knows the consequences of additional infractions. Progressive discipline provides due process for the employee, while incorporating disciplinary actions strong enough to stimulate change and effect correction of the employee's behavior or performance. The outcome of progressive discipline is discouragement of repeated offenses by employees and severing of relationships with irresponsible or noncompliant employees.

The best foundation for a progressive disciplinary approach is a set of well-defined institutional policies and procedures, or organizational rules. Such policies facilitate communication to employees and establish organizational norms. They describe management expectations of appropriate performance and behavior and the accepted methods to achieve those expectations. This protects employees and prevents a manager from looking at a case in terms of management needs of the moment. All policies should be understandable, written, easily accessible, and reviewed regularly by employees at specified time intervals. To be effective, policies must be reasonably capable of being attained in that particular institutional environment.

Institutional policies and procedures are often married to comprehensive published lists of penalties associated with types of infractions. This approach promotes consistency in application of disciplinary action throughout the organization over periods of time. It also assures that employees are informed as to what the consequence of a negative action will be. The published, public nature of this approach adds a feeling of legitimacy to a manager's actions, and it prevents a potentially vindictive supervisor from having an opportunity to invoke unfair, unusual, or unjust punishment.

The major disadvantage of publishing lists of infractions is that the circumstances of each case are different, and so extenuating circumstances could alter the nature of the most appropriate sanction. Thus, many institutions have developed a scale of penalties for managers' use that incorporates some latitude in selection and application. Using a scale of penalties provides general predictability in institutional discipline but allows managers discretionary authority to vary sanctions in light of surrounding circumstances. This enables the institution to balance situational individuality with consistency of action throughout the organization (Table 17.1).

There are five well-recognized steps in progressive discipline: counseling, verbal warning, written warning, suspension, and termination.

## Counseling

Ironically, progressive discipline can be both prevented and initiated by the same activity—individual counseling. The purpose of counseling is to coach or guide the employee so that he or she can bring behavior or performance to a minimal standard or beyond. Counseling as a preventive tool has the purpose of educating the employee and is the critical care nurse manager's greatest opportunity to effect real education and change in employee behavior and performance. The nurse manager can make clear to the staff member what behavior is required, what is acceptable, and what is unacceptable. In this modality, problems are discussed by the manager and the employee in a helpful, nonadversarial environment.

As the first step in the disciplinary process, counseling also has employee education as its primary purpose. However, it has the important secondary purpose of establishing the foundation for progressive disciplinary action as needed. This first step should be completely positive in nature. In an informal atmosphere, the employee should be encouraged to relate his or her view of the situation and to review the facts of the situation with the critical care nurse manager. The employee should be clearly shown any errors and also be shown that adherence to the rule or policy is important to the organization. In this situation the manager must make sure that the employee realizes he or she has made an error or broken a rule. The manager should privately reexplain the rule to the employee and emphasize the need for compliance.

After this type of counseling, the critical care nurse manager should write a brief anecdotal note describing the problem, what the employee was told, the employee's response, and the date and location of the counseling. This note should be signed by the supervisor and the employee, so that at a later date the nurse manager can prove, if necessary, that the counseling was given. Anecdotal counseling records should be kept on file by the nurse manager but not placed in the employee's official personnel record (see Fig. 17.2).

### Verbal Warning

Counseling sessions give the employee the time and opportunity to clarify expectations, realize the implications of his or her errors, and learn how to correct that behavior. If, however, the offense continues, formal discipline is initiated with a verbal warning. (Note that progressive discipline is appropriate for repetitions of similar offenses. An infraction of a different rule would result in counseling for the first infraction of that rule.) A verbal

**Table 17.1.**   Guide to Disciplinary Actions[a]

| | 1st Offense | | 2nd Offense | | 3rd Offense | | 4th Offense | |
|---|---|---|---|---|---|---|---|---|
| | Min. | Max. | Min. | Max. | Min. | Max. | Min. | Max. |
| Attendance/absence from work area/time records | | | | | | | | |
| 1. Chronic absenteeism and/or lateness | 1 | 1 | 2 | 2 | 3 | 3 | 5 | 5 |
| 2. Failure to provide proper notice of absence | 2 | 2 | 3 | 3 | 5 | 5 | | |
| 3. Abandonment of position (absence for 3 consecutive workdays without notification) | 5 | 5 | | | | | | |
| 4. Absence from work area without notification | 1 | 3 | 2 | 3 | 3 | 5 | 5 | 5 |
| 5. Stopping work before scheduled end of work time without authorization | 1 | 3 | 2 | 3 | 3 | 5 | 5 | 5 |
| 6. Extended break or meal time without authorization | 1 | 3 | 2 | 3 | 3 | 5 | 5 | 5 |
| 7. Deliberate signing/punching in or out of another employee's time record or asking another employee to sign or punch in for you | 3 | 5 | 5 | 5 | | | | |
| 8. Accidental signing/punching in or out of another employee's time record | 1 | 1 | 2 | 4 | 5 | 5 | | |
| 9. Failure to sign/punch in or out own time record | 1 | 1 | 2 | 2 | 3 | 3 | 5 | 5 |
| 10. Falsification of own or another employee's time record | 3 | 5 | 5 | 5 | | | | |
| 11. Abuse of sick leave | 1 | 5 | 2 | 5 | 3 | 5 | 5 | 5 |
| 12. Nonavailability when on call or when required by operational need | 1 | 5 | 2 | 5 | 3 | 5 | 5 | 5 |
| Performance | | | | | | | | |
| 13. Failure to meet reasonable standards/expectations of performance; unsatisfactory work performance | 1 | 1 | 2 | 2 | 3 | 3 | 5 | 5 |
| 14. Failure to use appropriate judgment | 1 | 5 | 2 | 5 | 4 | 5 | 5 | 5 |
| 15. Carelessness or inattention | 2 | 3 | 3 | 5 | 5 | 5 | | |
| 16. Gross neglect of duty; deliberate inattention to patient care | 4 | 5 | 5 | 5 | | | | |
| 17. Failure to fulfill the responsibilities of the job to the extent that might or does cause neglect to a patient or any other person, or cause damage, waste, or loss of material, supplies, equipment, time, facilities, or other hospital property. | 2 | 4 | 3 | 5 | 5 | 5 | | |
| 18. Performing non-work-related activities while on duty | 1 | 2 | 2 | 3 | 3 | 5 | 5 | 5 |
| 19. Loafing, loitering, or engaging in unauthorized personal visits | 1 | 2 | 2 | 3 | 3 | 5 | 5 | 5 |
| 20. Failure to carry out orders, instructions, or an assignment | 1 | 3 | 3 | 5 | 5 | 5 | | |
| 21. Refusal to carry out orders, instructions, or an assignment; insubordination | 5 | 5 | | | | | | |
| Demeanor/Conduct | | | | | | | | |
| 22. Rude or discourteous behavior; demeaner not in keeping with that expected of an employee; violation of "Hospitality House Rules" | 1 | 3 | 3 | 5 | 5 | 5 | | |
| 23. Inappropriate or unprofessional behavior | 2 | 4 | 3 | 5 | 5 | 5 | | |
| 24. Disorderly or disruptive conduct; behavior disruptive within work group | 2 | 5 | 3 | 5 | 5 | 5 | | |

**Table 17.1.** *Continued.*

| | 1st Offense | | 2nd Offense | | 3rd Offense | | 4th Offense | |
|---|---|---|---|---|---|---|---|---|
| | Min. | Max. | Min. | Max. | Min. | Max. | Min. | Max. |
| 25. Immoral conduct on hospital premises | 3 | 5 | 5 | 5 | | | | |
| 26. Engaging in activities that interfere with the operation of the hospital and/or services of patients | 4 | 5 | 5 | 5 | | | | |
| 27. Unauthorized sleeping on duty | 2 | 5 | 5 | 5 | | | | |
| 28. Actual or threatened violence or harm | 5 | 5 | | | | | | |
| 29. Profane or abusive languge to patient, visitor, another employee, supervisor, member of medical staff, or individual otherwise having a relationship to the medical center. | 2 | 4 | 3 | 5 | 5 | 5 | | |
| 30. Disclosure of confidential information to an unauthorized individual or accessing information without authority | 2 | 5 | 5 | 5 | | | | |
| 31. Unauthorized disclosure of confidential patient information or allowing access to such information by unauthorized persons | 3 | 5 | 5 | 5 | | | | |
| 32. Fraud, falsification of records, unauthorized removal or destruction of records NOTE: For falsification of own or another employee's time record, see no. 10 | 5 | 5 | | | | | | |
| 33. Fighting; assult on another individual | 3 | 5 | 5 | 5 | | | | |
| 34. Conduct of any illegal activity on hospital premises and/or during scheduled work hours | 3 | 5 | 5 | 5 | | | | |
| 35. Soliciting or accepting services, gifts, payments of any kind, or hospitality of more than nominal value from a patient, a member of patient's family, or any individual or organization with whom the medical center does business or has any other relationships; selling services to patients | 2 | 5 | 3 | 5 | 5 | 5 | | |
| 36. Illegal possession of, and/or unauthorized consumption of, use of, or being under the influence of an intoxicant or controlled substance | 3 | 5 | 4 | 5 | 5 | 5 | | |
| 37. Willful concealment of or refusal to provide current address, telephone number, or other pertinent personal information | 2 | 3 | 3 | 5 | 5 | 5 | | |
| 38. Unauthorized presence in a nonpublic area of the medical center | 1 | 2 | 2 | 3 | 3 | 5 | 5 | 5 |
| 39. Theft; unauthorized possession of property belonging to the hospital, other employees, patients, visitors, or others | 5 | 5 | | | | | | |
| 40. Misuse or damage to property belonging to the hospital, other employees, patients, visitors, or others | 2 | 4 | 3 | 5 | 5 | 5 | | |
| 41. Willful damage to, abuse of, or misuse of property belonging to the hospital, other employees, patients, visitors, and others | 5 | 5 | | | | | | |
| 42. Violation of a health, safety, parking, security, fire prevention, or related rule; failure to use prescribed safety precautions | 1 | 3 | 2 | 4 | 5 | 5 | | |
| 43. Possession of a firearm, explosives, or similarly dangerous substance on hospital premises | 5 | 5 | | | | | | |
| 44. Possession of deadly weapons (other than those in no. 43)[b] | 3 | 5 | 5 | 5 | | | | |

**Table 17.1.** *Continued.*

| | 1st Offense | | 2nd Offense | | 3rd Offense | | 4th Offense | |
|---|---|---|---|---|---|---|---|---|
| | Min. | Max. | Min. | Max. | Min. | Max. | Min. | Max. |
| 45. Negligence in reporting an injury or incident in which involved or a witness to | 1 | 2 | 2 | 3 | 3 | 5 | | |
| 46. Willful failure to report or concealment of any incident | 3 | 5 | 5 | 5 | | | | |
| 47. Unauthorized solicitation; unauthorized posting or distributing of printed matter | 1 | 5 | 3 | 5 | 5 | 5 | | |
| 48. Refusal to submit to a medical examination, when reasonably requested to do so by the hospital | 5 | 5 | | | | | | |
| 49. Disregard of hospital, departmental, or generally accepted standards of appearance, dress, uniform, or personal hygiene | 1 | 3 | 2 | 4 | 3 | 5 | 5 | 5 |
| 50. Discrimination against employees, patients, visitors, or others associated with the hospital on the basis of race, color, religion, sex, sexual orientation, national origin, age, or handicap | 1 | 5 | 2 | 5 | 3 | 5 | 5 | 5 |
| 51. Sexual harassment of employees, patients, visitors, or others associated with the hospital | 1 | 5 | 2 | 5 | 3 | 5 | 5 | 5 |
| 52. Actions or inactions that caused or could cause life-threatening situations | 3 | 5 | 5 | 5 | | | | |
| 53. Conduct or action contrary to the medical center's best interests | 1 | 5 | 3 | 5 | 5 | 5 | | |
| 54. An offense not specified in preceding | 1 | 5 | 1 | 5 | 1 | 5 | 1 | 5 |

[a]Reproduced with permission of Albert Einstein Medical Center, Philadelphia, Pennsylvania; copyright 1986 AEMC. Disciplinary action codes: 1, document counseling; 2, warning notice; 3, 1 to 2 days suspension; 4, 3 to 5 days suspension; 5, discharge.
[b]Deadly weapons include fixed blade knives of any size, switch blade knives, and any other illegal weapons.

warning is similar to counseling in that it is a private reexplanation of the rule and the need for compliance. However, the employee must understand that the disciplinary process has begun. The employee must understand that as a result of his or her behavior or performance, the individual is on a road that could lead to discharge. He or she must know what must be done to correct the behavior or error and in what time frame, how to avoid its repetition, and the consequences in failing to do so. A written summary of the disciplinary conference including all of the above should be signed by both the critical care nurse manager and the employee. A copy should be given to the employee for his or her records, and the original should be placed in the employee's file in the personnel department (see Fig. 17.3).

Before the critical care nurse manager decides that any discipline is warranted, he or she should undertake a thorough investigation of the situation. Objectivity is essential, and prejudging of a case before fact finding must not occur. The manager needs to talk with the employee, to hear his or her version of the situation. All facts leading to the situation must be uncovered and considered, including interviews with potential witnesses. The critical care nurse manager must review applicable hospital policy in light of the who, what, where, when, and why of the case. Thoughtful deliberation of all factors bearing on the situation is required to determine whether disciplinary action is indicated.

## Written Warning

If violation recurs after a verbal warning, formal discipline progresses to a written warning. This step includes all of the elements of a verbal warning but adds notation of prior disciplinary action on the warning notice. Thus a written warning includes a precise description of the problem, what rules were broken by whom under what circumstances, and what previous counselings or discipline have been undertaken on what dates for the same offense. The written warning also restates very clearly the desired standard, the corrective action expected from the employee in specified time frames, and future penalties that will result

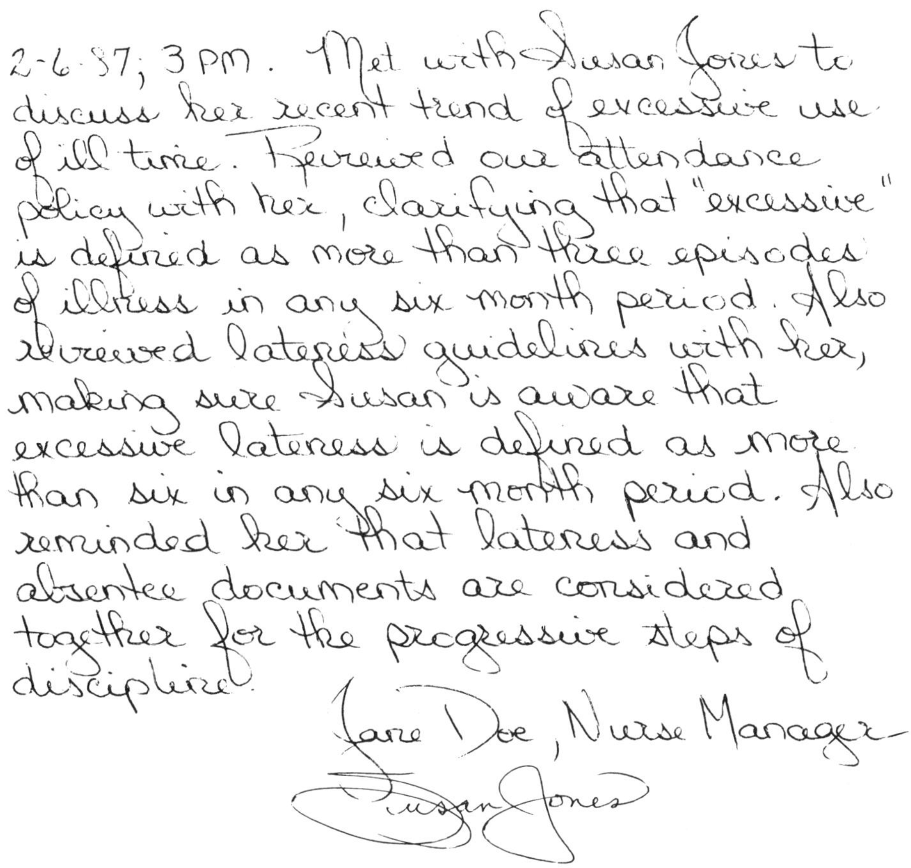
2-6-87; 3 PM. Met with Susan Jones to discuss her recent trend of excessive use of ill time. Reviewed our attendance policy with her, clarifying that "excessive" is defined as more than three episodes of illness in any six month period. Also reviewed lateness guidelines with her, making sure Susan is aware that excessive lateness is defined as more than six in any six month period. Also reminded her that lateness and absentee documents are considered together for the progressive steps of discipline.

Jane Doe, Nurse Manager

Susan Jones

**Figure 17.2** Counseling or anecdotal note.

if the corrective action is not taken or if another incident occurs. A summary of the written warning is dated and signed by both the critical care nurse manager and the employee. Copies are given to the employee and placed in the employee's file in the personnel department.

Before giving a written warning, the critical care nurse manager should check all facts bearing on the case. In addition, the nurse manager should review the discipline record of the employee, and past institutional responses to similar situations. Knowledge of the employee's history and organizational past practice will foster selection of sanctions that are appropriate and consistent with other actions previously taken (see Fig. 17.4).

## Suspension

Another breach of the rule brings the next step in the disciplinary process, suspension. Suspension is an appropriate sanction for minor violation only after a record of verbal and written warnings has been established. It can, however, be applied without the preceding steps of progressive discipline if there is a major infraction of the work rules. Suspension is most appropriately used when the critical care nurse manager believes there is still some hope for rehabilitating the employee. It is also appropriate in those situations wherein the manager feels that discharge would be overruled if the case were taken to arbitration or to outside regulatory agencies.

With suspension, the employee is removed from work without pay for a number of work days, varying in length from 1 day to 2 weeks. The length of the suspension is related to the severity of the infraction. Investigation and documentation are like written warnings. However, in the suspension documentation the suspension must be confirmed in writing, with clear specification of the number of dates of workdays involved,

| VERBAL WARNING | ABC HOSPITAL | Date      July 6, 1987 |
|---|---|---|
| Employee Name<br>  Susan Jones | Department<br>  Nursing - ICU | Job Title<br>  Staff Nurse |

Previous Discipline

  None

Reason for Verbal Warning

    Ms. Jones was absent from work March 25-27, April 17, May 26-27,
and July 3.  These four instances in a six month period constitute
excessive absenteeism as described in the Employee Handbook, page 23.
Frequent absenteeism hampers the Hospital's ability to render
quality patient care, and is detrimental to the function of the
Intensive Care Unit.

Action Required to Prevent Future Discipline

    In order to avoid moving to the next disciplinary step, you must
not exceed the following attendance standards:
1. Two episodes of absence within three months following issuance of
   this document.
2. Three episodes within any six month period.
3. Two episodes in conjunction with days off within any six month
   period.
4. Seven latenesses within any six month period, or four or more
   latenesses within two consecutive pay periods.

Employee Reaction to Warning

Recommended by:  *Jane Doe*          Date  7/6/87    Approved by (Dept. Head Signature): *Mary Johnson*   Date 7/6/87

This document has been discussed with me and a copy given to me.  My
signature does not necessarily signify agreement with this notice.

Employee Signature  *Susan Jones*                  Date   7/6/87

**Figure 17.3.**  Verbal warning documentation.

and written notice as to the day, date, and shift that the employee is to return to work. In addition, the suspension documentation should state that termination of the employee is the next probable step if the situation recurs or if there is inadequate improvement. It is imperative at this point that the employee understand the seriousness of the situation and that his or her employment is being jeopardized.

Suspension usually is instituted after full fact finding has been completed. However, at times it is essential to remove an employee from a situation

```
┌─────────────────────────────────────────────────────────────────────────────┐
│ WRITTEN WARNING          │    ABC HOSPITAL      │ Date December 29, 1987      │
├──────────────────────────┼──────────────────────┼────────────────────────────┤
│ Employee Name            │ Department           │ Job Title                  │
│   Susan Jones            │   Nursing - ICU      │   Staff Nurse              │
├──────────────────────────┴──────────────────────┴────────────────────────────┤
│ Previous Discipline                                                           │
│                                                                               │
│   July 6, 1987 - Verbal warning for excessive absenteeism                     │
│                                                                               │
│                                                                               │
├───────────────────────────────────────────────────────────────────────────── │
│ Reason for Written Warning                                                     │
│                                                                               │
│      Ms. Jones was absent from work October 1, November 9-13, Novem-          │
│   ber 27 and December 28. Four instances in a six month period constitute     │
│   excessive absenteeism as described in the Employee Handbook, page 23.       │
│   Frequent absences hamper the Hospital's ability to render quality           │
│   patient care, and are detrimental to the effective functioning of the       │
│   Intensive Care Unit.                                                        │
├───────────────────────────────────────────────────────────────────────────── │
│ Action Required to Prevent Future Discipline                                  │
│                                                                               │
│      In order to avoid moving to the next disciplinary step, you must         │
│   not exceed the following attendance standards:                              │
│   1. Two episodes of absence within three months following issuance of        │
│      this document.                                                           │
│   2. Three episodes within any six month period.                             │
│   3. Two episodes in conjunction with days off within any six month           │
│      period.                                                                  │
│   4. Seven latenesses within any six month period, or four or more            │
│      latenesses within two consecutive pay periods.                          │
├───────────────────────────────────────────────────────────────────────────── │
│ Comments and Explanation by Supervisor                                        │
│                                                                               │
│      Ms. Jones has received thorough explanations in the past of ABC          │
│   Hospital's attendance policy.  Failure to comply with these expecta-        │
│   tions will result in further disciplinary action.                          │
│                                                                               │
├───────────────────────────────────────────────────────────────────────────── │
│ Recommended by:                     │ Approved by (Dept. Head Signature):     │
│   [signature]    Date 12/29/87      │  [signature]          Date 12/29/87     │
├──────────────────────────────────────┴────────────────────────────────────── │
│ This document has been discussed with me and a copy given to me.  My          │
│ signature does not necessarily signify agreement with this notice.            │
├───────────────────────────────────────────────────────────────────────────── │
│ Employee Signature ── [signature]              Date                           │
│                                                  12/29/87                     │
└───────────────────────────────────────────────────────────────────────────── ┘
```

**Figure 17.4.** Written warning documentation.

in such an expeditious manner that opportunity for full fact finding does not exist. In this circumstance the employee is suspended pending investigation to provide time to determine whether disciplinary action is necessary. If after thorough review of the case it is determined that discipline was not war-

ranted, the employee must be compensated for all work time lost (see Fig. 17.5).

### Discharge

The final step in progressive discipline is termination of employment or discharge. Discharge

| SUSPENSION NOTICE | ABC HOSPITAL | Date      June 13, 1988 |
|---|---|---|
| Employee Name<br>  Susan Jones | Department<br>  Nursing - ICU | Job Title<br>  Staff Nurse |

Previous Discipline

  July 6, 1987 - Verbal warning for excessive absenteeism

  December 29, 1987 - Written warning for excessive absenteeism

Reason for Suspension

      Ms. Jones was absent from work February 13 and 14; April 14, 15 and 18; May 23 and June 10.  This continuing absenteeism impairs the Hospital's ability to provide quality patient care, and is detrimental to the functioning of the Intensive Care Unit.

| Date(s) of Suspension<br>     June 16, 1988 | Number of Work Days<br>     1 |
|---|---|

Action Required to Prevent Future Discipline

      In order to avoid moving to the next disciplinary step, you must not exceed the following attendance standards:
1. Two episodes of absence within three months following issuance of this document.
2. Three episodes within any six month period.
3. Two episodes in conjunction with days off within any six month period.
4. Seven latenesses within any six month period, or four or more latenesses within two consecutive pay periods.

      Ms. Jones is expected to return to work as scheduled on Wednesday, June 17 for the 3-11 shift.

| Recommended by:<br>*Jane Doe*            Date 6/13/88 | Approved by (Dept. Head Signature):<br>*Mary Johnson*      Date 6/13/88 |
|---|---|

Director of Personnel *Robert Smith*                Date June 13, 1988

This suspension notice has been discussed with me and a copy given to me. My signature does not necessarily signify agreement with this notice.

| Employee Signature<br>  *Susan Jones* | Date<br><br>    6/13/88 |
|---|---|

**Figure 17.5.** Suspension documentation.

is the supreme punishment and should be reserved for behavior that threatens operational effectiveness or the well-being of others. Discharge should be reserved for situations in which all other problem-solving and disciplinary efforts have been tried and proven unsuccessful. This is a grave punishment in that the employee loses ongoing employment, accumulated vacation, holiday and sick time, and pension and insurance benefits. Grounds for ''good cause'' discharge include poor performance, physical disability, inability to deal with peers, inability to get along with management, violation of major policy, supplying false employment information, insubordination, poor attendance, and threatening physical harm.

As in other steps of the disciplinary process, a full investigation must be completed before making a decision to terminate. The evidence to discharge the employee should be incontrovertible. All preceding steps in the disciplinary history of the employee should be reviewed to make sure that the steps in the process have been followed appropriately. If not, then termination is premature because the employee in question has not received progressive discipline applied correctly and in full accordance with institutional policies. Because of the serious economic and social implications of terminating an individual's employment, and because of the likelihood that the discharge will be grieved internally or to regulatory agencies, it is imperative that employees receive benefit of any doubt and that managerial action be fully justified.

During the conference terminating employment, the reasons for termination must be clearly stated and included in the written termination notice. The critical care nurse manager should exercise extreme caution in identifying these reasons, because the reasons he or she gives are the reasons the institution will have to prove if the discharge of the employee is challenged. Because of the seriousness of termination to the employee and the risk to the institution if employees are wrongfully discharged, terminations of employment usually must be preauthorized by the personnel director.

There are a few situations that stand as exceptions to the progressive nature of the disciplinary process. These include actions or behaviors so clearly wrong that everyone knows that they represent extremely unacceptable behavior or conduct and will result in immediate termination. Examples include theft, patient abuse, and threatening an employee with a lethal weapon. It is advisable to identify these extremely unacceptable behaviors in the institutional policies and employee handbook, so that there is consistent employee understanding that these actions constitute major offenses and that violators will not be given a second opportunity (see Fig. 17.6).

## WHEN TO DISCIPLINE

### To Discipline or Not?

The key to successful discipline lies in knowing when to discipline. Disciplinary action is taken for

unacceptable behavior that the employee has the capacity and ability to correct. The nurse manager must identify and understand the real problem being presented. Is the situation in question one in which the employee *cannot* or *will not* perform adequately? The most common reasons that employees *cannot* perform are incompetence, health problems, temporary personal problems, lack of self-motivation, work climate, and other factors that have an adverse effect on work performance (6). In these situations, nondisciplinary approaches are called for. Effective corrective approaches may include combinations of education and training, adjustments in work area or work assignment, counseling, and referral to employee assistance programs (6).

However, many situations arise in which the employee knows what is required on the job, has the capacity of carrying out what is expected, and chooses to perform in a manner other than that required. In these situations in which the employee *will not* perform adequately, providing additional education and counseling will not remedy the nonperformance. Disciplinary action is called for.

It is essential that the critical care nurse manager promptly take clear and unequivocal corrective action when counseling and assistance are ineffective. Situations that require disciplinary intervention should be brought to the employee's attention as soon as possible. Poor performance is more likely to be corrected if inappropriate behavior is discussed with the employee while the event is fresh. Also, the employee has the right to be made aware of his or her errors as soon as possible so there is full opportunity to correct the behavior. By dealing with a problem right away, the critical care nurse manager reduces the tension he or she may have related to the situation and to the employee. This will eliminate any tendency for the manager to build up resentment toward the employee or to develop a generalized poor opinion of the individual.

Two common errors in discipline should be avoided. First, behavioral problems or infractions should never be ignored; they should be addressed before they recur frequently or become too large. Situations tend to build if the manager ignores an event or just wishes it would go away. Moreover, a problem left uncorrected means that the manager allows the problem to regularly repeat itself. Overreaction is common when an overdue disciplinary action is finally taken. However, if an infraction has been ignored over a period of time, the critical care nurse manager cannot suddenly begin to enforce the rules without advance

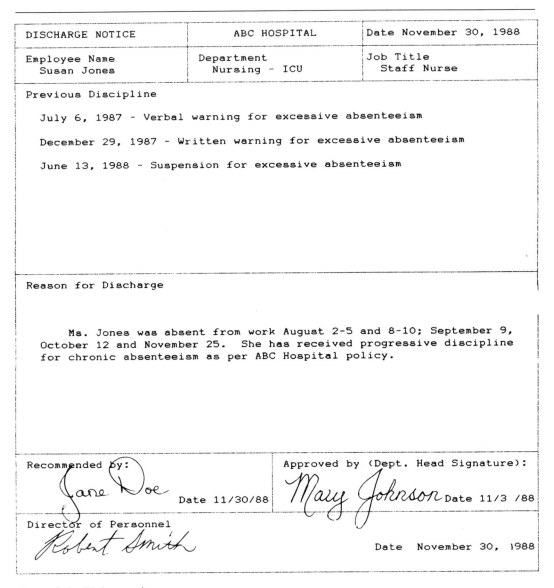

```
DISCHARGE NOTICE          ABC HOSPITAL        Date November 30, 1988

Employee Name          Department           Job Title
  Susan Jones            Nursing - ICU        Staff Nurse

Previous Discipline

   July 6, 1987 - Verbal warning for excessive absenteeism

   December 29, 1987 - Written warning for excessive absenteeism

   June 13, 1988 - Suspension for excessive absenteeism




Reason for Discharge


      Ms. Jones was absent from work August 2-5 and 8-10; September 9,
   October 12 and November 25.  She has received progressive discipline
   for chronic absenteeism as per ABC Hospital policy.




 Recommended by:                      Approved by (Dept. Head Signature):

      Jane Doe                           Mary Johnson
                  Date 11/30/88                        Date 11/3 /88

 Director of Personnel
      Robert Smith
                                         Date   November 30, 1988
```

**Figure 17.6.** Discharge notice.

notice. In this circumstance, each employee must be advised that as of a certain date, the rule will be strictly and consistently applied. This gives the employee due notice that expectations have changed and that the rule will be enforced.

Second, little things should not be allowed to linger. The employee has the right to be advised of any error or behavior that is less than desirable so that he or she knows to correct it. Also, little things tend to add up in time and may result in the manager having a negative impression of the employee. These feelings will not be well substantiated because recall of the detail will be lost in time. Often this negative information about an employee is expressed in the employee's performance evaluation, where it is a surprise to the employee and void of any substance due to lack of detail. It is more appropriate and effective for the critical care nurse manger to overcome the inertia of inaction and take disciplinary action when warranted.

## Timing

The disciplinary process should be instituted promptly whenever the critical care nurse manager first receives indication of a problem. Time is of course taken to allow for a full review of the situation in a deliberative, analytical fashion. This short passage of time also enables the nurse manager to adjudicate the situation free from an angry or reactive approach.

Once the critical care nurse manager has gathered the necessary information, he or she should consider the timing of the interview with the employee. If the manager anticipates that the employee will be highly upset or that the employee will return to the work area in a disruptive mood, it is best to meet with the employee at the end of the work period. (Note that the employee should be paid for time spent during the interview period, whether it is held during or after the employee's normal work hours).

Sanctions, when indicated, must be applied at the time of the offense, not at the convenience of the manager or of the unit schedule. Suspension periods are determined by when the offense occurred and when the investigation was completed, not by when it is convenient for the employee to be absent from work.

## STRATEGIES FOR EFFECTIVE DISCIPLINE

### Clear Communication

Clear communication to the employee is essential in both preventing the need for discipline and in administering discipline fairly. Employees have the right to have consistently received prior notice of all policies, standards, and expectations, because they must have knowledge of a rule before being held accountable to it. Thus a successful discipline program will include:

- a set of organization policies and procedures;
- guidelines for administering discipline for infractions;
- managers trained in implementing discipline;
- an orientation program that informs all new employees of management's expectations of appropriate performance and behavior;
- ongoing communication to employees of all changes and revisions in institutional policy or practice before those changes are put into effect (7).

In any dispute about discipline, management has the burden to prove actions taken were warranted, and it is advisable for the critical care nurse manager to develop the means to prove such communication took place. Thus it is common for employees to receive at the time of hire written copies of their individual job descriptions and the institution employee handbook that lists specific employment rules. Receipts for these documents should be signed by each employee and placed in the employee's file for future access as needed. Further, a written record should be available to document that a specific employee received both initial and ongoing communication as to policies, standards, expectations, and work practices. It is advisable to have each staff member sign copies of posted policies and memos so that the manager can verify that the employee received the information. These policies and memos can then be filed in binders and kept readily available and easily accessible to all employees for reference.

A written record of the critical care nurse manager's ongoing communication with employees is also needed. The content of staff meetings should be recorded, along with an accurate register of attendance. A sign-in sheet is very valuable as it offers proof that an individual was actually present. Minutes of group meetings should be distributed to all employees or posted in a readily accessible log. In either case, employees should sign indicating that they have read the minutes. Records of all signed minutes should be maintained by the critical care nurse manager for future access as needed.

Communication logs are helpful in encouraging communication, disseminating information equally to all staff, and recording that such communication did in fact take place. At the time of orientation, all employees should be informed that they are responsible for reviewing the log on a stated basis (daily, weekly) and for knowing the content of the log. These expectations should be communicated to the employee in a provable way. This makes future "I didn't know" defenses unacceptable.

Whenever the critical care nurse manager is dissatisfied with an employee's conduct or performance, the employee must receive an unequivocal message that his or her behavior is not acceptable and must be changed. The nurse manager provides a disservice to the employee if he or she hedges on the message. The employee must receive clear communication as to what the expectation is, what the offense was, how he or she can correct the situation, and the consequence in failing to do so.

The employee must understand his or her responsibility for whether the disciplinary process continues—that it is a chosen behavior that leads to secure employment or to progressive discipline.

## Equitable Discipline

The best means to administer discipline fairly and equitably is to follow the discipline and documentation procedures established by the organization. These are developed to protect both the rights of the employee and the needs of the institution. By following these established guidelines, equitable discipline for employees is fostered throughout the organization and over a period of time.

In order to be equitable, discipline must be administered consistently. Similar actions must result in similar responses. A manager cannot apply a sanction for an offense by one individual and ignore the same offense by another, and behavior cannot be monitored more for one group than another. To do so would be considered selective enforcement. If one employee receives a disciplinary action, then all others with similar behavior should receive similar discipline. Rules must be applied evenly to men, women, minorities, and nonminorities. Rules also must be applied evenly to professionals and nonprofessionals. As a professional, the critical care nurse manager may have a tendency to negate the need for corrective action for professional staff members, believing that it is unnecessary when dealing with educated, highly skilled employees. In addition, professional employees often believe that it is inappropriate for corrective disciplinary action to be applied to them. However, each employee must be held to preestablished rules, standards, and expectations. Rules must be applied equitably. Failure to do so represents selective enforcement and provides a disservice to the professional employee as well. Failure to equitably enforce institutional rules deprives the professional of clear communication about performance, and of the opportunity to adjust behavior and improve self-discipline and control.

Policies and work rules must be applied consistently throughout the organization. Selective enforcement can occur at the organizational level if different managers have different standards, tolerance limits, and views on what constitutes appropriate discipline. Thus the personnel department usually serves as a common resource to advise the manager as to what disciplinary action, if any, is indicated by an employee infraction.

Providing equitable discipline is made more difficult by the fact that no two situations are ever identical. The background and circumstances surrounding situations vary substantially. The critical care nurse manager must grant consideration to the full circumstances of the event in deciding the severity of the penalty, if any. Factors to consider when analyzing problems include:

- the seriousness of the infraction;
- extenuating circumstances, such as provocation by another;
- the frequency and nature of the problem;
- the degree of employee orientation to applicable rules, procedures, and consequences;
- the employee's past employment record; past discipline received quality of the employee's work performance the employee's work history;
- the implications for other employees, especially those of the employee's work unit;
- the history of discipline practices, both within the department and throughout the organization;
- management's ability to support the appropriateness of any disciplinary action (7).

Thus, because of the variety in situations, identical offenses will not necessarily indicate identical penalties, but similar infractions will result in similar disciplinary responses. Corrective discipline must be appropriate to the nature of the infraction and the employee's past record.

## IMPLEMENTATION OF DISCIPLINE

### Manager's Role and Response

The administration of a positive disciplinary program is not without its effect on the nurse manager. Managers must at all times function as good examples, and meet the policies, standards, and expectations established for the staff. Rules must be enforced equitably and fairly for all, including the manager. Disciplinary sanctions will not be upheld for a fault the manager shares with the employee.

To be an effective disciplinarian, the critical care nurse manager must (7):

- Deal with problems in a timely fashion.
- Know the topic and be prepared.

- Focus on facts and behavior.
- Dispassionately weigh the evidence.
- Believe the employee innocent until proven otherwise.
- See clearly what follows from the fact.
- Be willing to reconsider if indicated by new information.
- Have the courage to follow through.
- Seek the help of advisors as needed.
- Be conscious of the truth of the situation.
- Show regard for the feelings of others.
- Show concern for the employee as an individual.
- Be courteous yet assertive.
- Allow the employee dignity and to save face.

The critical care nurse manager must remain supportive of the employee throughout the disciplinary process. The nurse manager must guard against generalizing poor behavior to the whole individual or to all aspects of the employee's behavior. One aspect of the employee's behavior may be faulty, but not the whole individual. The manager must take care to maintain a working relationship with the employee in question. The critical care nurse manager must recognize and take responsibility for his or her own feelings. Often, there is a tendency for the manager to isolate or avoid the employee. It is the manager's continuing responsibility to regularly participate in two-way, work-related communication with each employee.

## Preparation

### Burden of Proof

The disciplinary process is directed toward correcting behaviors that have given just cause for complaint. Just cause for discipline is established by the merits of each situation. The burden of proof lies with the employer; in other words, the employee is presumed innocent of the charge of rule infraction until proven quilty of the offense. This means that the manager must prove that the employee committed the offense or breach of rule, the offense requires some corrective action, and the proposed sanction is appropriate to the offense. The critical care nurse manager must be able to prove that the employee did or did not do whatever is triggering the disciplinary process. For example, if the employee is charged with sleeping on the job, the critical care nurse manager must be able to satisfactorily prove that the employee *was asleep* (not just "resting his or her eyes") during *work

*time* (as opposed to break or meal times). In addition, management must be able to prove that the policy in question is applicable and that noncompliance is not caused by factors beyond the employee's control. For example, if a critical care nurse made a serious omission in caring for an assigned patient, the institution would need to show that the nurse had been made aware of the care requirement by the nursing care plan or other communication process, no other factors such as an excessive patient assignment contributed to the nurse's ommission of care, policies had been established to provide the nurse with additional temporary assistance if needed to meet the essential care requirements for assigned patients, and the nurse was familiar with such policies but did not avail him- or herself of them.

### Objectivity

As discussed earlier, objectivity is an essential element of a sound disciplinary system. Objectivity is the cornerstone of discipline that allows for thorough investigation, fair assessment of the need for penalty, reasonable selection of any discipline to be applied, and equitable treatment of all staff. Critical care nurse managers may encounter situations in which their responses to a given employee are biased by past or even cumulative nonrelated episodes with the employee in question. The nurse manager must have no favorites for good or bad issues. The manager must find a method to depersonalize any situation. One strategy for the critical care nurse manager to use is to mentally substitute another, average employee for the employee in question, and to then continue through the process to determine whether discipline is warranted. This simple substitution tends to promote a more reasoned response on the part of the manager and leads to more equitable administration of discipline.

### Confidentiality

A basic tenet for administering discipline is that information about employees must be safeguarded by the manager as confidential. A simple, effective guide for the critical care nurse manager is to praise in public but critique in private. Interviews and discussions about disciplinary actions must be held with the employee in a private environment where it is not possible to be overheard. This promotes exchange of information with the employee, reduces the employee's need to be defensive, and respects the rights of the individual (see Fig. 17.1).

## Guidelines for Implementing Discipline

*Correct the first error.* Do not allow the error to continue and perpetuate itself. Early notification optimizes the opportunity for the employee to improve behavior or conduct and reduces tensions with the employee. The manager's first approach to an employee problem should be that of providing assistance in problem solving: helping the employee to analyze the problem, identifying references or resources to the employee, and counseling or providing information to the employee as needed.

*If the undesirable behavior continues, perform a preliminary review.* Think through the nature of the problem at hand. Check institutional policies, procedures, and work rules to determine those that apply. Consistent, impartial, uniform application of the rules is essential. Review applicable legal standards and the employee's work record. Seek assistance as needed to ensure an equitable response that considers institutional precedence. Reasons for deviation from past precedence should be substantiated in writing in the employee's personnel record.

*Select the proper place and time to discuss behavior or conduct.* Intervention should take place soon after an error has occurred in order to heighten the effectiveness of the intervention. All discussions with employees should be held in confidence in a private setting.

*Maintain objectivity.* The critical care nurse manager should not be influenced by emotions when holding discussions with the employee. Selected behavior should be critiqued; care should be taken to not criticize the employee as a person.

*Verify information.* Undertake thorough fact-finding with all concerned, and eliminate assumptions, exaggerations, and gossip. Investigate all of the facts of the situation and the employee's version of it. The employee must have the opportunity to speak for him- or herself, and the employee's responses must be heard objectively. It is important for the critical care nurse manager to hear all relevant information about the situation before drawing any conclusions. The nurse manager must be alert for and fully explore any extenuating circumstances. Was this a willful mistake or something beyond the employee's control? Did the employee know this was unacceptable behavior? Did the employee attempt to comply? Was the situation provoked in any way? Who saw or heard what? Are all versions reconcilable? If not, which

versions are most credible? Keep an open mind until all information is obtained and all sides are heard. Consider a variety of alternatives and explanations of the situation.

*Be specific when identifying the offense or performance discrepancy.* Focus on facts and measurable behavior. Generalized statements without adequate examples may interfere with the employee's ability to receive the manager's comments and may prompt the employee to focus on defending the behavior under discussion.

*Avoid reacting to the employee's defenses.* It is human nature to try to defend or justify one's actions. The critical care nurse manager must not allow the employee to divert attention from the specific situation under review. Redirect the session as needed to maintain focus on the desired topic.

*Maintain the proper tone during discussions.* Be serious. The impact of progressive discipline can be of serious consequence to the employee. This should be imparted to the employee both in word and in tone. Do not threaten. The critical care nurse manager should maintain an assertive but caring approach in all discussions. The nurse manager should not make excuses or apologize to the employee for the administration of any disciplinary action. Any consequence to an employee is the result of employee behavior. It is the employee who controls whether discipline is indicated, and it is the manager's responsibility to respond to employee infractions. The employee has control over the eventual outcome of the disciplinary process.

*Analyze whether the intended disciplinary action is warranted and defensible if challenged.*

*Document all key elements of the situation thoroughly, including employee and witness versions.* Summarize and date all discussions, and have the summaries signed by the involved parties. Documentation by more than one observer reduces the risk of lack of objectivity. Provide copies of all disciplinary documents to the employee, and file original copies in the employee's personnel record.

*Leave the employee with a clear understanding of the situation.* Confront the situation firmly. Review the applicable standard or expectation, point out the employee's error, and indicate specifically what must be done, and when, to correct the situation or to avoid further disciplinary action.

*Elicit questions from the employee, and have him or her repeat back to confirm understanding of the situation*. Provide immediate feedback to the employee so as to fully correct any inaccurate interpretation of the situation.

## DEFENSIBLE DISCIPLINE

Although it is the manager's prerogative to administer disciplinary sanctions, internal institutional policy as well as federal and state laws restrict and regulate the employer/employee relationship. If an employee believes he or she has been treated unfairly, an appeal can be initiated through the internal grievance process of the organization, to an ombudsperson, to a fair hearing panel, or through the civil courts. The critical care nurse manager is less likely to place the institution in the position of having to defend itself against charges of injustice or discrimination if he or she uses a defensible disciplinary approach. Successful defensible discipline is characterized by discipline that:

- follows established institutional policy and practice;
- is based on the employee's advance knowledge of expectations and the consequences if the employee fails to meet them;
- is impartial. There are no favorites or exceptions;
- is administered promptly in relation to the offense, not at the convenience of the manager or the work area;
- is enforced equitably, throughout departments and all job categories;
- is fair. Applied discipline is based on factual information, with no assumptions or exaggerations;
- represents uniform application of the rules. Similar offenses stimulate similar disciplinary responses. Employees are not disciplined for faults they share with the manager;
- is consistently applied. Changes in expectations are communicated to employees before enforcement begins. Behaviors are not overlooked and then suddenly disciplined for without warning;
- treats the employee with courtesy and allows him or her to save face;

- includes an established internal grievance system to hear appeals of the disciplinary process.

## CONCLUSION

The purpose of the disciplinary process is to create a climate wherein employees regularly conform to the rules, regulations, and established norms of an organization. The most desirable means to accomplish this is prevention: creating an environment that reduces the occurrence of situations that require corrective action.

However, in any organization of more than a few people, there will always be some who break the rules. Consistent enforcement of the work rules through progressive discipline is required. The critical care nurse manager should administer progressive discipline with the intent of correcting deficient performance or conduct and securing compliance with established work rules. Because of its gradual application, progressive discipline gives the employee clear notice of the problem behavior and ample opportunity to correct it. Through the appropriate use of progressive discipline, the critical care nurse manager can stimulate the motivation of individual employees as well as enhance the productivity and contribution of the unit staff.

## REFERENCES

1. Trunzo TE. Toward developing sound disciplinary practices. Hosp Topics 1985;63(3):26–27.
2. *Webster's ninth new collegiate dicitionary*. Springfield, Massachusetts: Merriam-Webster Inc, 1983.
3. Beach DS. Personnel: the management of people at work. New York: Macmillan Publishing Company, 1985:372.
4. Henry KH. The health care supervisor's legal guide. Rockville, Maryland: Aspen Systems Corporation, 1984:2.
5. McConnel CR. The evolution of employee relations: a new look at criticism and discipline. Health Care Supervisor 1986;4(2):80–88.
6. Cameron D. The when, why and how of discipline. Personnel J 1984;63(7):37–39.
7. Rowland HS, Rowland BL. Hospital administration handbook. Rockville, Maryland: Aspen Systems Corporation, 1984:499–502.

# Chapter 18

# Applying Labor Relations in Critical Care Nursing

SUZETTE CARDIN

"What labor is demanding all over the world today is not a few material things like more dollars and fewer hours of work but a right to a voice in the conduct of industry."

Sidney Hillman, 1918 (1).

Nurses in today's health care society are becoming educated to labor relations and its impact on both patient care activities and how management interacts with staff in a health care system that is either unionized or threatening to unionize into a collective bargaining unit. Nurses in positions of authority will increasingly have to deal with employees represented by unions with collective bargaining agreements and thus will spend more time dealing with labor issues (2). The purpose of this chapter is to provide a framework for the critical care nurse manager on how to manage effectively in a setting where labor relations management exists or is threatening to exist. It is naive for any nurse manager to think union activity and/or collective bargaining cannot exist in his or her setting. Today's nurses in critical care want to be involved and are committed to quality patient care. A review of the history of unionization will reveal that it is these characteristics that have been the most apparent regarding union activity within nursing.

When nurses were polled regarding the generation gap in nursing, the biggest professional issue over which the generations differed was unionization (3). Most nurses over 45 say joining a union would make them less professional, they would not strike. The key lies not in the nurses' attitude toward their profession but toward life in general. Younger nurses are more inclined toward activism. If joining a union will also help gain salary increases and child-care benefits for instance, younger nurses appear to be for unionization (3). It then behooves a nurse manager of today to carefully assess the environment and determine whether a potential exists for unionization and if so, what is

my role before, during, and after a union drive? If a union does exist, how does one effectively manage? These questions will be answered in this chapter along with a review of the history of unionization in nursing, why nurses join unions, and an example of a management-labor conflict in critical care that will highlight the practical application of managing in a unionized setting.

## HISTORY OF LABOR RELATIONS IN NURSING

Labor relations refers to the relationship between management and employees within the work environment. This relationship is dependent upon the extent to which labor and management can agree on the conditions required in order to meet each other's needs. The goals of management are to produce a profitable service or product through the efforts of the workers. Labor is oriented toward safe working conditions, acceptable payment for work rendered, job security, and opportunity for growth and advancement (3). The most desirable circumstance is for those affiliated with labor and management to dialogue, confer, problem-solve, and negotiate to achieve mutual agreement.

Collective bargaining or the process by which health care employees elect an exclusive agent to represent them can be traced back to the 1920s in the San Francisco area; it was not until the late 1970s when the labor laws changed that collective bargaining reached significant proportions (4). Labor law initially did include most hospital employees. The Wagner Act (298 U.S. 238) passed in 1935 excluded public employees. All state and local hospitals operated by governmental units were exempt from coverage (4). The Wagner Act did not specifically exclude private/nonprofit hospitals. This changed in 1947 when the Taft-Hartley amendment to the Wagner Act exempted private, nonprofit health care facilities from federal collective bargaining laws (Public Law 101, 80th Congress, June 23, 1947) (4). In 1974 the Wagner Act was amended again and the Taft-Hartley exclusion was lifted. The amendment revisions allowed for 2 million employees and 3300 nonprofit hospitals to be protected under the collective bargaining guidelines (5). The amendment changes in 1974 had a positive effect on union activity as a whole. The health care industry is now considered the last frontier for organized union activity to occur within the labor market.

The American Nurses' Association (ANA) in 1946 received a mandate from its membership to act as the bargaining agent for nurses to improve the economic conditions and status of the profession (5). The review of the history of unionization also reveals that when the Brown Report was published in 1948, the issues that made nurses want to unionize were the following: little freedom in making clinical nursing judgments, minimal involvement in solving problems, and a highly authoritarian and unrewarding environment (5). Throughout history these conditions have been the driving force for employees to unionize. Nurses were found to work longer hours, do more shift work, and receive less pay and fewer fringe benefits than did most workers in comparable occupations. The average annual salary in 1948 was $2100. During the 1960s nurses began to make their concerns known, participating in demonstrations, picketing, sit-ins, call-ins, and slow-downs (5). Since the Taft-Hartley amendment in 1974, health care organizations have carefully examined their approach to employee relations programs. Most administrators routinely examine compensation packages for equity both within the organization and the marketplace. The advent of the nursing shortage has made this a high priority. Collective bargaining is not a national phenomenon. The geographical distribution of union activity is currently concentrated in New York, New Jersey, Massachusetts, Pennsylvania, California, and Michigan (5). The majority of nurses are represented by the economic and general welfare program of the American Nurses Association. One of seven nurses will join a union (6).

The term "professional collectivism" has been applied to nurses who want to participate in collective bargaining. Professional collectivism embraces the idea that the quality of patient care is inherently related to working conditions and that collective action is a professional responsibility (5). It is predicted that with the recent endorsement of the National Labor Board that supports all registered nurses' (RNs)

bargaining units, a significant impact on unionization will occur within nursing (7). Before this endorsement nurses could have been represented with other groups of health care employees.

## NURSING AND UNION ACTIVITY

Unionization in nursing is not a new movement. Nurses have been concerned with their economic and general welfare for sometime (4). Today's organizing and bargaining issues generally revolve around employees' desires to be compensated for their work, treated with dignity and respect, and be provided the opportunity to have an effective voice in decisions that affect the work and its environment (8). When compared to other employees, nurses' concerns are usually quite different. The concerns that nurses bring to the organizing drive or bargaining table revolve around the following themes (9):

1. inability to communicate concerns to management;
2. authoritarian behavior on the part of the management;
3. understaffing;
4. lack of respect from physicians;
5. lack of control over nursing practice;
6. lack of support from nursing administration;
7. dissatisfaction with shift assignments, rotations, weekend scheduling, and mandatory overtime.

A conceptual model of how employees will respond to the possibility of collective bargaining in the health care environment of the late 1980s and 1990s is illustrated in Figure 18.1. The implications for critical care managers can be drawn from the conceptual model. Structural/strategic responses can be formulated based on the 1988 American Association of Critical-Care Nurses (AACN) study on the supply and requirements for critical care nursing (10):

1. Patient acuity is increasing. By 1995 the range of RN hours required per intensive care unit (ICU) patient day will be 20–26.
2. The annual turnover rate for critical care nurses has been reported to be 25–50%.
3. The current vacancy rate for critical care units is 13.8%.
4. Critical care nurses require continuous expansion of specialized knowledge and experience to meet the increased nursing care requirements of critically ill patients.
5. Customized patient classification tools are needed

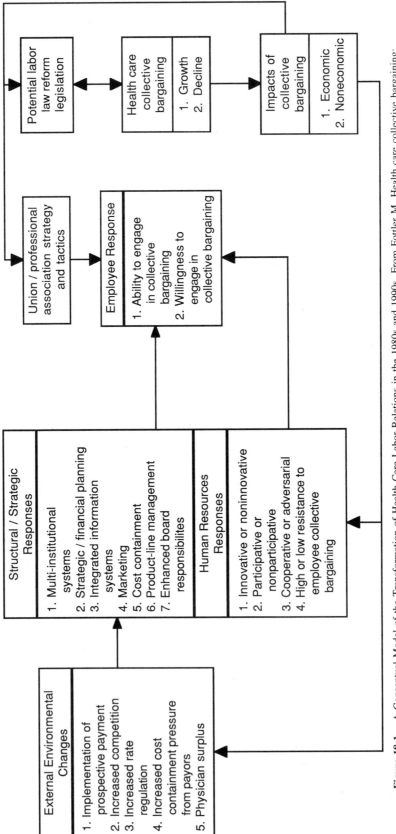

**Figure 18.1.** A Conceptual Model of the Transformation of Health Care Labor Relations in the 1980s and 1990s. From Fottler M. Health care collective bargaining: future dynamics and their impact. J Health Hum Resources Admin, 1987; 10(2):33–51.

to optimize staffing patterns, measure productivity of service provided, and project future requirements for critical care nurses.

The human resource responses in the conceptual model are a high priority for a critical care manager in any setting, be it unionized or nonunionized. Human resource responses to the conceptual model include the following (10):

1. Average annual salaries for critical care nurses range from $13,900 to $38,920 with a median of $25,000.
2. There is little incentive for job stability. Critical care nurses' salaries are compressed; experience and knowledge do not equal annual salary.
3. Most nurses who were surveyed by the American Association of Critical-Care Nurses in 1988 responded that their basic nursing education did not prepare them for critical care; 43% with an associate degree felt poorly prepared.
4. Critical care nursing requires considerable knowledge beyond basic nursing, however, the reality of the situation is that there are only brief, episodic continuing education programs that are offered.

Nurses of today are concerned with what the health care organization does or does not provide for them. The National Commission on Nursing in 1983 found that nurses are responding to the human resource component of their position in a number of ways: they leave nursing, they seek another position, they endure their present position, or they seek some form of collective bargaining (11). Table 18.1 illustrates the variables that have an impact on the utilization of collective bargaining. These trends and implications were based on recent trends in environmental, organizational, and human resource trends in the health care industry (11). It is estimated that 40–50% of all health care institutions and health care employees will be engaging in collective bargaining in 1995 (10). This estimate has serious implications for today's nurse manager. With the tremendous changes now occurring in the health care industry the nurse manager needs to carefully consider these trends in a proactive fashion.

## COLLECTIVE BARGAINING PROCESS

Employees have the right to organize and bargain collectively with management. Unionization usually occurs where management is weak, has poor communication styles, and does not understand the employees' needs and wants (5, 8). The most commonly stated reasons for nurses' involvement in collective bargaining have been: (a) to make management listen, (b) to improve pay and benefits, and (c) to have more say about patient care (12).

The stages of collective bargaining are outlined in Figure 18.2. The union drive originates in steps 1, 2, and 3. It has been stated that unions rarely organize employees, rather it is poor employee relations with administration that drives employees into unions (13). Frequently a disgruntled employee or a thwarted natural leader in the organization is the one who begins to plant the seeds of discontent. Behind the drive to organize employees is the union organizer who will be soliciting employees to join his or her particular union. The typical union organizer has a natural affinity for people, is a good listener, and knows how and at what level to communicate (13). In nursing, this is frequently a staff nurse. It is not uncommon for the organizer to be a critical care nurse and for the organizer to be bright, articulate, and dedicated to the union and what it represents.

The manager's role during a union drive is critical for it is the first line manager who is most dramatically affected by the organization of employees (13). Many nurse managers are unsure how to act during a union drive or when the contract has to be renegotiated. Section 7 of the National Labor Relations Act 157 (14) states: "Employees shall have the right to self-organization, to form, join, or assist labor organizations, to bargain collectively through representatives of their own choosing, and to engage in other concerted activities for the purpose of collective bargaining or other mutual aid or protection and should also have the right to refrain from any or all such actions." Employees are not allowed to unlawfully prevent or discourage unionization. Section 8 of the National Labor Relations Act describes two unfair labor practice prohibitions: to interfere with, restrain, or coerce employees in the exercise of the rights guaranteed in section 157 . . . (and) by discrimination in regard to hire or tenure of employment . . . to encourage or discourage membership in any labor organization (15). During a union drive there is conduct that is permissible or not permissible. What nurse managers can discuss during a union drive are the following:

**Table 18.1.**    Variables Affecting the Ability and Willingness of Health Care Employees to Use Collective Bargaining[a]

|  | Recent Trend 1980–1987 | Future Trend 1988–1995 | Implication For Collective Bargaining |
|---|---|---|---|
| Environmental factors | | | |
| 1. Health industry regulation | Increase | Increase | Positive |
| 2. Market competition | Increase | Increase | Negative |
| 3. Union organizing activity | Decrease | Increase | Positive |
| 4. NCRB organizing constraints | Increase | Decrease | Positive |
| 5. Effectiveness of union or association strategy/tactics | No change | Increase | Positive |
| Organizational factors | | | |
| 1. Management resistance to unions | Increase | No change | Neutral |
| 2. Organizational complexity | Increase | Increase | Positive |
| 3. For profit facilities | Increase | Increase | Negative |
| 4. For profit and nonprofit goal differentiation | Decrease | Decrease | Negative |
| Perceptions of the work environment | | | |
| 1. Pace of change | Increase | Increase | Positive |
| 2. Job dissatisfaction | Decrease | No change | Positive |
| 3. Working conditions | Decrease | Decrease | Positive |
| 4. Job insecurity | Increase | Increase | Positive |
| 5. Interpersonal conflict | Increase | No change | Positive |
| 6. Adequacy of economic and noneconomic rewards | Decrease | Decrease | Positive |
| 7. Inequity perceptions | Increase | Increase | Positive |
| Perceptions of influence | | | |
| 1. Gap between desired and actual influence | Increase | Increase | Positive |
| Beliefs about Collective Bargaining | | | |
| 1. Belief collective bargaining instrumental in goal attainment | Increase | Increase | Positive |

[a]From Fottler M. Health care collective bargaining: future dynamics and their impact. J Health Hum Resources Admin 1987; 10(2):33–51.

(*a*) advantages of remaining nonunion, such as current wages and benefits and how they compare to unionized compensation as well as a comparison of benefits both existing and what the union is proposing; and (*b*) disadvantages of unionization that include dues, loss of income during strikes, possibility of being required to serve on the picket line. During a strike hospital services will be interrupted and patient care may be adversely affected. There is also an inability to discuss problems directly with the supervisor and employer (16). Table 18.2 outlines the activities that are unlawful during the union certification process. If these activities occur, either management or the union can be charged with an unfair labor practice. The previously mentioned activities also pertain to the nurse manager's role once the contract has been voted in.

The majority of nurse managers in a unionized setting will have access to a labor relations department that will actively assist the nurse manager in implementation of the contract or memorandum of understanding that is the collective bargaining agreement. The contract defines rights, responsibilities, and benefits to both management and the union. The role of the nurse manager is not to interpret the contract to the staff but to abide by the agreements that were made at the bargaining table. It is the union representative who interprets the contract for staff. An example would be the following contract agreement for the nurse manager. The contract grants a certain number of educational hours per year for each staff nurse. It is the staff nurse's responsibility to monitor how many hours are being used for educational classes and to know when they expire. The manager may keep

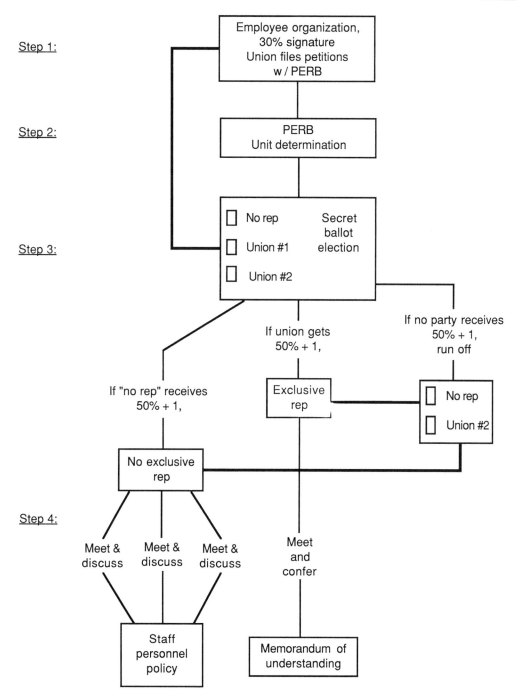

Step 1:

Employee organization,
30% signature
Union files petitions
w / PERB

Step 2:

PERB
Unit determination

Step 3:

☐ No rep          Secret
                        ballot
☐ Union #1      election

☐ Union #2

If "no rep" receives
50% + 1,

If union gets
50% + 1,

If no party receives
50% + 1,
run off

Exclusive
rep

☐ No rep

☐ Union #2

No exclusive
rep

Step 4:

Meet &
discuss

Meet &
discuss

Meet &
discuss

Meet
and
confer

Staff
personnel
policy

Memorandum of
understanding

**Figure 18.2**    The Stages of Collective Bargaining.

**Table 18.2.**  Unlawful Activities during the
Union Certification Process[a]

Management
1. Management cannot promise pay increases, promotion, improved benefits, betterment, or special favor for voting against a union.
2. Management cannot say the organization will close if unionized.
3. Employees cannot be fired, laid off, given a less favorable job, or otherwise discriminated against because of union activities.
4. Employees cannot be interrogated about union activities or encouraged to withdraw from the union.

Union
1. The union cannot use threats or actual violence against employees who refuse to participate or cooperate with the union.
2. Union members cannot interfere with, restrain, or coerce employees in forming, joining, or assisting labor organizations.
3. The union cannot use surveillance or questioning concerning employee interest or activities related to unions.

[a]From Othman JE, Chaney H. Labor relations in union and nonunion environments in Vestal K, ed. *Management Concepts for the New Nurse.* Philadelphia: JB Lippincott, 1987; 310.

his or her own records to prevent overbudgeting of class hours, however, it is the staff nurse's responsibility to know to what he or she is entitled. The union contract gives both the union and management certain rights. The union rights are related to the grievance procedures, dues, and access to a central communication area. The nurse manager can expect a management rights provision as well as a no-strike clause for the duration of the contract (5). The contract is valid for a specific period of time and there may be portions of the contract that may be negotiated at certain periods of time during the agreement. Salary is usually one item that is a reopener item during the length of the agreement.

Nurses in general are usually concerned with and have many questions regarding the possibility of striking. A strike only occurs when there is no contract, the original contract has expired, and both the union and management were unable to agree to another memorandum of understanding. If nurses strike with a contract in place, it is considered a wildcat strike. In some states, these types of strikes are considered illegal. Each nurse manager needs to be familiar with her individual state regulations. The right to strike may be defined as the right, moral or political, of workers to withdraw or with-

hold labor to gain concessions (17). Nurses believe that they possess the ethical right to strike when no other means are available to resolve problems affecting the quality of nursing care (17). This kind of thinking generated the withdrawal of the no-strike policy by the ANA in 1968 (8). Established in 1950, the no-strike pledge, for all its 18-year existence, conflicted with the ability of the association to conduct effective collective bargaining with nurses (8). Nurses are now the most frequent strikers in the health care field (18). Elaine Betzer, a past president of the New York State Nurses' Association, has pointed out why nurses have changed their stance regarding the decision on whether to strike or not (18):

Nurses' reluctance to maximize their bargaining power has paralleled other professional groups. However, increasing collective bargaining sophistication, changing norms within professional groups and society at large, the impact of the womens' liberation movement, and increased professional consciousness have resulted in nurses' increased commitment to the visible demonstration of bargaining power in the labor-management relationship.

The 1974 congressional amendments to the National Labor Relations Act contained a special section (8g) that requires the union to give in writing adequate notice of at least 10 days before engaging in any strike, picketing, or other concerted refusal to work at a health care institution (18). It is during this 10-day period that both the nurse manager and medical director need to develop a strike contingency plan for the proposed strike. The plan should include all of the details of the day-to-day operations and what mode and type of patient care delivery system will be implemented. Once the strike begins, it is the individual staff nurse's decision whether he or she strikes. The nurse manager's role at this time is one of visibility, communication with staff, and troubleshooting potential problems that arise before and after the strike occurs.

The decision to vote in a union and become unionized is a tedious process at best. The result is a contract to which all parties mutually agree. The nurse manager in a critical care setting can expect to manage according to the following guidelines:

1. The nurse manager's major responsibility is to administer the contract.
2. Consistency and parity are essential traits for

the nurse manager to possess, especially in the evaluation and promotion process.

3. The work conditions are clearly stated in the contract, i.e., hours of work, pay structure, overtime, vacation and holidays, and leave status.

4. The nurse manager does not interpret the contract for the staff; this is the responsibility of the union.

5. The labor relations department is your ally in the day-to-day operation of contract administration.

6. No union activity is allowed at the bedside, and only on breaks away from the patient is discussion of union activity permitted.

7. Nurses can request to have a union representative present for any discussion with a nurse manager; conversely the nurse manager does not have to talk to the union unless his or her representative from labor relations is also present.

8. Do not personalize the contract. The memorandum of understanding is a mutually agreed upon document.

9. Patient care assignments can be subject to union review. It is not uncommon for the union to insist upon a patient care committee, which will be stated in the contract.

10. Nurse managers need to be versed in the grievance and arbitration process.

11. Seniority is an important aspect of unionization and needs to be carefully adhered to in a unionized setting.

12. Never overestimate the loyalty of employees. Employees may be angry, bitter, bored, or discouraged and can use the union in order to achieve their own personal needs.

13. Be positive and realistic in your approach with your staff. Keep communications open with staff to prevent an atmosphere of distrust.

14. Visibility is a key management trait.

## LABOR MANAGEMENT CONFLICTS

In the collective bargaining process there is an inherent assumption that conflict is natural between management and employees. The contract establishes a framework to deal with this conflict in a rational, peaceful, and predictable manner. The nurse manager needs to be aware of the fact that collective bargaining is a continuous process, adversarial in nature, that begins with contract negotiation, flows through the resolution of disputes

under the agreement, and extends to the negotiation of successor agreements (19). The mechanism by which management and the union interact is the grievance-arbitration procedure. It is essential that the nurse manager be fluent with the grievance procedure and its application to his or her role as a manager. The grievance procedure functions as a system of industrial jurisprudence. There is a formal set of rules and procedures to identify disputes between the parties, process them, and provide for final resolution through the arbitration procedure (19). A grievance can be whatever the parties say that it is. The nurse manager can be influenced by this definition and create a management style that is very threatened by the presence of the union. Some staff will use the grievance process as leverage against the manager. As described earlier, consistency and parity in management style need to be exercised by the nurse manager. If all staff nurses are treated equally, the leverage will not be utilized. Critical care nurses are bright and know when there is favoritism and lack of consistent application of the contract agreements. Most union contracts in nursing, for example, specify what constitutes the Christmas/New Year holidays and what the staff nurse can expect to work or not expect to work. If the manager grants both Christmas and the New Year off to one nurse and all of the other staff work either Christmas or the New Year as stated in the contract, she is setting herself up for a grievance by the staff nurse who had to work the holiday.

The nurse manager should have the contract readily accessible to provide clarification. A staff nurse is on call for the coronary care unit (CCU) and the unit is notified by the emergency department (ED) that a cardiac arrest has just arrived. The on-call nurse is called in, however, the patient expires immediately upon arrival in the CCU. Because this is an infrequent occurrence, the nurse manager cannot remember the call-back pay allowance. She refers to the contract that states 3 hours, and failure to pay the 3 hours could result in a grievance.

Each staff has his or her copy of the contract; some staff are very cognizant of the contract, others are very indifferent. The perceptive nurse manager will be very familiar with the contract. If clarification is needed, she will contact labor relations. A phone call is much easier and more expedient than a filed grievance against the nurse manager.

The grievance-arbitration procedure provides a mechanism for resolution of disputes regardless of the cause. The reasons for or causes of particular grievances frequently influence how the procedure will be carried out (19). Reasons for grievances can be any one or all of the following: (*a*) unclear contract language, (*b*) interpersonal relationships that will allege unfair treatment or lack of parity, (*c*) inconsistent implementation of the contract by the nurse manager, and (*d*) the union itself that must take an active role in upholding employee grievances (19).

Most negotiated grievance procedures are basic in structure; they may vary in the number of steps. Each contract will state the grievance procedure as it was agreed upon at the time that the contract was signed. Figure 18.3 illustrates the structure of a model grievance procedure. Time limits for each step in the grievance procedure are specified in each contract. The employee cannot file a grievance until management takes some action against the employee or the contract. Once action is taken by management, the employee notifies the union (steward) and the grievance process is initiated. In the model the word steward is used interchangeably with the term union.

The majority of grievances are usually resolved at step one. The role of the nurse manager cannot be overemphasized at this stage. Step one is a meet and confer process. It is here that the nurse manager defends her actions and listens with an open mind to the allegations that the grievant is stating. There is either a mutual resolution of the grievance at this stage or the grievance moves on to step two. At step two of the grievance process there are specific references made to the contract by the grievant, specifically where in writing the nurse manager took action that resulted in either disparity of treatment, inconsistent application of the terms of the agreement, or unfair treatment to the grievant. Nurse managers need to be cognizant of the fact that the union may decide that this particular grievance is one in which they will be the champion of all staff nurses. If neither party can agree to the grievance being resolved, it moves to step three. At this step the manager of labor relations will become involved and decide the merits of the case. The union and management will be notified of the decision. If neither party agrees, the grievance will then move onto the union committee. It is at this step that the union decides whether they want to go onto arbitration, which is binding in

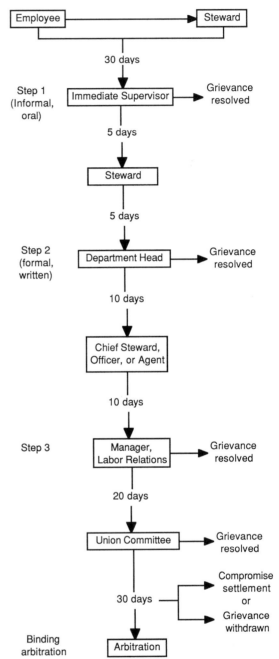

**Figure 18.3.** Model grievance procedure. From McPherson D, Gates C, Rogers K. Resolving grievances, a practical approach. Reston, Virginia: Reston Publishing Co, Inc, 1983.

nature. The arbitrator will make the decision based on the merits of the case. This decision cannot be reversed. Management and the union are then involved in a significant amount of risk taking for one side will win, one side will lose. Most arbitration hearings usually cost several thousand dollars. Both parties need to consider the following when deciding to proceed with arbitration (19):

1. Are we convinced that our interpretation of agreement is correct?
2. Is the issue important enough to risk arbitration?
3. What would be the effect of winning?
4. What would be the effect of losing?
5. Can we afford the cost and delay in final resolution?
6. Based on known arbitration principles and what we know about the case of the other party and our own, can we win?

If involved in a labor management conflict, the nurse manager needs to consider the following points when handling a grievance:

1. Employees deserve a complete and emphatic hearing of all grievances they present.
2. Look for the hidden agenda. Look beyond the selected incident and then judge the grievance in context.
3. The grievance should be given your full consideration and the following questions should be asked: What actually happened; where did it happen; what should have happened; when did it happen; who was involved; were there any witnesses, and why did the problem develop?
4. Utilize the labor relations or human resources departments to assist in fact finding.
5. The decision that is made is based on the fact finding, therefore the ownership rests with the nurse manager.
6. Written documentation is required. It serves as a review for the nurse manager to ensure consistency and provide the nurse manager with a record of the events.
7. Once the grievance is settled follow-up with the staff nurse is essential. It is a way of ensuring that the employee has received due recognition.

The following case study is an example of applying labor relations in the critical care setting.

The grievance procedure will be outlined from step one through binding arbitration.

The nurse manager was approached by one of her staff concerning the time schedule. The staff nurse was scheduled to work the Friday night (19-0730) before the AACN certification examination that was to be held on Saturday at 8:00 A.M. The time schedule request change was made 2 weeks before the date of the examination. The nurse manager informed the staff nurse that she would be unable to grant her the night off because it would lower the staffing standard to an unacceptable level. The staff nurse was told she could switch her schedule with someone else or ask one of the staff not scheduled to work for her. Three days before the examination the staff nurse approached the nurse manager and told her she could not find anyone to work for her. The nurse manager reviewed the options for the staff nurse to consider. The day before the examination the staff nurse called and said she could not find anyone to work and could she just have the night off. The nurse manager was unable to grant the request and on the night shift two additional nurses were already required secondary to high census and acuity. If the staff nurse was granted the time off, a total of three supplemental staff nurses would be required. When considering the schedule change, the nurse manager did not see a request in the time request book and the time schedule request was made 2 weeks after the schedule was posted. The staff nurse did call in sick for the 19-0730 shift secondary to a headache. The nurse manager did not pay the staff nurse for her sick call and issued a counseling memo to the staff nurse.

The staff nurse filed a grievance with the union. The claim was alleged disparity on the part of management and failure to abide by the contract agreement that states when sick time pay will be granted. In the step one process a review of the merits of the case was discussed. Management was unwilling to resolve the grievance. The staff nurse alleged that other staff members would frequently be granted time off once the time schedule was posted, and the fact that she was black and the nurse manager was caucasian was the basis for disparity of treatment. The nurse manager believed that the sick call was circumstantial in origin and therefore did not warrant sick pay. The previous department of nursing decisions in situations was the precedent that the nurse manager used to support her decision.

At step two, management responded to written, formal allegations by the union. Management was not willing at this step to settle. In the step three process, the manager of labor relations decided there was no disparity in treatment and management was justified in not paying sick time. The union committee reviewed the merits of the case and decided to proceed with arbitration. Management denied the grievance at this step and decided to also proceed with arbitration.

The arbitration hearing was held 2 years after the incident occurred, and the decision that was made was binding. Management won on the merits of the case. The staff nurse was not awarded sick time pay, and it was also decided that there was no disparity in treatment at the time. The counseling memo was removed from the personnel file, so the union won in this area of the grievance.

As the nurse manager reviewed the case after the arbitration decision was made, the following suggestions should be considered by any manager who may be involved in the grievance-arbitration process (9):

1. Treat each other with mutual respect and courtesy. The nurse manager and staff nurse have to work with one another throughout and after the grievance procedure.
2. The role of bargaining in good faith is implicit in the process; do not withhold any facts or information.
3. Stay objective especially during the hearings; once subjectivity occurs the nurse manager's stance may be threatened.
4. Know the strengths and weaknesses of the issue for either side; the labor relations department should assist the nurse manager in handling the grievance procedure.
5. Know your bottom line as a nurse manager for compromise, and at what level you will not accept agreement.
6. Observe the time limits of the grievance procedure. If the time limits are exceeded, the grievance can be discontinued.
7. Get all of the facts, information, witnesses, and documentation. Find out whether any similar situations have occurred and what the outcome has been.

The nurse manager in this case study did follow these suggestions and found that she had the most difficulty with remaining objective, particularly when the falsehood of disparity in treatment was the issue on which the union decided to mount its attack. As with any experience in management

there were lessons to be learned, particularly in a unionized setting. The nurse manager realized the importance of thorough documentation, consistency in treatment, and the value of upholding a staffing standard.

## SUMMARY

Sidney Hillman was astute in his statement in 1918 regarding the demands of labor (1). In today's health care environment the nurse manager needs to be aware of the issues surrounding unionization and the impact these issues may or may not have on the implementation of the role. The health care industry has been called the last frontier for organizing collective bargaining. The conceptual model that was described supports the current changes in the health care industry and provides a framework for the nurse manager to conceptualize the impact of unionization. The nurse manager in any setting also needs to reflect on the variables that were described in Table 18.1 and realize the impact they have on collective bargaining for the future. The movement in nursing supports some of these variables. It is the informed, visionary, and prepared nurse manager who will survive in the future, particularly if the setting is unionized or is threatening to become unionized. As stated by Debs (1) in 1914, "Intelligent discontent is the mainspring of civilization. Progress is born of agitation. It is agitation or stagnation."

## REFERENCES

1. Hillman S. Taft-Hartley ammendments: implications for the health care field. Chicago, 1975.
2. Moylan L, Implications of the National Labor Relations Act. Nurs Management 1988;19:80.
3. Wilson D. How wide is the generation gap in nursing. RN, 1985;25–29.
4. Decker P. Nursing associations and collective bargaining. In Sullivan E, Decker P, eds. Effective management in nursing. Menlo Park, California: Addison-Wesley Publishing Company, 1988.
5. Othman JE, Chaney H. Labor relations in union and nonunion environments. In Vestal K, ed. Management concepts for the new nurse. Philadelphia: JB Lippincott Company, 1987.
6. Ballman C. Union busters. Am J Nurs, 1985;10:96–966.
7. News. Am J Nurs, 1988;13:1409.
8. Fennel K. The unionization of the health care industry: general trends and emerging issues. J Health Hum Resources Admin. Summer 1987;10(2):66–81.
9. Metzger N, Ferentino J, Fruger K, eds. When health care employees strike. Rockville, Maryland: Aspen Systems Corporation, 1984.
10. Fottler M. Health care collective bargaining: future dy-

namics and their impact. J Health Hum Resources Admin. Summer 1987;10(2):33–51.

11. American Association of Critical-Care Nurses. Summary analysis of critical care nurse supply and requirements. Newport Beach, California: American Association of Critical-Care Nurses, 1988.

12. Hunter K, Bamberg D, Castiglia P, et al. Job satisfaction: is collective bargaining the answer? Nurs Management, 1986;17:56–60.

13. Metzger N. The health care supervisor's handbook. Rockville, Maryland: Aspen Systems Corporation, 1982.

14. 29 USC, 157 (1982).

15. 29 USC, 158 (A) (1982).

16. Henry K. Health care union organizing: guidelines for supervisory conduct. Health Care Supervisor, 1985:4:14–26.

17. Colvin C. Conflict and resolution: strikes in nursing. Nurs Admin Q, 1987;12:45–51.

18. Rothman W. Strikes in hospitals. J Health Hum Resources Admin. Summer 1987;10(2):7–19.

19. McPherson D, Gates C, Rogers K. Resolving grievances, a practical approach. Reston, Virginia: Reston Publishing Company, Inc, 1983.

# Index

Page numbers in *italics* denote figures; those followed by "t" denote tables.

## A

Addiction syndromes (*see* Chemical dependency)
Administration levels, responsibilities, 30–31, 31t
Administrative justice, 191–192
Administrative supervisor position in decentralized
    management, 36
Advertising in recruitment, 13–14
Agency personnel, 55
Aggressive behavior in communication, 81–82
Alcohol abuse (*see* Chemical dependency)
American Association of Critical-Care Nurses
    certification, 66–67
    competence testing, 19
    cost effectiveness study, 121
    nurse involvement in, 67–68
    nurse manager role expectations, 3, 6–7
    scope of practice, 3, *4–5*
    standards of care, 19–20, 146
American Nurses Association as bargaining agent,
    209
Ancillary personnel utilization, 16–17, 17t
Arbitration in labor grievance, 215–218, *216*
Autonomous staffing, 53–54, 94, 96–97

## B

Bargaining (*see* Collective bargaining; Negotiation)
Basic Knowledge Assessment Tool, 19
Benefit programs
    in recruitment, 14
    in staff retention, 105–106
Body language, 80–81
Burnout (*see* Stress)

## C

Career mobility, mentoring and, 112, 118–119, 121
Career transition matrix, 101, 101t
CCRN certification, 66–67
Centralization of staff, 53
Certification, 66–67
Change (*see also* Motivation)
    principles, 126, 126t
    resistance to, 126–128, 127t–129t
    theories, 124
Chemical dependency, 176–188
    action plans for, 185–187
    confrontation in, 185
    crisis situation handling, 186–187
    definitions, 177–178
    discipline in, 178–179, 185–187
    documentation, 184–185
    education and, 178–179

    employee assistance program, 185
    hiring and, 22
    history, 176–177
    identification, 178–184, 180t–181t
    ignoring, 178
    interview in, 182t
    legal aspects, 178
    proactive approach, 178
    recovery from, 177, 182t, 187
    signs and symptoms, 181t
    statistics, 177
    substances misused/abused, 180t
    termination in, 187
Child care in staff retention, 105
Clinical ladder in professional development, 68
Cognitive theories of motivation, 133–134, *134*
Collaboration model of practice, 73, 74t
Collective bargaining, 211–215
    employee response to, 209, *210*, 211, 212t
    grievance handling, 215–218, *216*
    stages, 211, *213*
Communication, 78–91
    accuracy, 86–87
    aggressive, 81–82
    assertive, 81–82
    barriers to, 85–89
    chain of command and, 86
    channels for, 79–81
    crisis and, 87–88
    distortion, 87–88
    employee signing of, 203
    formal, 79–80, 81t
    grapevine in, 80
    humor in, 90–91
    importance, 78–79
    in discipline, 203–204
    in shared governance system, 41–42
    informal, 79–81, 81t
    interdivisional, 83
    intradivisional, 83–84
    intrastaff, 84
    job threat and, 88
    listening and, 91
    meetings, 80, 85
    memoranda, 80
    nonassertive, 81–82
    nonverbal, 81–82
    optimal level, 84
    perceived homophyly in, 85–86
    presentation, 88
    productivity and, 89–91
    receiver perceptions, 89

Communication—*continued*
  simplicity in, 90
  skills for, 22, 26–27, 79
  spoken, 80–82
  style, 89
  validation, 90
  variation in, 90
  with ancillary departments, 35–36
  with different levels, 82–85
  with family, 79–80, 84
  with patient, 84
  with physician, 84–85
  workplace climate and, 89–90
  written, 80–81
Community involvement assessment in hiring, 22, 27
Competence
  definition, 19, 161
  measurement, 19–20
Competence levels
  novice to expert, 60–62, 62t, 108–109, 165–167, 166t, *167*
  staff turnover effects on, 92
Competency-based education, 160–175 (*see also* Professional development)
  administration support, 163–164
  characteristics, 160–163, 162t
  committees for, 165
  competency definitions, 167–168, 167t
  competency statements, 162, 162t, 168–174, 171t–174t
  cost savings, 161
  criteria statements, 163, 168, 170, 171t–173t
  critical incident technique, 168
  design techniques, 164–168, 166t–167t, *167*, 169t
  evaluation tools, 170, 173, 174t
  field testing, 170, 173
  flexibility, 163
  history, 161
  human resources department support, 164
  mastery learning in, 162–163
  nursing practice levels, 165–167, 166t, *167*
  peer evaluation in, 173–174
  preceptors in, 102, 164, 165t
  priority matrix, 168, 169t
  risk management, 164
  skills checklist in, 170, 174t
  staff retention and, 102
Competitive negotiation, 142, 143t
Confidentiality in discipline, 205
Contingency plans for staffing, 54–55
Contracts
  for recovering chemically dependent nurse, 182t
  in labor relations, 212, 214–215
Cooperative negotiation, 142, 143t
Costs
  competency-based education, 161
  shared governance and, 43–44
  staffing and scheduling and, 49, 57
  versus nurse experience, 120–121
Counseling in discipline, 193, *197*
Crisis, communication problems in, 87–88
Criterion-referenced evaluation (*see* Competency-based education)

Criticism, constructive, 191
Cyclical scheduling, 57

**D**

Darling Measuring Mentoring Potential tool, 119, 120t
Decentralization (management), 30–36
  ancillary department communication in, 35–36
  case study, 33–35, 35t
  definition, 30
  education for, 32
  effects, 33
  evaluation, 32–33
  geographical, 30
  management levels in, 31–32, 31t
  motivation for, 30
  organizational, 30
  outcome, 33
  structuring approaches, 30–33, 31t
Decentralization (staff), 32, 53
Decision making in shared governance system, 41
Delphi technique in competency-based education, 168
Demand strategies in recruitment, 15–16
Discharge (*see* Termination)
Discipline, 189–207
  autocratic approach, 189–190
  burden of proof in, 205
  chemical dependency and, 178–179, 185–187
  communication in, 203–204
  confidentiality in, 205
  constructive criticism in, 191
  counseling in, 193, *197*
  criteria for, 201–202
  defensible, 207
  definition, 189
  discharge in, 199–201, *202*
  due process procedures, 192
  employee rights in, 190, 190t
  errors in, 201–202
  fairness in, 191, 204
  guidelines for, 206–207
  implementation, 204–207
  in probationary period, 191
  individual differences in, 191
  infraction-penalty list for, 193, 194t–196t
  legal aspects, 191–192
  objectivity in, 205
  policy definition and, 193
  preparation for, 205
  preventive, 190–191
  progressive, 192–201, 194t–196t, *197–200*
  purpose, 189–190
  relationships and, 191
  self-control in, 190
  strategies for, 203–204
  suspension in, 197–199, *200*
  timing, 203
  verbal warning in, 193, 196, *198*
  work rules and, 190–191
  written warning in, 196–197, *199*
Discrimination, discipline and, 192

Distributive bargaining (competitive negotiation),
    142, 143t
Documentation
    chemical dependence, 184–185
    counseling, 193, *197*
    employment termination, 201, *202*
    performance appraisal, 153–154
    suspension, 197–198, *200*
    time consumed by, 56
    verbal warning, 196, *198*
    written warning, 196–197, *199*
Drug abuse (*see* Chemical dependency)

**E**

Education
    competency-based (*see* Competency-based
        education)
    decentralized management and, 32
    interview questions on, 25
    nurse manager, 7–9
    professional development and, 65–66
    recruitment problems and, 15
    staff retention and, 102–103, 105
Empirical-rational change strategy, 124–125
Employee relations (*see* Labor relations)
Employee rights, discipline and, 190, 190t
Equity theory of motivation, 133, *134*
ERG theory in motivation, 131–132
Ethics rounds as staff retention strategy, 98
Evaluation
    of chemical dependency (*see* Chemical dependency)
    of job performance (*see* Performance appraisal)
Expectancy/valence theory of motivation, 133, *134*
Experience
    assessment, 20–21, 25
    competence/development and, 60–62, 62t, 108–
        109, 165–167, 166t, *167*
    nurse manager, 9
    versus expertise, 119
Expert nurse as mentor, 108–109
Expertise versus experience, 119

**F**

Fairness
    in discipline, 191, 204
    in negotiation, 141–142
Family
    communication with, 79–80, 84
    negotiation with, 142
Feedback
    in performance appraisal, 155–157
    in shared governance, 42
Financial incentives in recruitment, 14
Functional nursing, 52

**G**

Getzels-Guba model of social behavior, 135–136,
    *135–136*
Goal-setting theory of motivation, 133, *134*
Gray gorilla syndrome, 121
Greenhalgh's career transition matrix, 101, 101t
Grievance-arbitration procedure, 215–218, *216*
    discipline and, 192

**H**

Harvard Negotiation Project, 138–140, 140t
Herzberg motivation-hygiene theory, 132
    in staff retention, 104
Hiring, 19–28 (*see also* Recruitment)
    communication skill assessment, 22, 26–27
    community involvement assessment, 22, 27
    competence measurement, 19–20
    desired characteristics, 20–22
    evaluation of process, 27–28
    experience assessment, 20–21, 25
    human relationship skill assessment, 21–22
    intellectual assessment, 21
    interview in, 23–27, *25*
    knowledge assessment, 20, 25–26
    motivation assessment, 21, 26
    orientation after, 96
    personality assessment, 21, 26
    procedure for, 22–23
    professional involvement assessment, 22, 27
    undesirable characteristics, 22
Hospitals
    generalized versus specialized units in, 75, 75t
    rural versus urban, 71–73, 72t
    teaching versus nonteaching, 73–75, 74t
Human relationship skills assessment, 21–22

**I**

Integrative bargaining (cooperative negotiation), 142,
    143t
Intellectual assessment, 21
Internship program, 121–122
Interview
    chemical dependence problems, 182t, 185
    disciplinary, 203, 206–207
    evaluation, 27–28
    hiring, 23–27, *25*
    nurse manager selection, 7
    performance appraisal, 155–157, *155*
    questions for, 23–27
    scoring sheet for, 23, *24*
    structure for, 23, *25*
    team, in hiring, 23–24
    termination, 100

**J**

Job application review, 23
Job description
    in hiring, 20
    in performance appraisal, 147, 148t–151t
Job performance (*see* Performance appraisal)
Job satisfaction
    decentralized management and, 30
    professional development and, 60
    versus turnover, 92–95, 95t
Joint Commission on Accreditation of Health Care
        Organizations, job description, 146
Jujitsu in negotiation, 141

**K**

Knowledge assessment in hiring, 20, 25–26

## L

Labor relations, 208–219
  collective bargaining in (*see* Collective bargaining)
  conflict in, 215–218, *216*
  contracts, 212, 214–215
  definition, 208
  discipline and, 191–192
  dissatisfaction responses, 211
  grievance procedure, 216–218, *216*
  history, 208–209
  professional collectivism, 209
  strikes, 214
  union activity, 209, *210*, 211–215, 212t
Language in communication, 81–82
Leadership (*see also* Mentor(ing))
  in change process, 128–129, *130*, 131t
Lecturing in professional development, 67
Legal aspects
  chemical dependency, 178
  discipline, 191–192, 207
  staffing and scheduling, 49

## M

Marketing in recruitment, 13–14
Maslow's needs hierarchy in motivation, 130–131
Mastery learning (*see* Competency-based education)
Measuring Mentoring Potential tool, 119, 120t
Meetings, 80, 85
Memoranda, 80
Mentor(ing), 107–123
  action requirements, 114
  affect in, 114
  aspects not included, 110
  attraction in, 114
  boss as, 114
  career assistance/mobility and, 112, 118–119
  characteristics, 119, 120t
  clinical career ladder and, 121
  definition, 107
  feedback in, 113
  for new graduates, 108
  for nurse manager, 111–116, 115t
  functions, 109–110, 109t, 112–113, 115t
  informational stage, 114, 115t
  internship programs and, 121–122
  invitational stage, 114, 115t
  mentee responsibilities, 111
  mentor-mentee relationship, 110–111
  need for, 116
  nurse manager as, 116–119, 117t
  orientation programs and, 121
  potential for, 119, 120t
  proficiency levels and, 108–109
  promotion, 121
  questioning stage, 114, 115t
  selection, 114–116
  self esteem and, 112
  staff nurses as, 119–122
  success tips, 122
  termination, 116
  "The Dream" in, 109

  time considerations in, 110
  transitional stage, 114, 115t
  value, 107–108
  versus apprenticeship, 110
  versus role model, 110, 113
Motivation, 124–137
  agent for, 124–126
  Alderfer modified need theory, 131–132
  assessment, in hiring, 21, 26
  change theory and, 124
  cognitive theories, 133–134, *134*
  delegated power approach, 129, 130t
  empirical-rational strategy, 124–125
  equity theory, 133, *134*
  expectancy/valence theory, 133, *134*
  Getzels-Guba social behavior model, 135–136, *135–136*
  goal-setting theory, 133, *134*
  Herzberg motivation-hygiene theory, 132
  in decentralized management, 30
  in staff retention, 93, 104
  in unionization, 209
  leadership style and, 128–129, *130*, 131t
  Maslow's need hierarchy, 130–131
  Murray manifest need theory, 132
  need theories, 130–133
  normative-reeducative strategy, 125–126, 126t
  organizational climate for, 128–129, 130t
  Planned Change Model, 128, 128t–129t
  power-coercive strategy, 125
  reinforcement theories, 134–135
  resistance to change, 126–128, 127t
  shared power approach, 129, 130t
  theories, 129–135, *134*
  unilateral approach, 128–129, 130t
Murray manifest need theory in motivation, 132

## N

Need theories of motivation, 130–133
Negotiation, 138–144
  bargaining in, 139
  best alternative in failure, 140–141, 141t
  competitive (win-lose), 142, 143t
  cooperative (win-win), 142, 143t
  definition, 138
  in grievance-arbitration procedure, 215–218, *216*
  interdepartmental, 142
  interests in, 139
  jujitsu in, 141
  mutual gain options, 139–140
  objectivity in, 140, 141t
  parties in, 142
  people versus problem, 140
  positions in, 139
  principled, 138–139, 139t
  salary, 140–141, 141t
  unfair tactics in, 141–142
  with family, 142
  with patient, 142
Normative-reeducative change strategy, 125–126, 126t

Nurse manager
  decentralized management responsibilities, 32
  desirable characteristics, 5, 7, 8t–9t
  educational level, 7–9
  evolution of role, 2–3
  experience requirements, 9
  functions, 2–3, 4–7
  professional development, 69
  Queen Bee syndrome in, 9
  selection, 3, 7
  staff retention responsibilities, 95–99
  undesirable characteristics, 9–10
  versus head nurse, 2
  visionary, 5, 7
Nursing Gestalt theory, 121

**O**

Objectivity in discipline, 205
Organizational climate in motivation, 128–129, 130t
Organizations (*see also* American Association of
      Critical-Care Nurses)
  in professional development, 67–68

**P**

Patient
  communication with, 84
  negotiation with, 142
Peer review, 151–153, 155
  in competency-based education, 173
Performance appraisal, 146–159
  anecdotal review in, 151
  behavior checklist in, 147, 151
  computers in, 153–154
  delegation, 155
  delivery, 155–157, *155*
  documentation, 153–154
  feedback in, 155–157
  graphic rating scale in, 147
  hostile reaction to, 156
  in competency-based education, 170, 173, 174t
  job description and, 147, 148t–151t
  management by objectives technique, 151
  methods for, 147, 151
  multiple raters in, 151
  peer review in, 151–153
  preparation for, 155–156
  problems with, 157–158
  production output in, 147
  purpose, 146
  rank ordering in, 147
  rating scale in, 147t–151t, 153–154, 154t
  standards for, 146–147
  tools for, 153–154, *154*
Performance-based education (*see* Competency-based
      education)
Personality assessment in hiring, 21, 26
Physician
  communication with, 84–85
  negotiation with, 141–142
  responsibility delegation by, 74–75
Planned Change Model, 128, 128t–129t
Politics, mentoring and, 113
Power-coercive change strategy, 125

Preceptors for competency-based education, 102, 164,
      165t
Primary nursing, 52–53
  staff retention and, 92–93, 101–102
Principled negotiation, 138–140, 140t
Priority matrix in competency-based education, 168,
      169t
Probationary period, critique during, 191
Productivity, communication and, 89–91
Professional development, 59–70 (*see also*
      Competency-based education; Mentor(ing))
  advantages, 59–60
  association involvement in, 67–68
  avenues for, 59
  career matrix for, 101, 101t
  certification in, 66–67
  clinical ladder in, 68
  continuum, 60–62, 62t
  education in, 65–66
  evaluation, 64
  hospital activities in, 65
  in-service programs in, 66
  job satisfaction and, 60
  journal club in, 65
  lecturing in, 67
  manager support of, 68
  need assessment in, 62–63, *63*
  nurse manager, 69
  objectives, 64
  opportunities, 64–68
  options for, 63–64
  overcommitment to, 68–69
  pitfalls in, 68–69
  plan implementation, 64
  publishing in, 67
  research conduct/utilization in, 65
  responsibility for, 59, 68
  results, 59–60
  self-assessment in, 62–63
  staff retention and, 93–94, 102–103
  steps for, 62–64, *63*
  unit activities in, 65
  versus other priorities, 68–69
Professional growth, organizations for, 67–68
Professional involvement assessment in hiring, 22, 27
Progressive discipline, 192–201, 194t–196t, *197–200*
Protege (*see* Mentor(ing))
Publishing in professional development, 67
Punishment (*see* Discipline)

**Q**

Queen Bee syndrome in nurse manager, 9

**R**

Reality shock, mentoring and, 108
Recruitment, 11–18
  advertising, 13–14
  ancillary personnel use, 16–17, 17t
  benefit programs, 14
  demand strategies for, 15–16
  educational assistance programs, 15
  feeder mechanisms, 14–15
  financial incentives, 14

Recruitment—*continued*
   foreign nurses, 17
   from affiliated nursing schools, 14
   from within hospital, 15
   future trends, 17–18
   marketing, 13–14
   marketplace factors, 11–12
   nursing shortage and, 11–12
   retention program participation, 94
   salaries and, 11
   strategies, 13–16, 13t
   supply versus demand, 12
   turnover rates and, 12
   work-study programs and, 14–15
Registered Care Technologist, 17
Reinforcement theories of motivation, 134–135
Research conduct/utilization, 65
Resume review, 25
Retention of staff, 92–106
   autonomous practice in, 96–97
   benefit packages, 105–106
   career transition matrix in, 101, 101t
   caring environment in, 97
   child care provision, 105
   competency-based education, 102
   cost advantages, 92
   earned-time programs, 105
   educational needs/programs, 102–103, 105
   ethics rounds in, 98
   factors in, 92–95
   flexible scheduling, 105
   goal setting in, 96
   job satisfaction and, 92–95, 95t
   morale and, 92
   motivation-hygiene theory, 104
   new employee handling, 96
   nurse manager role, 95–99
   nursing shortage and, 92
   preceptor-guided orientation, 102
   primary nursing, 101–102
   professional development programs, 103–104
   recruitment and, 12
   research activities, 104
   salary policies, 104–105
   scheduling flexibility in, 97–98
   strategies, 101–106
   stress control in, 94, 98
   team building in, 98
   turnover data assessment, 99–101
   unit competence level and, 92
Risk management in competency-based education,
   164
Rural settings for critical care, 71–73, 72t


**S**

Salary
   certification and, 67
   negotiation, 140–141, 141t
   performance and, 155–156
   staff retention and, 104–105
Scheduling (*see* Staffing and scheduling)

Self-discipline, 189–190
Self-esteem, mentoring and, 112
Self-governing system (*see* Shared governance)
Self-instruction (*see* Competency-based education)
Self-perception in negotiation, 140
Settings for critical care, 71–76
   collaboration and, 73, 74t
   general units, 75, 75t
   nonteaching hospitals, 73–75
   nurse demographics and, 72
   nurse specialization and, 73
   opinion leaders and, 74
   patient population and, 72–73
   physician availability and, 74–75
   rural, 71–73, 72t
   specialized units, 75, 75t
   teaching hospitals, 73–75
   urban, 71–73, 72t
Shared governance, 37–46
   action pathway in, 38–39
   autonomous staffing in, 53–54
   commitment to, 39–40
   communication in, 41–42
   cost considerations in, 43–44
   decision making definitions, 41
   evaluation, 45–46
   feedback in, 42
   information pathway in, 38
   leadership development in, 45
   nursing congress in, 43
   nurturing, 44–45
   participative structures in, 42–43
   problems, 39
   professional nursing organization in, 43
   results, 37
   role ambiguity in, 41–42
   societal changes favoring, 37–38
   support for, 40–41
Social behavior model of Getzels-Guba, 135–136,
   *135–136*
Specialization versus type of hospital, 73, 75
Staffing and scheduling, 47–58
   acuity needs, 49–50
   agency personnel in, 55
   autonomous, 53–54, 94, 96–97
   centralized, 53
   checklist, 51t
   collaboration model of practice and, 73, 74t
   contingency plans, 54–55
   cost considerations, 49, 57
   creative environment for, 56
   cyclical, 57
   decentralized, 53
   definitions, 47
   efficiency, 50
   elements, 58
   external factors in, 47–49, 48t
   flexible, 57, 105
   floating system, 53
   for functional nursing, 52
   for managed care, 52–53
   for nonteaching hospital, 73–75
   for primary nursing, 52–53

for professional development promotion, 66
for rural settings, 71–73, 72t
for staff retention, 105
for teaching hospital, 73–75
for team nursing, 52
for urban settings, 71–73, 72t
goals, 55–56
internal factors in, 47
legal aspects, 49
needs assessment, 47–50, 48t
nurse demographics and, 72
nurse specialization and, 73
nursing care hours in, 49–50
nursing dependency systems in, 49
patient population and, 72–73
patterns, 56–57
physician availability and, 74–75
program evaluation, 57–58
skill mix in, 51–52
staff retention and, 98
standards, 47–49, 48t
turnover problems (*see* Retention of staff)
unit activity trends and, 50, 51t
unit specialization and, 75, 75t
unit workload and, 50–51
Standards
discipline and, 190–191
for performance appraisal, 146–147, 148t–151t
for staffing, 47–49, 48t
in competence measurement, 19–20
in staff retention, 96
Stress
nurse manager and, 3
staff retention and, 94, 98
Strikes, 214
Substance abuse (*see* Chemical dependency)  ared
Supervisor responsibilities, 32
Suspension as discipline, 197–198, *200*

T
Taft-Hartley Amendment, 208–209
Team nursing, 52
Temporary agency personnel, 55
Termination
chemical dependency and, 187
job satisfaction investigation and, 100
management right to, 192
procedure, 199–201, *202*
Training (*see also* Education; Mentor(ing))
ancillary personnel, 17

U
Unionization
contract in, 212, 214–215
employee attitudes, 209, *210*, 211, 212t
history, 209
manager role, 211–212
motivation for, 209, 211
organizers, 211
process, 214–215
strikes, 214
unlawful activities during, 211–212, 214t
Urban settings for critical care, 71–73, 72t

V
Verbal warning as discipline, 193, 196, *198*

W
Wagner Act, 208–209
Work rules explanation, 190–191
Work-study programs in recruitment, 14–15
Written warning as discipline, 196–197, *199*